Rapid ECG Interpretation

Rapid ECG Interpretation

Fourth Edition

(Late) M Gabriel Khan
MD FRCP (London) FACC FRCPC MB BCh (Queen's Belfast)
Former Associate Professor
Department of Medicine and Division of Cardiology
University of Ottawa
The Ottawa Hospital
Ottawa, Ontario, Canada

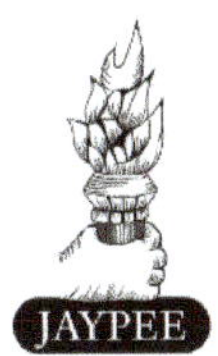

JAYPEE BROTHERS MEDICAL PUBLISHERS
The Health Sciences Publisher
New Delhi | London

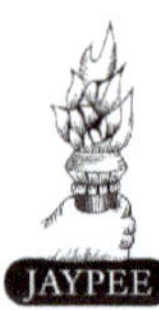

Jaypee Brothers Medical Publishers (P) Ltd

Headquarters
EMCA House
23/23-B, Ansari Road, Daryaganj
New Delhi 110 002, India
Landline: +91-11-23272143,
+91-11-23272703
+91-11-23282021, +91-11-23245672
E-mail: jaypee@jaypeebrothers.com

Overseas Office
JP Medical Ltd.
83, Victoria Street, London
SW1H 0HW (UK)
Phone: +44-20 3170 8910
E-mail: info@jpmedpub.com

Corporate Office
Jaypee Brothers Medical Publishers (P) Ltd.
4838/24, Ansari Road, Daryaganj
New Delhi 110 002, India
Phone: +91-11-43574357
Fax: +91-11-43574314
E-mail: jaypee@jaypeebrothers.com

EU GPSR Authorised Representative
Logos Europe, 9 rue Nicolas Poussin
17000, La Rochelle, France
Phone: +33 (0) 6 67 93 73 78
E-mail: Contact@logoseurope.eu

Website: www.jaypeebrothers.com
Website: www.jaypeedigital.com

Rapid ECG Interpretation

Third Edition: 2008, Springer (Humana Press)

Fourth Edition: 2020, Reprint: **2025**

ISBN: 978-93-89188-58-5

Contents

Electrocardiogram Basic Concepts Must be Mastered

ELECTRICAL ACTIVITY OF THE HEART

Each contraction of the heart is preceded by excitation waves of electrical activity that originate in the sinoatrial (SA) node. Figure 1.1 depicts the radial spread of activation from the SA node. The waves of electrical activity spread through the atria and reach the atrioventricular (AV) node. Note that the SA node tracing shows no steady resting potential, as does the ventricular muscle tracing. The SA node's spontaneous depolarization and repolarization provides a unique AV node, which conducts the activation current down the bundle branches to activate the ventricular muscle mass. Cardiac cells outside the SA node must be activated.

Depolarization

In a resting cardiac muscle cell, molecules dissociate into positively charged ions on the outer surface and negatively charged ions on the inner surface of the cell membrane; the cell is in an electrically balanced or polarized resting state (Figs. 1.2A to C).

- When the cell is stimulated by an excitatory electrical wave, the negative ions migrate to the outer surface of the cell and the positively charged ions pass into the cell; this reversal of polarity is called depolarization (*see* Figs. 1.2A to C).

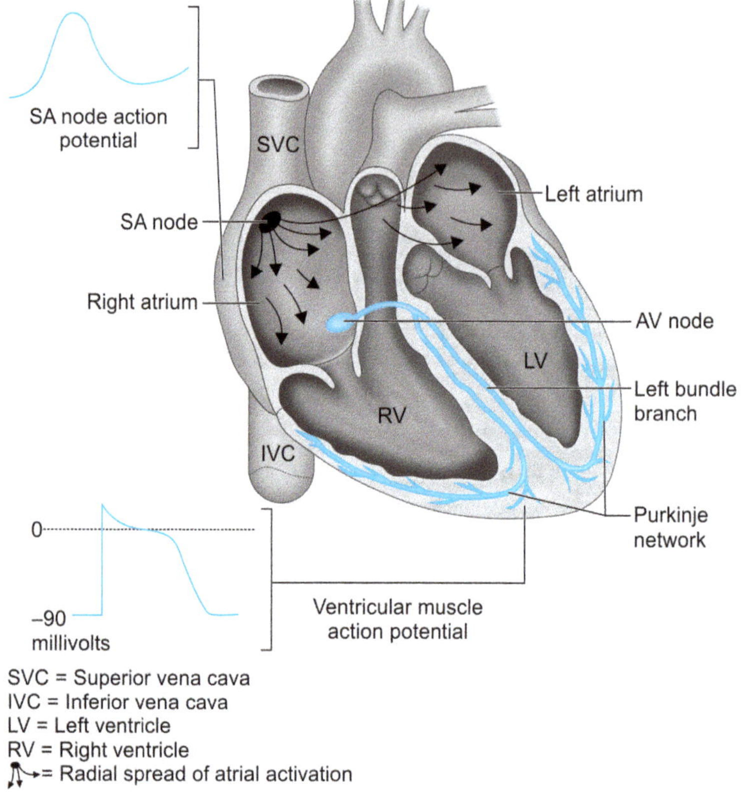

Fig. 1.1: Electrical activation of the heart by the sinoatrial (SA) node. The current of activation (arrows) spreads radially from the SA node across the atria to the atrioventricular (AV) node and down the bundle branches to the ventricular muscle and Purkinje network. The SA node tracing shows no steady resting potential and is characterized by spontaneous depolarization.

- If an electrode is placed so that the depolarization wave flows toward the electrode, a galvanometer will record an upward or positive deflection (Figs. 1.2A to C and Fig. 1.3A to C).
- When a depolarization current is directed away from an electrode, a negative or downward deflection is recorded (*see* Figs. 1.2A to C).

Repolarization

- During a recovery period, positively charged ions return to the outer surface and negatively charged ions move into the cell. The electrical balance of the cell is restored; this process is called repolarization (*see* Figs. 1.2A to C).
- The transfer of sodium (Na^+) and potassium (K^+) ions across the cell membrane plays an important role in generating cardiac electrical activity. In Figure 1.4, the relative magnitudes of the concentration of Na^+ and K^+ ions are indicated. Intracellular concentration of K^+ is 30 times greater than extracellular K^+. Na^+ concentration is 30 times less inside the cell than outside. Because of this ionic composition, the membrane of the resting cardiac fiber is in

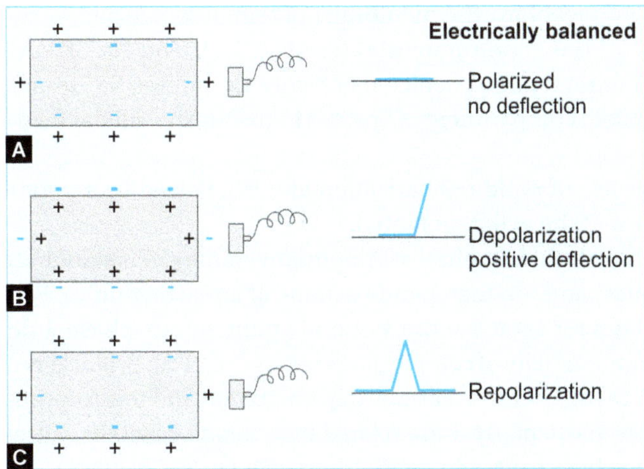

Figs. 1.2A to C: (A) Resting cell: positive ions on the outer surface and negative ions inside equal an electrically balanced or polarized cell; (B) Depolarized cell: negative ions on the outer surface and positive ions inside; (C) Repolarization of cell: positive ions return to the outside.

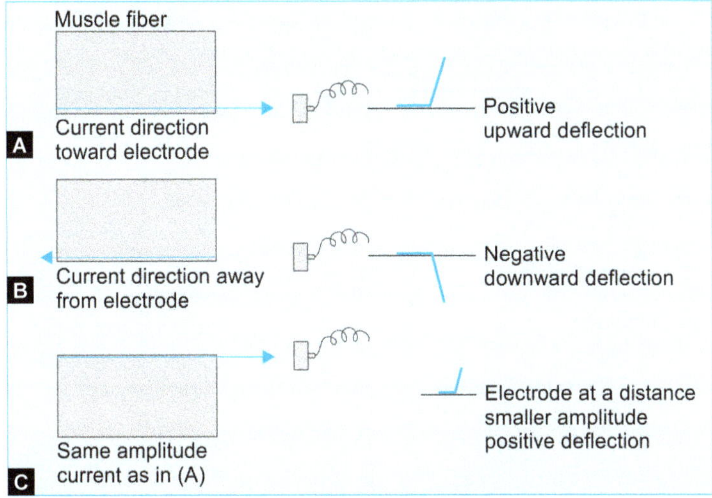

Figs. 1.3A to C: Recording of the effects of electrical activation process. (A) Current flows toward the electrode produce a positive upward deflection; (B) Current flows away from the electrode produce a negative downward deflection; (C) Current flows toward an electrode placed at a distance produce a positive but smaller amplitude deflection than in (A).

an electrically balanced or polarized state. The potential difference across the cell membrane can be measured by a microelectrode and is observed on an oscilloscope to be –90 mV.

Action Potential

- The inward Na^+ current results in a change in transmembrane potential; results in depolarization; and is shown as the upstroke, phase 0 of the action potential. With a decrease in Na^+ and K^+ permeability, the membrane potential remains close to 0; this represents phases 1 and 2 of the action potential (*see* Fig. 1.4). The Na^+-K^+-ATPase (adenosine triphosphatase) sodium pump, depicted in Figure 1.4, pumps Na^+ from the intracellular to the extracellular fluid compartment; K^+ passes from the extracellular fluid to the intracellular fluid.

- Phase 3 is the phase of rapid repolarization and is followed by a period of stable resting potential, phase 4 of the action potential.

The appreciation of these four phases is important for the understanding of abnormal heart rhythms (arrhythmias) and the therapeutic actions of antiarrhythmics. For example, digoxin or excess catecholamines increase the slope of spontaneous phase 4 depolarization and therefore increase automaticity of ectopic pacemakers (Fig. 1.5); β-blockers cause inhibition or depression of spontaneous phase 4 diastolic depolarization and thus suppress catecholamine-induced arrhythmias, particularly those related to ischemia. Digitalis causes inhibition of the cellular Na^+ pump, which causes increased intracellular Na^+, which is then exchanged for

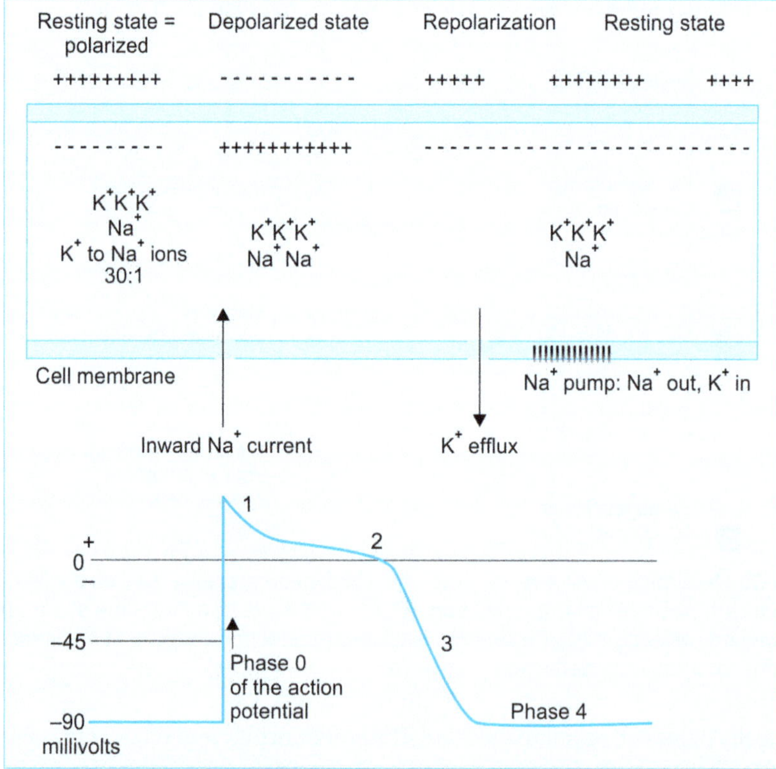

Fig. 1.4: A simplified concept of ionic exchange; the polarized, depolarized, and repolarized state of a myocardial cell; and the action potential. An electrical current arriving at the cell causes positively charged ions to cross the cell membrane, which causes depolarization, followed by repolarization, which generates an action potential: phases 0, 1, 2, 3, and 4. This electrical event traverses the heart and initiates mechanical systole, or the heartbeat (*see also* Fig. 1.7).

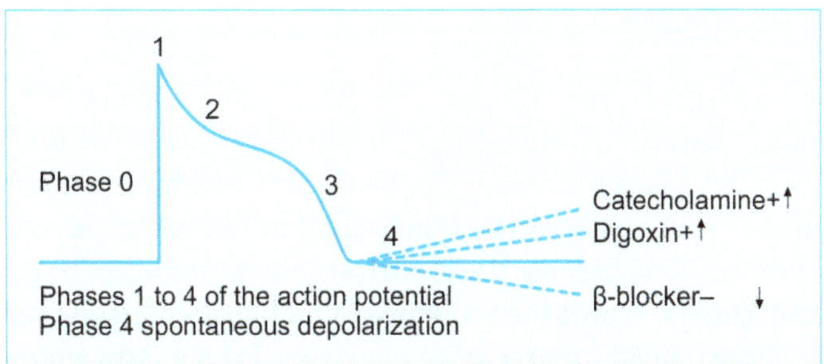

Fig. 1.5: Effects of catecholamines, digoxin, and β-blockers on spontaneous phase 4 depolarization. β-blockers inhibit or decrease spontaneous phase 4 depolarization caused by catecholamines, especially that caused by ischemia.

calcium via the Na^+-calcium exchanger. Increased intracellular calcium during cardiac systole increases myocardial muscle contractility. Digitalis toxicity causes cellular calcium overload that potentiates arrhythmias.

Sinoatrial Node

The SA node is unique and has no steady resting potential. After repolarization, slow, spontaneous depolarization occurs during phase 4 that causes the automaticity of the SA node fibers (*see* SA node waveform in Fig. 1.1). Thus, the unique pacemaker provides individuals with an automatic infinitesimal current that sets the heart's electrical activity and contractions. The SA discharge rate, usually 50–100/minute, is under autonomic, chemical, and hormonal influence.

Atrioventricular Node

The AV node provides a necessary physiologic delay of the electrical currents, which allows the atria to fill the ventricles with blood before ventricular systole.
- From the AV node and bundle of His, the excitatory electrical current rapidly traverses the right and left bundle branches, the specialized conductive tissues of the ventricles, and the Purkinje system, and the entire ventricular muscle is depolarized (*see* Fig. 1.1).
- Depolarization spreads down the intraventricular septum toward the apex of the heart and then along the free wall of the left ventricular myocardium; it always proceeds from the endocardium toward the pericardium. The specialized fine arborization of branches that constitute the Purkinje network spreads over the endocardial surfaces of the ventricles.
- The transient halt and slowing of conduction through the specialized AV node fibers play an important protective role in patients with atrial flutter and atrial fibrillation. In these common conditions, a rapid atrial rate of approximately 300–600 beats/minute reaches the AV node; this AV "tollgate" reduces the electrical traffic that reaches the superhighway that traverses the ventricles to approximately 120–180 beats/minute, and serious life-threatening events are prevented.

ELECTROCARDIOGRAM

The heart muscle is made up of several thousand muscle elements, about 10^{10} cells. Each instant of depolarization or repolarization represents different stages of activity for a large number of cells. The electrical activity of each element can be represented by a vector force.

- A vector is defined as a force that can be represented by direction and magnitude. The sum total of cardiac vectors is considered the electrical activity of the entire heart (Fig. 1.6). The electrocardiogram (ECG) records the sequence of such instantaneous vectors.
- The heart muscle is arranged in three muscle masses: (1) the intraventricular septum, (2) a large left ventricular muscle mass, and (3) a small right ventricular muscle mass. The magnitude or amplitude of the deflections recorded is influenced by the size of the muscle mass depolarized and the distance from the recording electrode (*see* Figs. 1.3 and 1.6).

The graphic representation of the heart's electrical activity recorded through electrodes positioned at strategic points on the body constitutes the ECG. The recording of the electrical currents, their direction, and their magnitude, as well as the rate of the heart's contractions, is made by the machine and electrocardiograph, which is essentially a galvanometer whose deflections are recorded on moving, specially prepared paper.

The ECG is the recording obtained, and to simplify interpretation, it suffices to state that the ECG displays the following:

- Three major deflections or waves: (1) the P wave, (2) the QRS complex, and (3) a T wave (Fig. 1.7).
- Two time intervals of clinical importance: (1) the PR interval, and (2) QRS duration (*see* Fig. 1.7).
- The ST segment, a most important ECG component. The study of abnormalities of the ST segment reveals the early diagnosis of acute myocardial infarction (MI) and myocardial ischemia. Thus, this text devotes an in-depth chapter to abnormalities of the ST segment

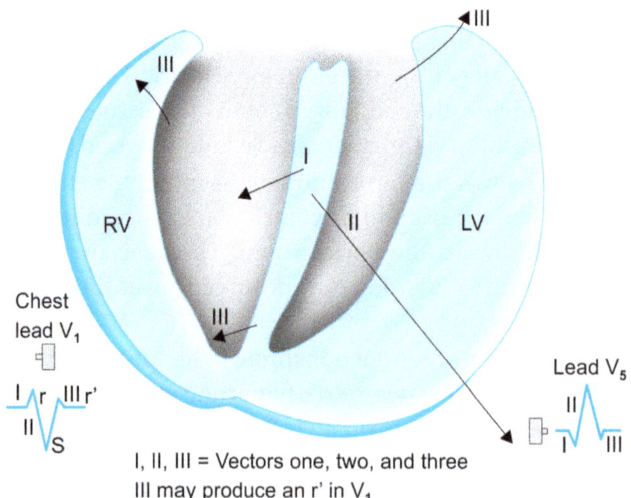

Fig. 1.6: Electrical activation of the heart: resultant vector forces. Vector III may produce an r' in V₁.

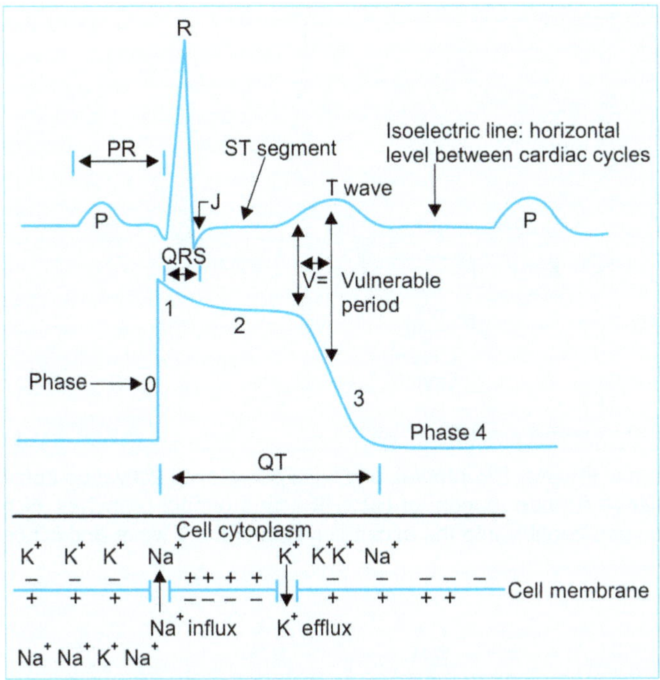

Fig. 1.7: Sodium influx, potassium efflux, the action potential, and the electrocardiogram.

Source: Adapted with permission from Khan MG. On Call Cardiology, 3rd edition. Philadelphia: WB Saunders, Elsevier Science; 2006.

and does so early in the interpretive sequence; that is, before analysis of abnormalities of the P wave, ventricular hypertrophy, QRS abnormalities, and the electrical axis. This approach simplifies ECG interpretation and is a strategy that is now embraced by physicians who render acute care to patients with acute MI and those with myocardial ischemia.

HOW ARE THE WAVES OF THE ELECTROCARDIOGRAM PRODUCED?

P Wave

The early part of the P wave represents the electrical activity generated by the right atrium; the middle portion of the P wave represents completion of right atrial activation and initiation of left atrial activation; and the late portion is generated by the left atrium. The P wave is the first deflection recorded and is a small, smooth, rounded deflection that precedes the spiky-looking QRS complex (Fig. 1.8). (See Chapter 3 for an in-depth discussion of P waves.)

PR Interval

The PR interval involves the time required for the electrical impulse to advance from the atria through the AV node, bundle of His, bundle branches, and Purkinje fibers until the ventricular muscle begins to depolarize (*see* Figs. 1.7 and 1.8).

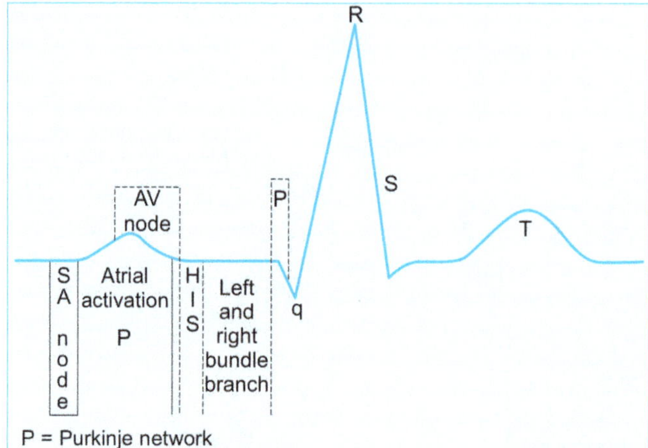

Fig. 1.8: Relationship of P wave, PR interval, and QRS complex to activation from the sinoatrial (SA) node, atrioventricular (AV) node, bundle of His (HIS), and bundle branches. Note that the normal ST segment curves imperceptibly into the ascending limb of the T wave and is not a horizontal line.

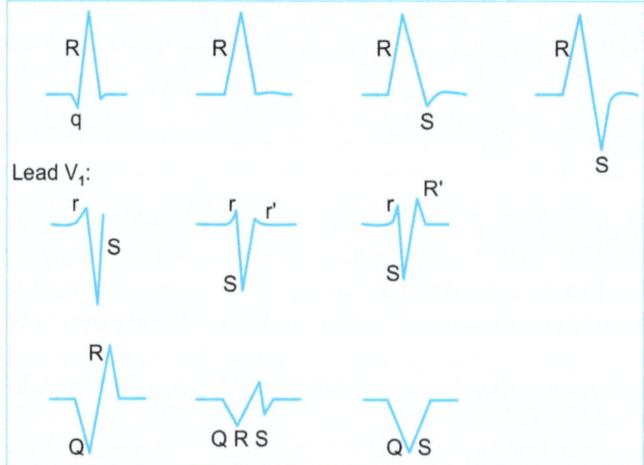

Fig. 1.9: Variation in QRS waveform. Uppercase letters are used to denote large deflection; R or r is used for first positive deflection; and R' or r' for second positive wave. Q or q is used for negative deflection before an r or R wave.

QRS Complex

The QRS complex represents the spread of electrical activation through the ventricular myocardium; the resultant electrical forces generated from ventricular depolarization are recorded on the ECG as a spiky deflection (*see* Figs. 1.7 and 1.8). The sharp, pointed deflections are labeled QRS regardless of whether they are positive (upward) or negative (downward).

Figure 1.9 indicates the conventional labeling of the QRS complex: q or Q, r or R, s or S, depending on the size of the components that may be recorded (i.e. those influenced by the electrode position) and the direction of the resultant vector forces. Large deflections are labeled with uppercase letters.

The genesis of the QRS complex is intricate and is better understood after the reader has been presented with information on leads and lead positions and why 12 leads are used to capture 12 views of the heart's electrical activity. Thus, the genesis of the QRS complex is discussed at the end of this chapter.

ST Segment

The ST segment is the segment that lies between the end of the QRS complex and the beginning of the T wave (*see* Figs. 1.7 and 1.8). It represents the period when all parts of the ventricles are in the depolarized state or a stage in which the terminal depolarization and the starting repolarization are superimposed and thus neutralize each other. Early repolarization may encroach on the ST segment to a variable degree. The part at which the ST segment takes off from the QRS complex is called the J, or the junction point. The ST segment normally curves imperceptibly into the ascending limb of the T wave and should not form a horizontal line or form a sharp angle with the proximal limb of the T wave. The student must be aware of this important diagnostic point.

T Wave

The T wave represents electrical recovery, repolarization of the ventricles, and is a broad, rounded wave (*see* Figs. 1.7 and 1.8). The T wave follows each QRS complex and is separated from the QRS by an interval that is constant for that ECG. Because ventricular recovery proceeds in the general direction of ventricular excitation, the polarity of the resultant T vector is similar to that of the QRS vector. The T wave is recorded during ventricular systole, whereas the QRS occurs immediately before mechanical systole.

- The T wave process is energy consuming, but the QRS process is not. During repolarization, cellular metabolic work and energy consumption occurs to accomplish the ionic flux associated with repolarization. Thus, several metabolic, hemodynamic, and physiologic factors may affect the repolarization process and alter the morphology of the T wave. The student or clinician interpreting ECGs should be aware of the normal variations in T wave morphology and the influence of a host of factors that may alter the T wave and lead to erroneous diagnoses.
- Levine listed approximately 67 causes for T wave changes, which include the patient drinking ice water, eating, exercising, or fasting or having infections, fever, tachycardia, anoxia, shock, electrolyte derangements, acidemia, alkalemia, hormonal imbalances, subarachnoid hemorrhage, or drug or alcohol abuse.

Because of the unreliable diagnostic yield derived from the scrutiny of T waves, further details on this topic are relegated to Chapter 8.

U Wave

The U wave is a wave that follows the T wave and is observed only in the ECG tracings of some individuals. It is a small, often indistinct wave, and its source is uncertain (*see* Chapter 8).

WHY USE 12 LEADS TO RECORD THE ELECTROCARDIOGRAM?

Einthoven's discovery in 1901 was of paramount importance. His landmark paper was published in 1901, and a further paper on the galvanometric registration of the human electrocardiogram was published in 1903. However, the initial work of Galvani (1791), Muller (1856), and Waller (1887) initiated Einthoven's accomplishment. Einthoven recognized that the heart possessed electrical activity, and he recorded this activity using two sensors attached to the two forearms and connected to a silver wire that ran between two poles of a large permanent magnet. He noted that the silver wire moved rhythmically with the heartbeats, but to visualize the small movements Einthoven shone a light beam across the wire, and the wavy movements of the wire were recorded on moving photographic paper. Einthoven recorded the waves and spiky deflection and labeled the first smooth, rounded wave, P; the spiky deflection, QRS; and the last recorded wave, T.

- Einthoven labeled the waves P, Q, R, S, and T; his lettering obeyed the convention used by geometricians: curved lines were labeled beginning with P, and points on straight lines were labeled beginning with Q.

Einthoven, Sir Thomas Lewis, and others correlated the ECG waves with the contracting heart and correlated that the P wave was related to atrial contraction and that the QRS deflection was associated with ventricular contraction. Improvements in the quality of recordings resulted from the immense work and technique of Frank Wilson, who studied with Lewis and, in Michigan (1934), described the unipolar leads that include the precordial V leads and VR, VL, and VF.

LEADS AND ELECTRODES

Why are 12 Leads Necessary?

Figure 1.10 shows the infinite number of electrode positions arranged in a continuous circle, at the center of which is the origin of the depolarization wave. The illustration indicates that the electrode position has a profound influence on the size, or amplitude, of the recording.

- Twelve ECG leads are used to obtain 12 views of the heart's electrical activity. The heart may be considered to lie at the center of an equilateral triangle (Fig. 1.11). The leads attached to the limbs, the limb leads, act as linear conductors and have virtually identical voltages at all points along their lengths. The limbs can be regarded as extensions of a lead wire. Thus, the left arm electrode placed at the wrist, arm, or shoulder displays the same ECG record. Because the limb leads act as linear conductors, the effective sensing points and electrode locations are at the left and right shoulders and left groin, but are usually positioned and labeled as follows:
  - R = right arm lead
  - L = left arm lead
  - F = foot = left leg lead.

These leads lie along the frontal plane of the body and display action potential only in the frontal plane. (See discussion of frontal plane axis in Step 9 in Chapter 2 and in Chapter 9.) Two important concepts must be re-emphasized:

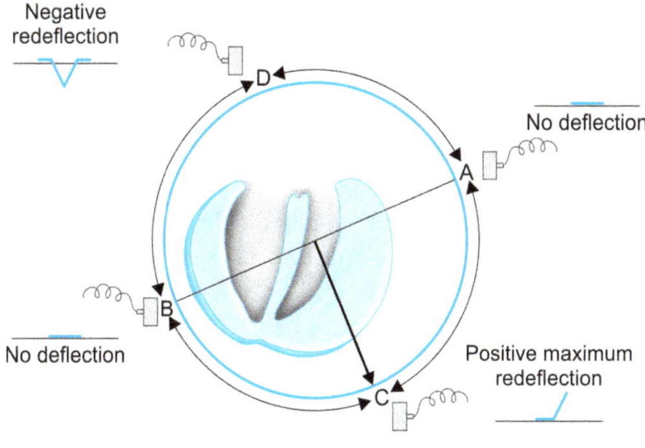

Fig. 1.10: Effect of varied electrode positions on the amplitude and direction of deflections recorded: leads between C and A or C and B give positive deflection less than at C. Leads at D and A or D and B record negative deflection of varying size. The line AB is perpendicular to the electrical current.

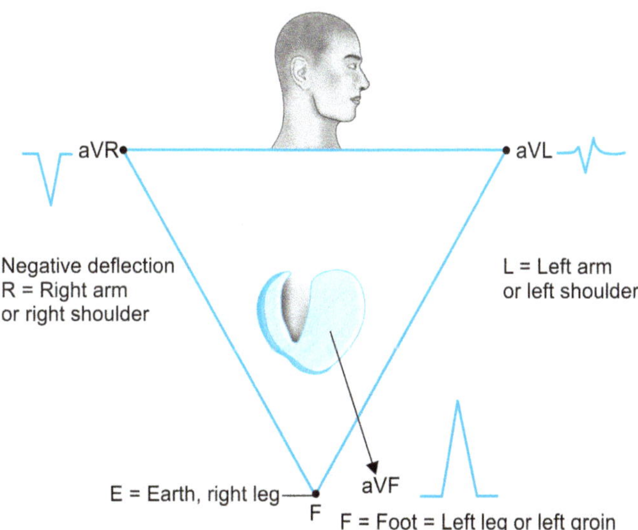

Fig. 1.11: The heart depicted as a three-muscle mass that lies in the center of an equilateral triangle. The two shoulders and left groin are sensing positions.

- If the excitatory depolarization head of the current (vector force) flows toward a unipolar electrode, a galvanometer will record an upward or positive deflection (*see* Figs. 1.3A to C).
- When an excitatory depolarization process is directed away from the electrode, a downward or negative deflection is recorded (*see* Fig. 1.3B).
- Figure 1.11 displays deflections that can be recorded by limb leads R, L, and F. The main electrical current of activation flows toward the F (left leg) electrode and records an upward

or positive deflection of large amplitude. The current flows away from the right shoulder (R) electrode and records a downward deflection. The right shoulder lead (R) looks into the interior of the heart toward the endocardium, and as mentioned previously, the current of activation flows from the endocardium and traverses the myocardium toward the pericardium and thus displays a negative deflection. The student should notice that aVR is always relatively negative and aVF is always relatively positive.

- Lead L at the left shoulder or left arm usually displays a small positive or equiphasic deflection, but the heart hangs in the chest and is subject to rotational changes, and the main current direction may be altered; thus, this lead may show a large-amplitude positive deflection in some individuals, and a negative deflection if the heart's position is vertical.

Why Augmented Leads?

- Why is a V added to the R, L, and F? These leads are termed unipolar limb leads, but voltage measurements are virtually never unipolar. The connection formed by attaching the R, L, and F electrodes together acts as a reference connection, and the lead formed is termed a V lead (V = voltage); thus the convention VR, VL, and VF, and the V is also used for the leads positioned on the chest, V_1 to V_6.
- Goldberger (1942) augmented Wilson's unipolar extremity leads that gave low-amplitude records; Goldberger's strategy increased the amplitude of the deflections by 50%. Thus, the letter a is used to denote the augmented lead [e.g. aVL = augmented-voltage left arm lead (V = voltage)].

Standard Bipolar Limb Leads I, II, and III

Figure 1.12 shows the views of the heart obtained by leads I, II, and III.

- Lead I connects the two arms and is formed by connecting L to the positive terminal and R to the negative terminal of the galvanometer; thus, I = aVL – aVR. Lead I looks at the heart from the left, inferior to lead aVL, the lead of the left shoulder (arm), and displays the electrical tracing produced by a combination of the right arm and left arm electrodes. The right leg electrode is an earth (or ground) and minimizes interference.
- Lead II looks at the heart from a position to the left of the left groin, foot lead F (see Fig. 1.12).
- Lead III looks at the heart from a position to the right of the left groin, foot lead F. Thus, leads II, III, and aVF look at the inferior surface of the heart from different angles, and they usually show some similarities. Lead III is the most unreliable of the leads II, III, and aVF. Thus, many errors are made from the observation of the QRS and T wave in lead III. Normal yet pathologic-appearing Q waves and T wave inversion may be observed frequently in lead III as a normal variant.
- The six leads display six photographs of the heart's electrical activity taken from six angles (one every 30°). The six leads can be visualized as traversing a flat plane over the chest of the patient (i.e. the frontal plane). Importantly, if only two of the six leads are recorded, the most informative pair is I and aVF.

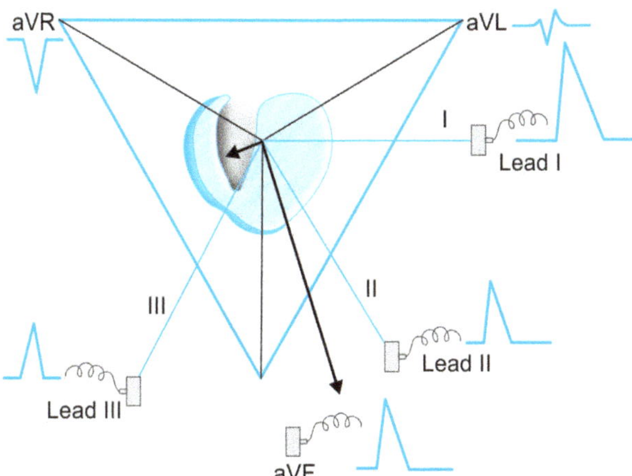

Fig. 1.12: Standard bipolar limb leads I, II, and III. Note that aVF leads II and III look at the inferior surface of the heart and deflections show minor variation. Leads I and aVL look at the anterolateral aspect of the heart. Lead aVF is always relatively positive, aVR is always relatively negative, and aVL is variable.

Vertical versus Horizontal Heart Position

Figures 1.13A and B show the changes in QRS waveform caused by alteration of the position of the heart.

- Both aVR and aVL face the ventricular cavity and show a QS complex.
- A qR complex in lead aVL indicates a horizontal heart position, and the QRS morphology in aVL resembles that in V_5.
- A qR complex in aVF and a QS complex in aVL indicate a vertical heart position, and the QRS morphologies in leads aVF and V_5 resemble each other.
- The position of the heart varies between horizontal and vertical.

Chest Leads/Precordial or V Leads

The six chest leads give six more views of the heart's electrical activity and vector forces; they are positioned around the anterior and left chest wall in a horizontal plane. Figures 1.14 and 1.15 indicate the position of the precordial chest leads that overlie the right and left ventricles.

V_1 and V_2 face and lie close to the wall of the right ventricle. V_2 and V_3 lie near the intraventricular septum. V_4 and V_3 look at the anterior parts of the left ventricle, with V_4 close to the apex. V_5 and V_6 (leads I and aVL) view the anterolateral region of the left ventricle and often appear similar to each other. The recording in lead aVL, however, varies depending on a horizontal or vertical heart position. If V_7 is taken, it is positioned in the posterior axillary line.

The precordial electrodes V_1 to V_6 are so close to the electrical currents of the heart that no augmentation is necessary. Lead V_6 is far around (in the axilla) and is separated from the free wall of the left ventricle by a significant distance.

Figure 1.15 re-emphasizes that the position of leads aVL and aVF and other limb leads are in the same frontal plane. The chest leads V_1 to V_6 encircle the left thorax in a horizontal plane.

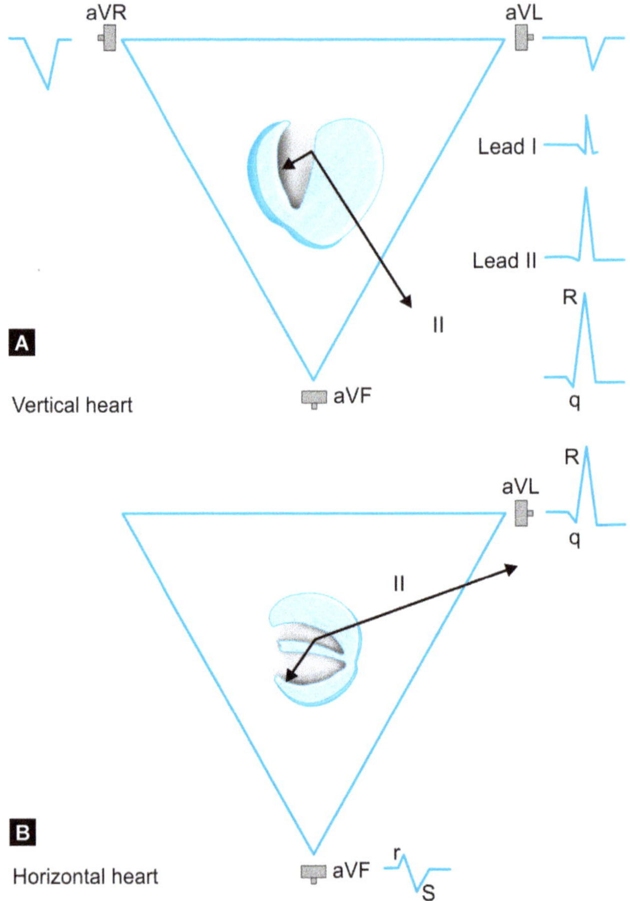

Figs. 1.13A and B: Changes in deflections with the heart in: (A) a vertical and (B) a horizontal position. (A) In the vertical position, both the aVR and aVL face the cavity of the ventricles and record a QS complex; (B) A QRS complex in aVF indicates a heart that is positioned close to vertical; qRS in aVL indicates a horizontal heart position.

Caution: The entire chest, with the heart within it, acts as a volume conductor, and thus voltage varies appreciably at locations only a centimeter apart. Therefore, the leads placed on the chest wall V_1 to V_6 must be positioned meticulously so that when the ECG is repeated days or years later, accurate comparison can be made. Caution is required so that the V_5 and V_6 electrodes are not placed too anteriorly. V_5 must be placed in the anterior axillary line; V_6 should be placed in the midaxillary line at the level of V_4 in the fifth intercostal space or in line with the apex beat.

If lead V_3 is placed too close to V_2 or is positioned near the left third intercostal space, no positive deflection or a reduced-amplitude R wave may be recorded, which can falsely simulate an anterior MI. If lead V_2 is positioned too close to V_1, no R wave may be recorded in lead V_2, and the erroneous diagnosis of anteroseptal MI may be made. These errors are made commonly

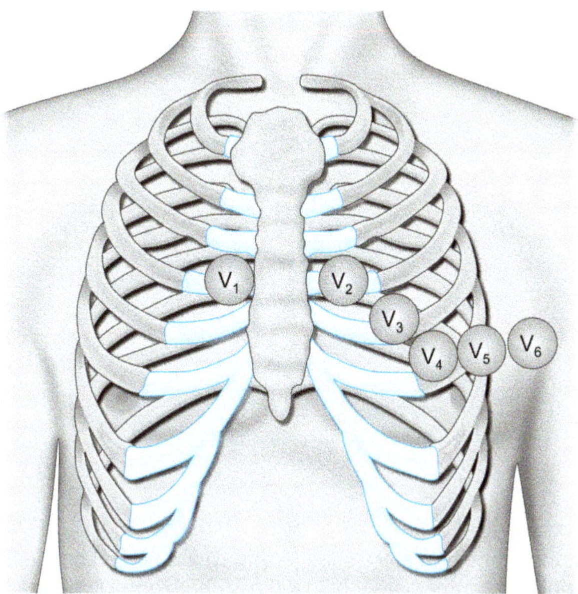

Fig. 1.14: Position of precordial chest leads.

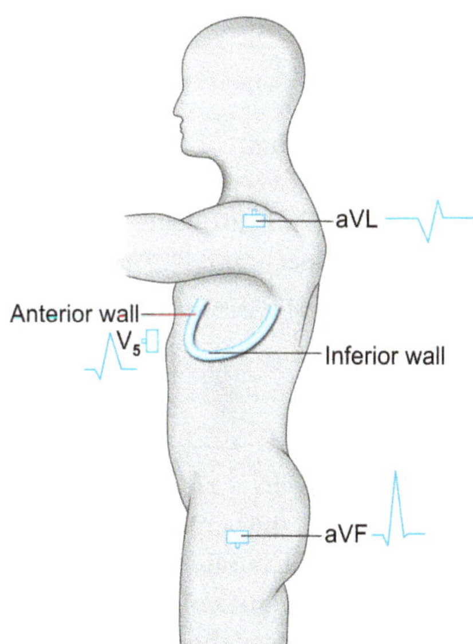

Fig. 1.15: aVF and aVL are in the same frontal plane. The chest leads encircle the
left thorax in a horizontal plane.

in the ECGs of females, and they may be interpreted as "loss or poor R wave in V_3, consider anteroseptal MI". An ECG with faulty recording may lead to serious errors in interpretation.

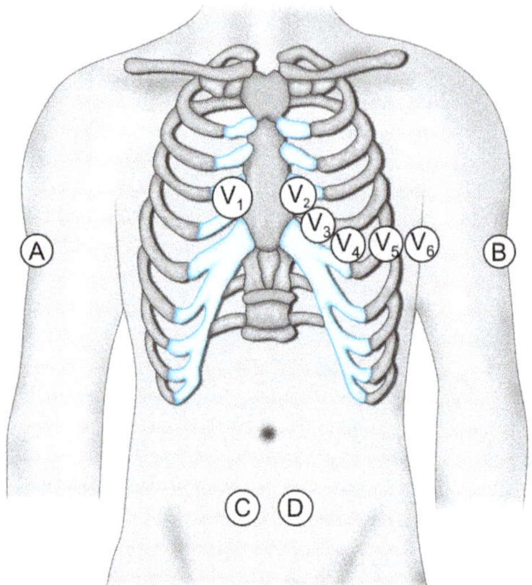

Fig. 1.16: The Khan method. The arm electrodes (A and B) are placed on the mid-arm, on the lateral or medial aspect of the biceps, immediately below the V_4 horizontal line. The abdominal electrodes (C and D) placed 7–7.6 cm (~2.5–3 inches, ~3 fingerbreadths) below the umbilical horizontal line, and 5 cm (~2 inches) on either side of the umbilical vertical line. The distance between these two electrodes to be 10 cm (~4 inches).
Source: Khan GM. A new electrode placement method for obtaining 12-lead ECGs. Open Heart. 2015;2:e000226.

NEW PLACEMENTS FOR LIMB LEADS

The author has shown in a study that placement of the limb lead electrodes on the upper arm and lower abdomen gives better quality ECGs with removal of artifacts produced by the old wrist and above than ankle placements (Khan 2015).

Figure 1.16 shows the new electrode placement (NEP) for the extremity leads that have been placed on the wrist and ankles since 1946 and are now on the upper arm and abdomen (Khan 2015).

GENESIS OF THE QRS COMPLEX

Understanding the genesis of the QRS complex is a fundamental step. Knowledge of the normal sequence of activation or depolarization of the ventricles is crucial to an understanding of the normal and abnormal QRS complex. The accurate diagnosis of acute and old MI, right and left bundle branch block, hemiblocks, and ventricular hypertrophy depends on knowledge of resultant vectors that dictate the components of the QRS complex.

The electrical impulse that proceeds from the SA node activates the atria, producing the P wave, the first wave of the ECG. The electrical impulse is briefly slowed in the AV node, then progresses rapidly down the bundle of His, the right and left bundle branches, and the Purkinje fibers of the ventricular myocardium. The spread of the electrical impulses through the septum and ventricular muscle is called depolarization, which produces the QRS complex of the ECG.

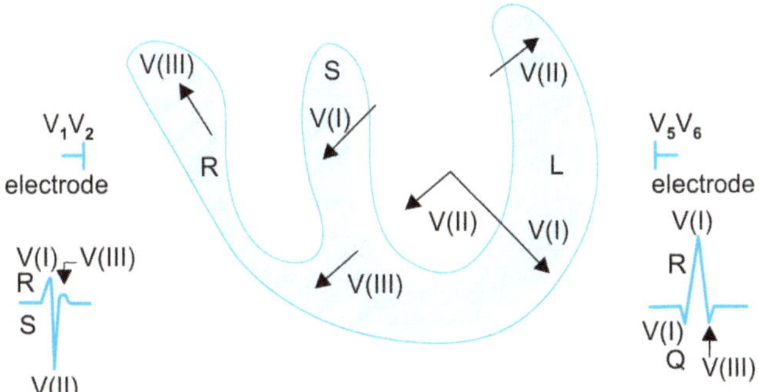

Fig. 1.17: Genesis of the normal QRS complex. V(I), vector I produces a small r wave in leads V_1 and V_2, Q in leads V_5 and V_6; V(II), vector II produces an S wave in lead V_1 and an R wave in lead V_5 or V_6; V(III), vector III produces the terminal S in leads V_5 and V_6 and the terminal r or r′ in V_1, V_2, and aVR; V_1, lead V_1 electrode; V_6, lead V_6 electrode; R, right ventricle muscle mass; L, left ventricle muscle mass; S, septum.
Source: Adapted with permission from Khan MG. On Call Cardiology, 3rd edition. Philadelphia: WB Saunders, Elsevier Science; 2006.

VECTOR FORCES

The electrical impulses that activate each area of heart muscle have direction and magnitude and can be represented by a vector force. The direction of the resultant force can be represented by an arrow, the length of which represents the magnitude of the force. The term *vector* does not imply vector cardiography.

Three Caveats

A vector describes a force in terms of its duration and magnitude.

The following three caveats must be considered:

1. An electrical impulse traveling toward an electrode causes a positive deflection or R wave (Fig. 1.17).
2. When the impulse is traveling away from the electrode, a negative deflection occurs (i.e. an S, a small Q, or a QS wave is recorded).
3. Three resultant vectors dictate the inscription of the QRS complex.

Vector I

- The ventricular septum is activated from left to right; electrodes or leads positioned over the right ventricle (V_1 or V_2) face the wave of depolarization and inscribe a positive wave, a small R wave (*see* Fig. 1.17).
- Because the force of the activation impulse (vector I) is small, the positive deflection is small; the R wave recorded in V_1 and V_2 is small and ranges from 1 mm to 4 mm in V_1 and from 1 mm to 7 mm in V_2 in normal individuals older than age 30 years (*see* Table 2.1). Incorrect lead placement of V_1, V_2, and V_3, especially in women, may cause the ECG tracing to falsely show diminished or loss of R or r waves in V_2 and V_3, which is often incorrectly interpreted as anteroseptal MI.

- The initial depolarizing current travels away from leads V_5 and V_6 and thus inscribes a small negative deflection, a small Q wave in leads V_5, V_6, and I.

Vector II

- After septal depolarization, both ventricular walls are activated simultaneously.
- The impulse depolarizes the thin-walled right ventricle; however, the magnitude of the forces is small in comparison with the forces that activate the thick left ventricular free wall. Thus, the resultant force, vector II, is directed toward and through the left ventricular free wall (*see* Fig. 1.17).
- The resultant force, vector II, is indicated by an arrow directed toward the left; the electrodes V_5 and V_6 face the left ventricle and show a positive wave, an R wave, the height of which depends on the thickness of the left ventricular muscle. The height of the R wave in V_4 through V_6 ranges from 10 mm to 25 mm and may exceed 30 mm in individuals with left ventricular hypertrophy and in normal subjects younger than age 25 years. The R wave in V_4 through V_6 is lost or is reduced to less than 3 mm in height in patients with anterior MI.
- Because the electrical current represented by vector II travels away from an electrode overlying the right ventricle, V_1 and V_2 record a negative deflection, an S wave.
- The larger the left ventricular muscle, the deeper the S wave in V_1 and V_2.

Vector III

- Activation of the posterobasal right and left ventricular free walls and the basal right septal mass, including the crista supraventricularis, represents vector III.
- The resultant force is directed to the right, is small in magnitude, and may record a small S wave in V_5 and V_6 and a terminal r′ wave in lead V_1 or V_2; thus, an Rsr′ pattern in V_1 may occur in normal individuals.

NORMAL ELECTROCARDIOGRAM, QRS NORMAL VARIANTS AND ABNORMALITIES

Figures 1.18 to 1.23 show normal ECGs.

Lead I shows an upright (positive) deflection; the entire QRS complex is positive (upright), the P wave is upright. R waves increase in height from V_1 to tallest in V_5-V_6, note that aVR is the only lead that has totally negative deflections for P wave, QRS complex and T waves. Lead aVR normally records a negative QRS or QS complex because aVR looks into the cavity of the ventricle and faces the endocardial surface; the activating current flows from endocardium to pericardium (see Figs. 1.24 and 1.25).

Figure 1.24 shows a tracing with reversed arm leads.

Normal Q Waves

- Normal Q waves are less than 0.04 second in duration and are less than 3 mm deep. These small Q waves are recorded when a small activation current is directed away from the

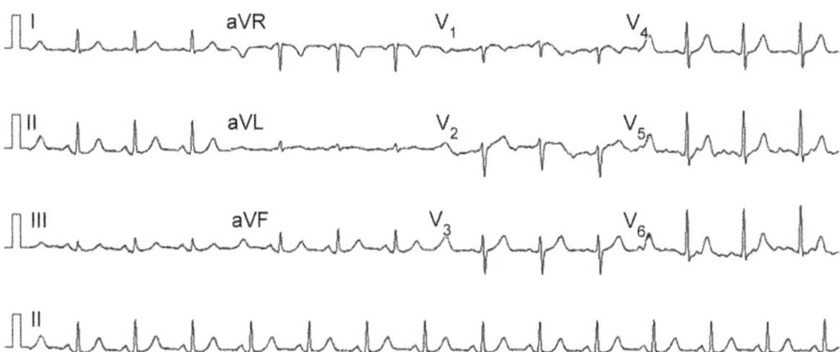

Fig. 1.18: Normal ECG. Note in lead aVR, all waves are negative: P inverted, QRS negative deflection; T wave negative. These all become positive, upright if the arm leads are reversed, a common technical error.

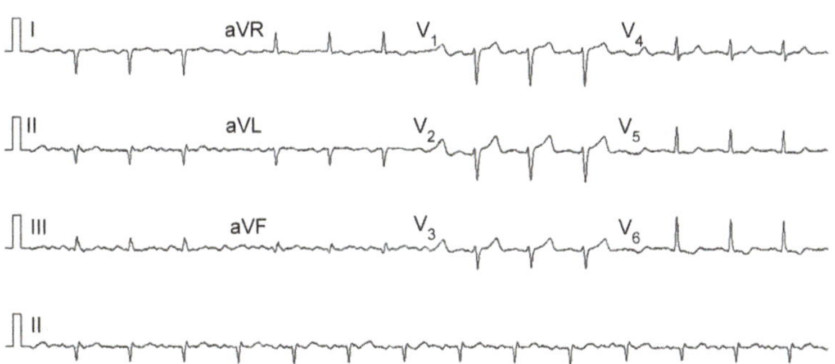

Fig. 1.19: Reversed arm leads, otherwise ECG within normal limits. Left electrode placed on right wrist or arm lead I and aVL show negative P, QRS and T waves. Note lead I and V_6 QRS are dissimilar; with dextrocardia, they are similar.

electrode. Small Q waves are found normally in leads V_5, V_6, and I (*see* Fig. 2.2) (*see* Figs. 1.18 to 1.23). Changes in the position of the heart may cause small Q waves in leads II, III, aVF, and sometimes in leads I and aVL. With extreme counterclockwise rotation, small Q waves occur in V_1 through V_6.

- Leads III and aVL may record narrow Q waves up to 10 mm deep in normal individuals. In lead III, the Q wave can be normally less than or equal to 0.04 second wide (*see* Fig. 2.2D). In all other leads, Q waves should be considered normal if they are less than 0.04 second wide and less than 3 mm deep. If Q waves are not observed in leads II or aVF, a Q wave in lead III should be considered normal (*see* Table 2.1).

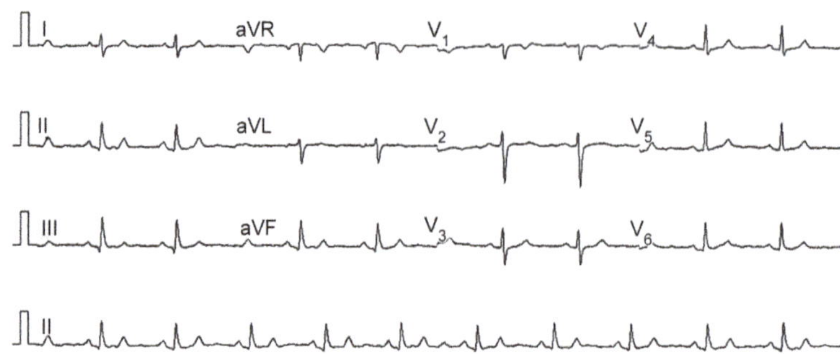

Fig. 1.20: Normal ECG. Note small narrow, normal Q waves in leads III and aVF, occasionally Q also in leads II and V_6.

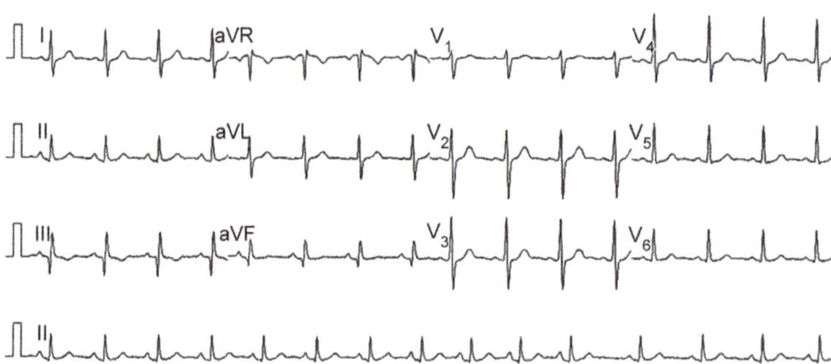

Fig. 1.21: A 31-year-old male; computer diagnosis: old inferior MI. Corrected: sinus arrhythmia; nondiagnostic inferior Q waves noted: 35 <Q <40 ms in aVF with Q in II, III; Q/R >1/3 in aVF. Borderline ECG—clinical correlation required.

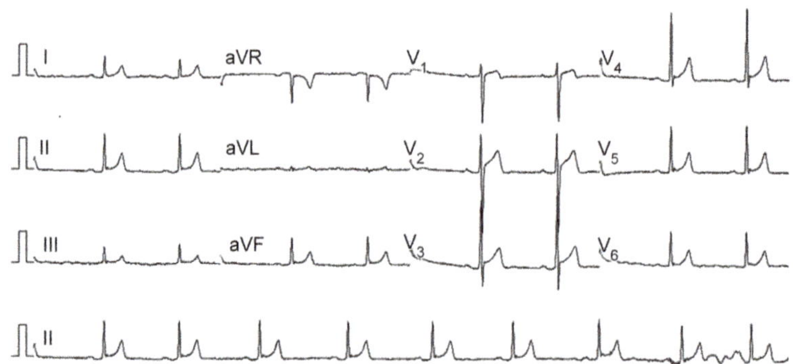

Fig. 1.22: ST segment elevation V_2-V_4 in a healthy 26-year-old male. Note a little notch at the end of the QRS complex as it merges into the ST segment: "fish hook", sometimes more obvious and is typical for normal variants ST elevations.

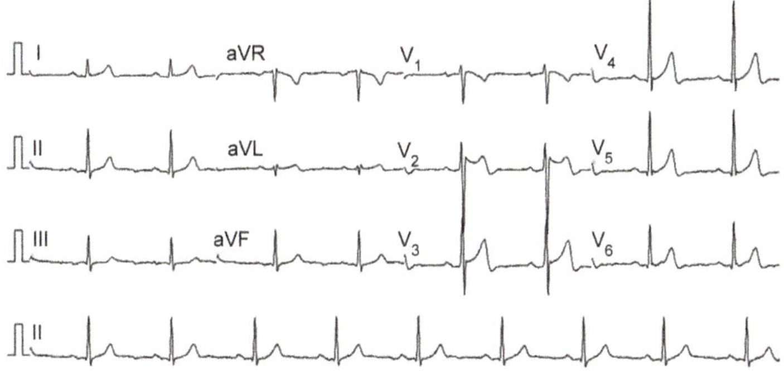

Fig. 1.23: ST segment elevation V_2-V_3 in a healthy 21-year-old male (this feature is less commonly seen in females).

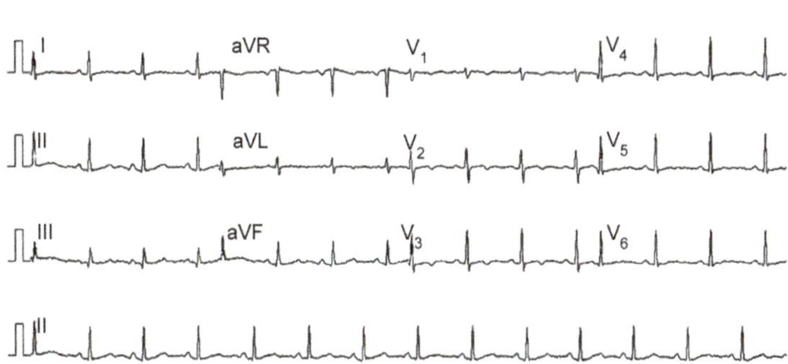

Fig. 1.24: A 40-year-old female T inversion V_1-V_3; normal variant; T inversion occurs in approximately 5% of females and is described by some as female variant.

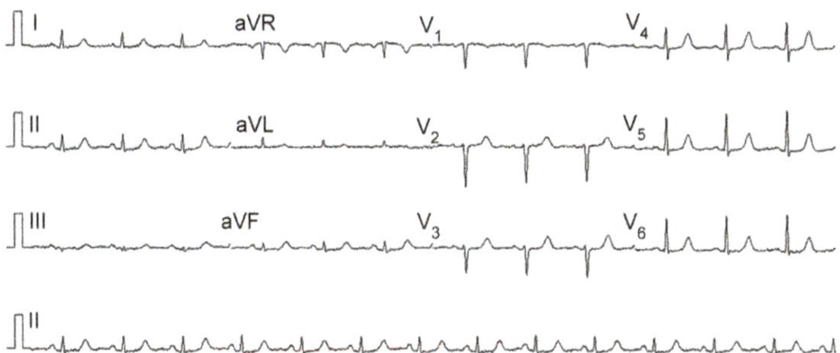

Fig. 1.25: Note poor R wave progression in V_2 and V_3; R waves should grow taller from V_2 to V_3, V_4 and in V_3 are expected to be taller than 10 mm. Lead placement in females may cause poor R wave progression in V_2-V_3. This is a common error made by technicians and causes many misdiagnosis and repetition of ECGs.

- Hypertrophy of the interventricular septum occurs in hypertrophic cardiomyopathy, and the ECG often reveals deep Q waves that can mimic MI (see discussion of pathologic Q waves and QS patterns given in Chapter 6).
- Infarction of the ventricular septum causes the loss of vector I, as well as loss of the normal R wave in leads V_1 and V_2 (i.e. pathologic Q waves), indicating anteroseptal infarction (*see* Figs. 1.26 to 1.30).
- Replacement of ventricular muscle by tumor; fibrosis; or amyloid, sarcoid, or other granuloma may cause an electrical window and Q waves that simulate infarction.

Nondiagnostic Inferior Q Waves (Figs. 1.26 to 1.33)

- Electrocardiograms showing these nondiagnostic inferior Q waves (Q, inferior leads II, III, aVF, not Q = deep and wide) are often incorrectly interpreted as probable old inferior infarction (see Figs. 1.31 and 1.32).

Nondiagnostic inferior MI—a common finding and often interpreted as probable old inferior MI.

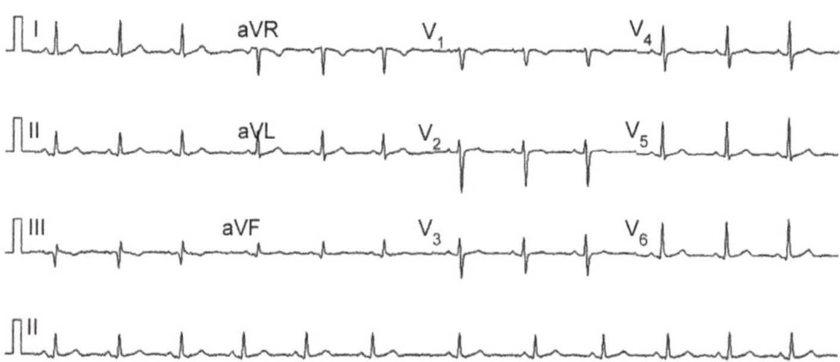

Fig. 1.26: Nondiagnostic Q waves inferior leads, commonly reported by computer as probable old inferior MI causing repeat ECGs over several years.

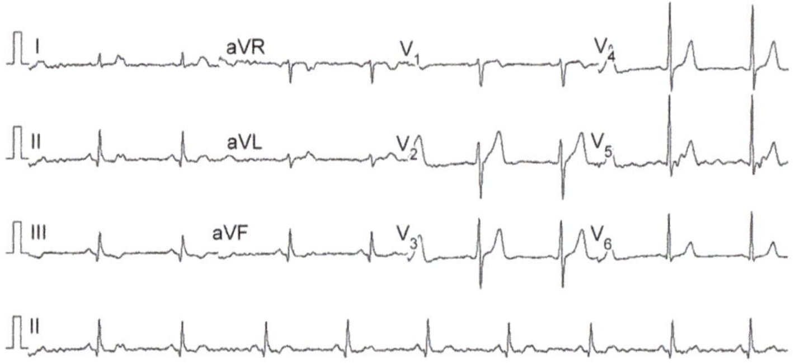

Fig. 1.27: Normal Q waves II, III, aVF, V_6. Other examples of normal Q waves that are over-read by computer diagnosis; see Fig. 1.28 to 1.33.

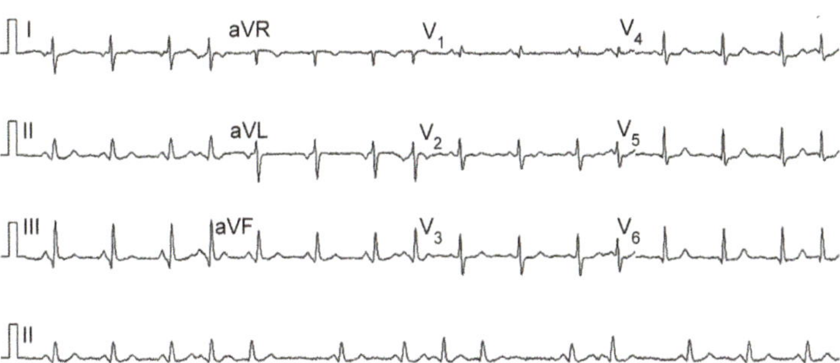

Fig. 1.28: Abnormal Q waves. Infarction of the ventricular septum causes the loss of vector I, as well as loss of the normal R wave in leads V_1 and V_2 (i.e. pathologic Q waves), indicating anteroseptal infarction (see Fig. 2.18A).

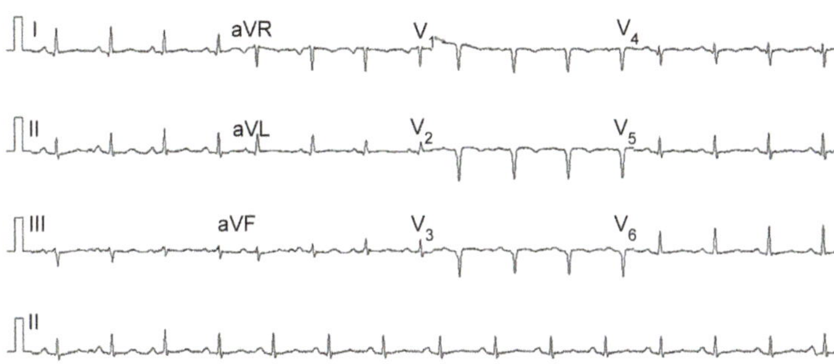

Fig. 1.29: Deep wide Q waves V_1-V_3: anteroseptal MI.

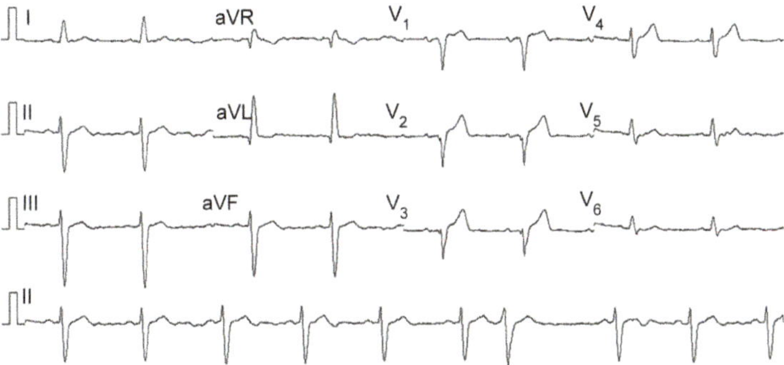

Fig. 1.30: Deep wide Q waves V_1-V_3; old anteroseptal MI.

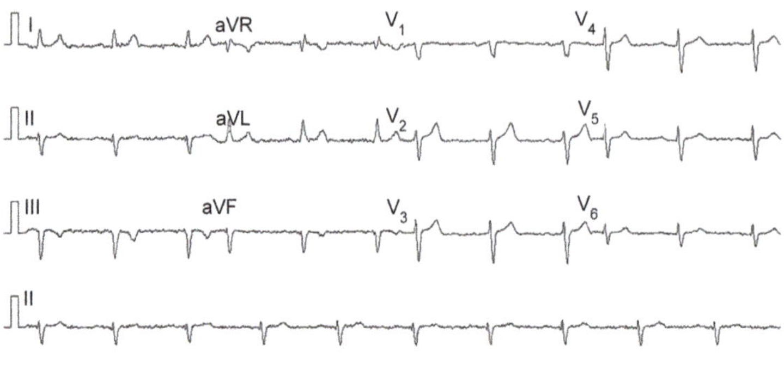

Fig. 1.31: Old inferior MI.

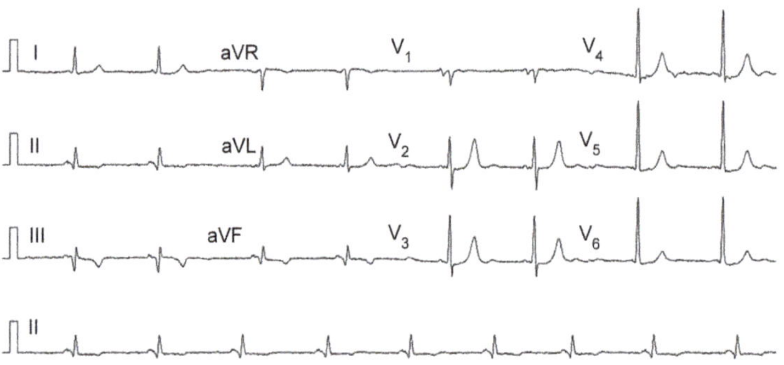

Fig. 1.32: Deep wide Q waves, inferior leads II, III, aVF. Proven old inferior MI.

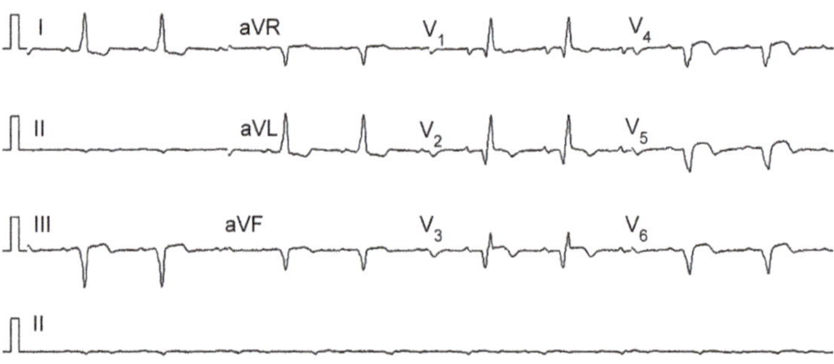

Fig. 1.33: Deep wide Q waves III, aVF, V_2, V_6 old inferior and anterior MI. Wide complexes—
right bundle branch block (RBBB).

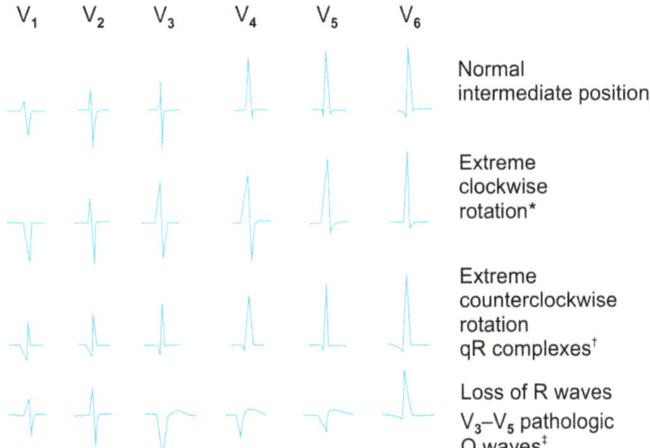

Fig. 1.34: Variations in the normal precordial QRS configuration and correlations with abnormals.
*With clockwise rotation, the V_1 electrode, like aVR, faces the cavity of the heart and records a QS complex; no initial q in lead V_6.
† qR complexes: q <0.04 second, less than 3 mm deep; therefore not pathologic Q waves.
‡ Loss of R wave in leads V_3 through V_5; pathologic Q waves: signifies anterior myocardial infarction.
Source: Adapted with permission from Khan MG. On Call Cardiology, 3rd edition. Philadelphia: WB Saunders, Elsevier Science; 2006.

Clockwise and Counterclockwise Rotation

- Variations in the normal QRS configuration are shown in Figure 1.34. If the heart undergoes strong clockwise or counterclockwise rotation, changes in QRS morphology occur. Failure to recognize these normal variants may result in incorrect interpretation of the ECG.
- With clockwise rotation, the V_1 electrode, like aVR, faces the cavity of the ventricle and records a QS complex; therefore, Q waves can occur as a normal finding if there is extreme clockwise rotation of the heart (*see* Fig. 1.34). The normal Q wave in V_6 disappears because the resultant force of the initial vector I is not directed toward the electrode V_1.

ECG Interpretation: A New Method

INTRODUCTION

Conventional Sequence Regarding Interpretation

The time-honored advice to students and staff is as follows: In every electrocardiogram (ECG), the following features should be examined systematically:

- Rate
- Rhythm
- P wave morphology
- PR interval
- QRS interval, QRS complex morphology

- ST segment
- T wave
- Electrical axis
- U wave and QT duration.

Some authors advise the following sequence:

Assess: Rate, rhythm, axis, hypertrophy, infarction but this is not the conventional teaching of cardiology tutors.

New Sequence for Interpretation

This text departs somewhat from the conventional sequence and gives a new approach consistent with the changes in cardiology practice that have evolved over the past decade. The early diagnosis of acute myocardial infarction (MI) depends on astute observation for abnormal changes in the ST segment. Determination of creatine kinase MB (CK-MB) and troponins is not relevant in the early phase of acute MI, because these cardiac enzymes are not elevated and are nondiagnostic within the crucial first hour of onset of MI. The door-to-needle or balloon time must be minimized if maximal lifesaving is to be achieved. Diagnosis depends on symptoms and ST segment changes. Thus, this text rushes the interpreter to the assessment of ST segment morphology and suggests an *11-step method* or sequence for the rapid yet accurate interpretation of ECGs.

BRIEF HIGHLIGHTS OF AN 11-STEP METHOD

Figure 2.1 defines the ECG waveform; Figures 2.2A to F show features of the normal ECG; and Table 2.1 gives normal ECG intervals and parameters.

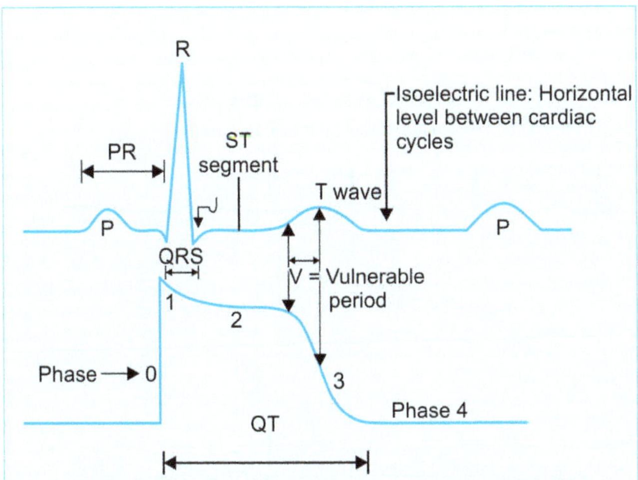

Fig. 2.1: Sodium influx, potassium efflux, the action potential, and the ECG.
Source: Adapted with permission from Khan MG. On Call Cardiology, 3rd edition. Philadelphia: WB Saunders, Elsevier Science; 2006.

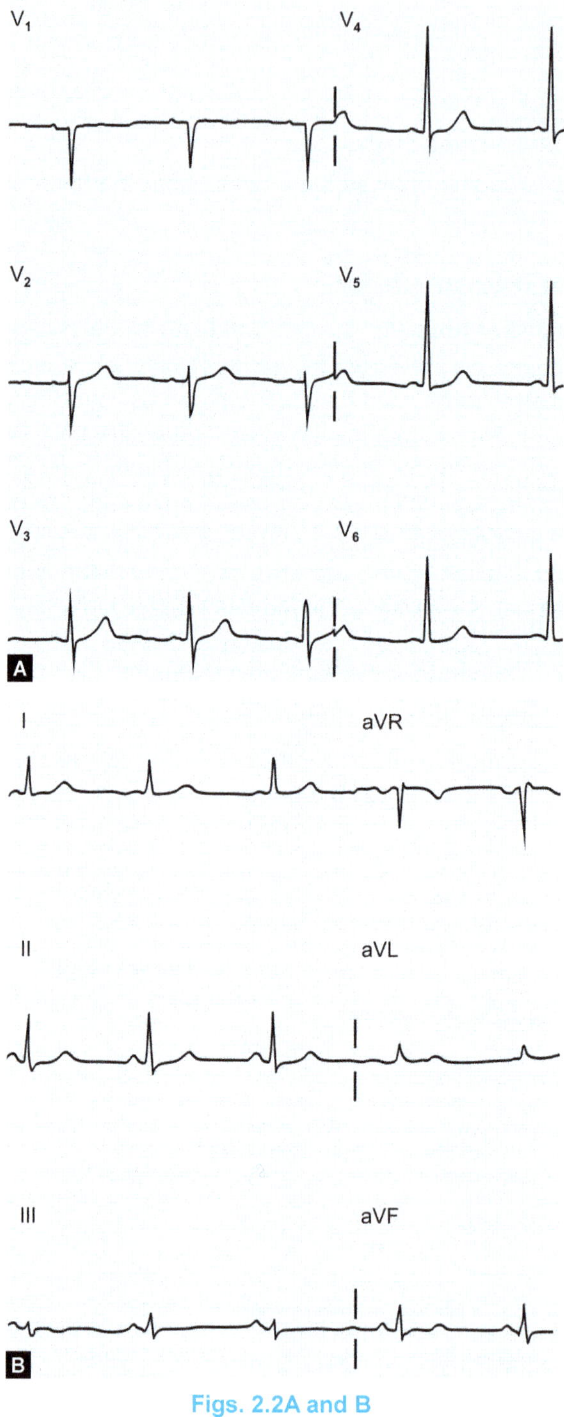

Figs. 2.2A and B

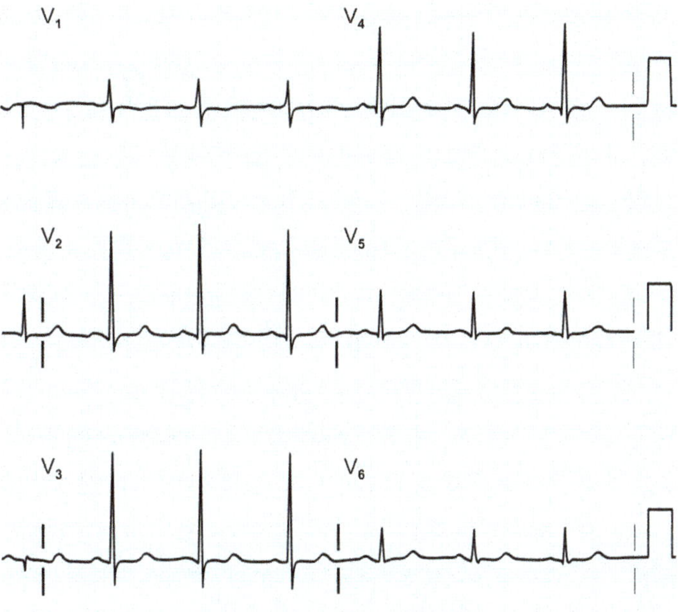

Fig. 2.2C

Figs. 2.2A to C: (A) Chest leads V₁ through V₆; (B) Limb leads I through aVF. Sinus rhythm, rate 65 beats/minute; PR interval, 0.14 second; QRS duration, 0.08 second; QT interval, 0.36 second; axis, +30°; (C) Chest leads of a normal ECG with a QRS complex in V₂ that is positive, indicating early transition. Compare with Figure 2.2A, in which transition is normal, occurring in lead V₃; tall R waves in V₁ and V₂ are not caused by posterior infarction (see Table 2.3). Heart rate, 75 beats/minute (see Table 2.2). Note normal small Q wave in V₄ through V₆.

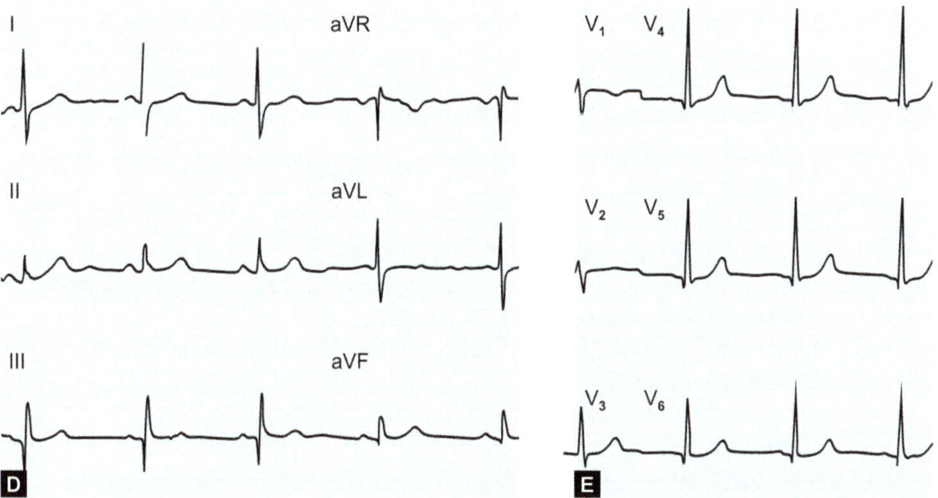

Figs. 2.2D and E: (D) Limb leads of a normal ECG showing a deep but normal Q wave in lead III (see Table 2.1 for normal parameters); (E) Leads V₄ through V₆ show small, normal Q waves less than 4 mm deep; leads V₁ through V₃ show normal R wave progression.

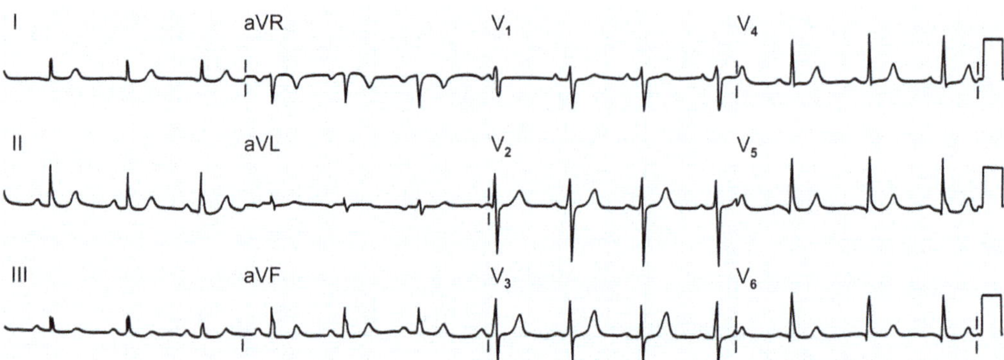

Fig. 2.2F: Normal ECG, sinus rhythm 75 beats/minute; PR interval, 0.16 second; QRS duration, 0.08 second; normal QRS axis +60°; QT interval, 0.35 second. The small notch on the R wave of leads II, III, and aVF is a normal finding in some individuals and does not indicate intraventricular conduction delay (see Chapter 4).

TABLE 2.1: Important normal ECG intervals and parameters.*	
PR interval	0.12–0.2 second (up to 0.22 second in adults)
P waves	<3 small squares (0.12 second) in duration, and amplitude
	<3 mm. Upright in lead I, inverted in aVR (if opposite, suspect reversed arm leads[†] or dextrocardia) (*see* Step 6, Figs. 2.21 and 2.36)
QRS duration	0.05–0.1 second; ≥0.1 second, consider incomplete LBBB, incomplete RBBB, or WPW syndrome (*see* Steps 2 and 3, Figs. 2.4, 2.9, and 2.10)
Q waves	Normally present in aVR; occasionally in V_1 or in aVL (vertical heart) (*see* Chapter 6)
	Often present in lead III: should be ≤0.04 second duration
	Other leads except lead I: <0.04 second duration and ≤3 mm deep; lead I ≤1.5 mm in patients older than age 30. Q waves may be up to 5 mm deep in several leads in individuals age <30
R waves	V_1: 0–15 mm, age 12–20 (*see* Table 2.3)
	0–8 mm, age 20–30
	0–6 mm, age >30[‡]
	V_2: 0.2–12 mm, age <30[‡] (*see* Step 5)
	V_3: 1–20 mm, age >30[‡]
ST segment	Isoelectric or <1 mm elevation in limb leads and <1 mm in precordial leads except for normal variant (*see* Step 4)
T wave	Inverted in aVR; upright in I, II, and V_3 through V_6. Variable in III, aVF, aVL, V_1, and V_2 (*see* Step 8)
Axis	0° to +110° age <40. −30° to +90° age >40 (*see* Step 9)
QT interval	See Table 2.5

*ECG paper speed 25 mm/s.

[†]Precordial leads remain normal.

[‡]Age >30 is relevant to the diagnosis of myocardial infarction (*see* Fig. 2.20 and compare with Fig. 2.18, poor R wave progression).

An 11-step method is advised to ensure accurate, yet rapid, interpretation of the ECG. Algorithms, illustrations, and many sample ECGs make the 11 steps easy to understand and apply. The 11 steps are briefly outlined in this chapter, and each step receives in-depth coverage in later chapters, which also give advanced diagnostic features for postgraduates.

Step 1 (See Fig. 2.3)

Assess:
- Rhythm, then the rate.
- Note that rhythm is assessed before rate, because it is clinically more important, and a normal rate of 60–100 beats/minute is easily spotted.

Step 2 (See Fig. 2.4)

Assess:
- PR and QRS intervals for blocks.
- Widening of the QRS duration suggests right bundle branch block (RBBB) or left bundle branch block (LBBB) (*see* Table 2.1 and Fig. 2.4).

Step 3 (See Fig. 2.9)

If the QRS duration is increased in the absence of LBBB or RBBB, assess:
- For nonspecific intraventricular conduction delay (IVCD), a cause of which is Wolff-Parkinson-White (WPW) syndrome (*see* Fig. 2.9).
- Although WPW syndrome is uncommon, it is an important diagnosis that may be missed by computer analysis and by physicians. Because WPW syndrome is a cause of widening of the QRS complex, it is logical to consider this diagnosis in the same frame as bundle branch blocks; this approach avoids the embarrassment of missing the diagnosis. No other text considers WPW syndrome in the assessment of the 10 essential ECG features, and conventional teaching does not give the approach outlined in Step 3.
- Most importantly, it is imperative to exclude mimics of MI early in the assessment sequence. WPW syndrome may mimic MI. RBBB may reveal Q waves in leads III and aVF that may be erroneously interpreted as MI. The diagnosis of LBBB must be documented quickly, because the presence of LBBB obviates many diagnoses, particularly ischemia and hypertrophy, and the diagnosis of MI is difficult.
- Because ECG changes of bundle branch block may be observed in V_1 and V_2, the reader is requested to first focus on V_1 and V_2. Importantly, V_1 usually reveals the morphology of P waves and is an excellent lead for the assessment of sinus rhythm and arrhythmia. Thus, sinus rhythm or rhythm disturbances can be rapidly documented; in addition, the PR interval can be assessed, and left atrial enlargement may be revealed.
- The thorough assessment of V_1 and V_2 provides considerable information.
- In addition, the assessment of V_1, V_2/V_3 may assist with the diagnosis of Brugada syndrome and right ventricular dysplasia, which may display particular forms of RBBB and have been shown to be causes of sudden death in young adults. We should not fear to divulge rare

syndromes at an early stage to students, because these topics may serve to motivate them to higher levels of excellence. The steps that discuss these rare but important topics are directed to senior trainees and internists. It is logical to discuss basics mixed with advanced material because this may appeal to students and medical residents.

Step 4 (See Fig. 2.12)

Assess:
- The all-important ST segment.
- The early diagnosis of acute MI depends on observation for ST segment changes. New terms have emerged: ST elevation MI (STEMI) and non-ST elevation MI (previously termed non-Q wave MI). The ST segment holds the key to the diagnosis. This text describes ST segment abnormalities in detail in this chapter and provides further discussion in Chapter 5.

Step 5 (See Fig. 2.16)

Assess:
- For pathologic Q waves, which, with the prior assessment of the ST segment should determine the presence or absence of new or old MI.
- Search the V leads for the loss of R waves or poor R wave progression, which may indicate MI, lead placement errors, or other cause (*see* later discussion, Figures 2.16 and 2.18 in this chapter, and Chapter 6).

Step 6 (See Figs. 2.21 and 2.22)

Assess:
- P waves for atrial hypertrophy.

Step 7 (See Fig. 2.24)

Assess:
- For left ventricular hypertrophy (LVH) and right ventricular hypertrophy (RVH).

Step 8 (See Fig. 2.27)

Assess:
- T waves for inversion, which can have many causes (*see* later discussion in this chapter and Chapter 8).

Step 9 (See Fig. 2.30)

Assess:
- The axis and for fascicular blocks.
- The axis provides no specific diagnosis and is of ancillary assistance only. In the 21st century, I believe conventional teaching should change a little. We should not lose sight of the fact that medical students and interns are bright individuals who desire to move quickly to

clinical problem solving. Thus, boring topics, particularly difficult ones to grasp such as axis determination, which provides little diagnostic yield, should be assessed after most others. Thus, determination of the axis is relegated to Step 9.

Step 10 (See Fig. 2.32)

Assess:
- Miscellaneous conditions, such as long QT, pericarditis, pacing, and pulmonary embolism (*see* later discussion and Chapter 10).

Step 11 (See Fig. 2.37)

Assess:
- For arrhythmia.
- Step 11 is indeed Step 1 if an abnormal rhythm is revealed in Step 1: assessment of rhythm (*see* later discussion in this chapter and detailed coverage in Chapter 11).

Switching the Sequence

Most importantly, these steps can be switched. After the assessment of the important ST segment in Step 4 and for Q waves indicative of acute or old MI in Step 5, Step 7 can switch with Step 9. Thus, the conventional approach is restored, with assessment of the P wave followed by that of the T wave, axis, hypertrophy, and miscellaneous conditions. Therefore, in essence, this text covers the 11 ECG features systematically with minor changes to the conventional approach and offers relevant and important diagnoses during the sequence, which allows the readers to interpret ECGs with greater accuracy.

Close attention to the 11 steps for ECG interpretation outlined in this chapter and reference to detailed explanations given in subsequent chapters should allow students, staff, and practicing clinicians to be competent interpreters of most ECGs. Accurate, yet rapid, interpretation of the ECG requires a methodical approach.

NORMAL ELECTROCARDIOGRAM

Figures 2.2A to F show normal ECG tracings. Figure 2.1 and Table 2.1 list important ECG intervals and parameters. The ECG interpretation should end with one of the following statements:
- Normal ECG
- ECG within normal limits
- Borderline ECG
- Abnormal ECG.

STEP 1: ASSESS RHYTHM AND RATE (FIG. 2.3)

Focus on leads V_1, V_2, and II (*see* Figs. 2.2A to F). Leads V_1 and II are best for visualization of P waves to determine the presence of sinus rhythm or an arrhythmia, and V_1 and V_2 are best to observe for bundle branch block. If P waves are not clearly visible in V_1, assess them in lead II,

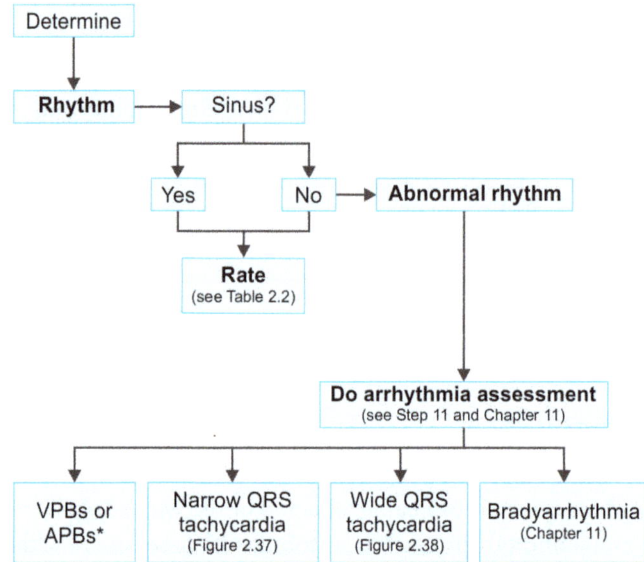

Fig. 2.3: Step-by-step method for accurate ECG interpretation. Step 1: assess rhythm and rate. *Ventricular premature beats, atrial premature beats

which usually shows well-formed P waves. Identification of the P wave and then the RR intervals allows the interpreter to discover immediately whether the rhythm is sinus or other and to take the following steps:

- Confirm, if the rhythm is sinus, that the RR intervals are equidistant (*see* Fig. 2.2A), that the P wave is positive in lead II, and that the PP intervals are equidistant and equal to the RR interval.
- Do an arrhythmia assessment if the rhythm is abnormal [*see* Fig. 2.3, Step 11 (Fig. 2.37), and Chapter 11].
- Determine the heart rate (Table 2.2).

STEP 2: ASSESS INTERVALS AND BLOCKS (FIG. 2.4)

- Determine the PR interval; if it is abnormal (>0.2 second), consider first-degree atrioventricular (AV) block (*see* Table 2.1).
- Assess the QRS duration for bundle branch block; if it is more than or equal to 0.12 second, bundle branch block is present; assess both V₁ and V₆. Understanding the genesis of the QRS complex is an essential step and clarifies the ECG manifestations of bundle branch blocks (*see* Figs. 2.5 to 2.8 and Chapter 4).

TABLE 2.2: Determination of heart rate.

Heart rate (bpm)

Number of large squares (bold boxes) in one RR interval*	
1	300
1.5	200
2	150
3	100
4	75
5	60
6	50
7	42
8	38
9	33
10	30
Number of QRS complexes in 6 seconds[†]	
5 × 10	50
6	60
7	70
10	100
15	150
20	200

*Normal paper speed 25 mm/s. One large box or five small squares (0.2 second) = 300 bpm (see Fig. 2.2C); four large boxes = 75 bpm.

[†]If the ECG paper has markers at 3-second intervals, count the number of QRS complexes in two of these 3-second periods (6 seconds) and multiply by 10 (see Fig. 2.2C). This method is advisable if there is bradycardia or irregular rhythm. For 5-second interval, multiply the number of QRS complexes by 12. *For regular rhythm:* Start with a complex that lies on a bold vertical grid line. Rate = 300 bpm ÷ number of large boxes (0.2 second) in one RR interval.

Normal rate is between 60 bpm (five boxes) and 100 bpm (three boxes); therefore, no need to calculate exact rate.

Or: rate = 1,500 ÷ number of small (1 mm, 0.04 second) squares in one RR interval.

Right Bundle Branch Block

The ECG criteria for RBBB are as follows:

- QRS duration more than or equal to 0.12 second.
- M-shaped complex in V_1 and V_2.
- Slurred S wave in leads I, V_5, V_6; and an S wave that is of greater amplitude (length) than the preceding R wave (*see* Figs. 2.4, 2.6 and 2.7, and Chapter 4).

Left Bundle Branch Block

The ECG criteria for LBBB are as follows:

- QRS duration more than or equal to 0.12 second.
- A small R or QS wave in V_1 and V_2.
- A notched R wave in leads I, V_5, and V_6 (see Figs. 2.4 and 2.8).

In the presence of LBBB, vector forces are deranged and the ECG cannot be used for the diagnosis of ischemia or ventricular hypertrophy. The diagnosis of acute MI in the presence of LBBB is difficult to make and can be erroneous.

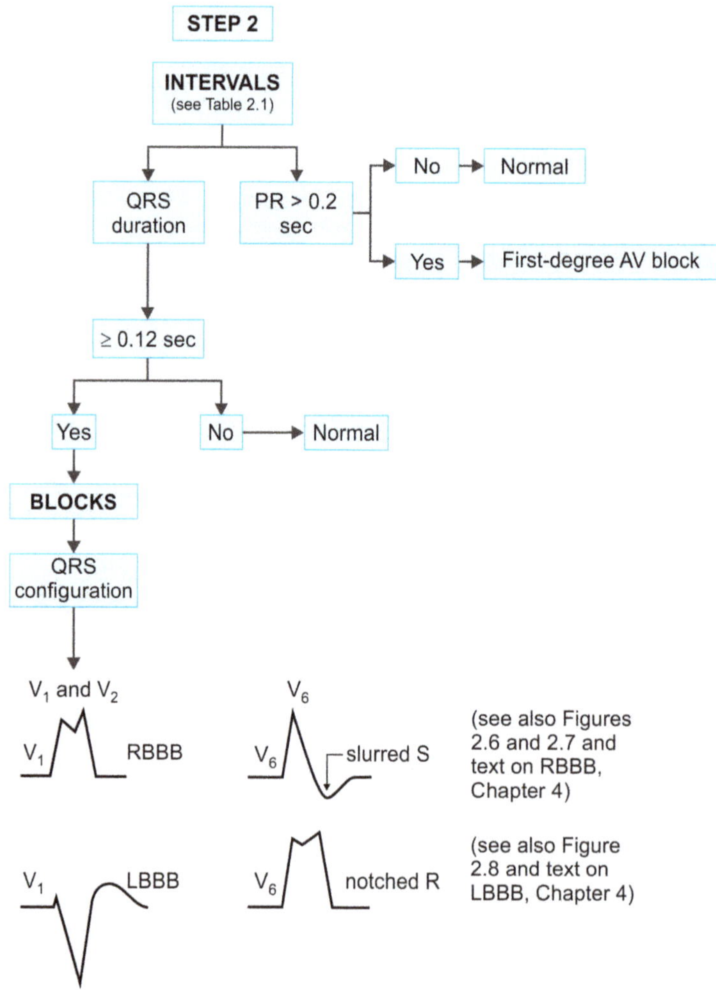

Fig. 2.4: Step-by-step method for accurate ECG interpretation. Step 2: assess intervals and blocks.

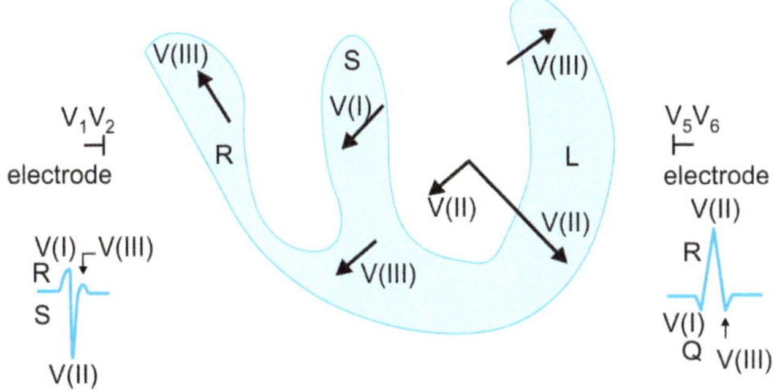

V(I) = Vector I produces a small r wave in leads V_1 and V_2, Q in leads V_5 and V_6.

V(II) = Vector II produces an S wave in lead V_1 and an R wave in leads V_5 or V_6.

V(III) = Vector III produces the terminal S in leads V_5 and V_6 and the terminal

      r or r' in V_1, V_2, and aVR.

V_1 = Lead V_1 electrode.

V_5 = Lead V_5 electrode.
R   = Right ventricle muscle mass.
L   = Left venticle muscle mass.
S   = Septum.

Fig. 2.5: Vectors I, II, and III, labeled V(I), V(II), and V(III), underlie the genesis of the normal QRS complex.
Source: Adapted with permission from Khan MG. On Call Cardiology, 3rd edition. Philadelphia: WB Saunders, Elsevier Science; 2006.

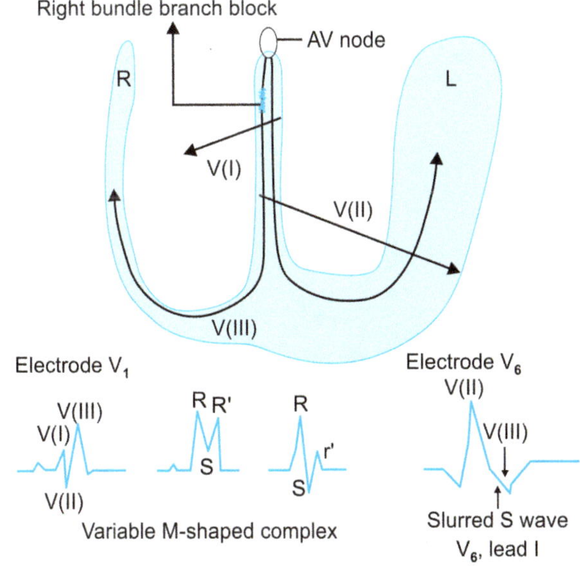

Fig. 2.6: Genesis of the QRS complex in right bundle branch block.
Source: Adapted with permission from Khan MG. On Call Cardiology, 3rd edition. Philadelphia: WB Saunders, Elsevier Science; 2006.

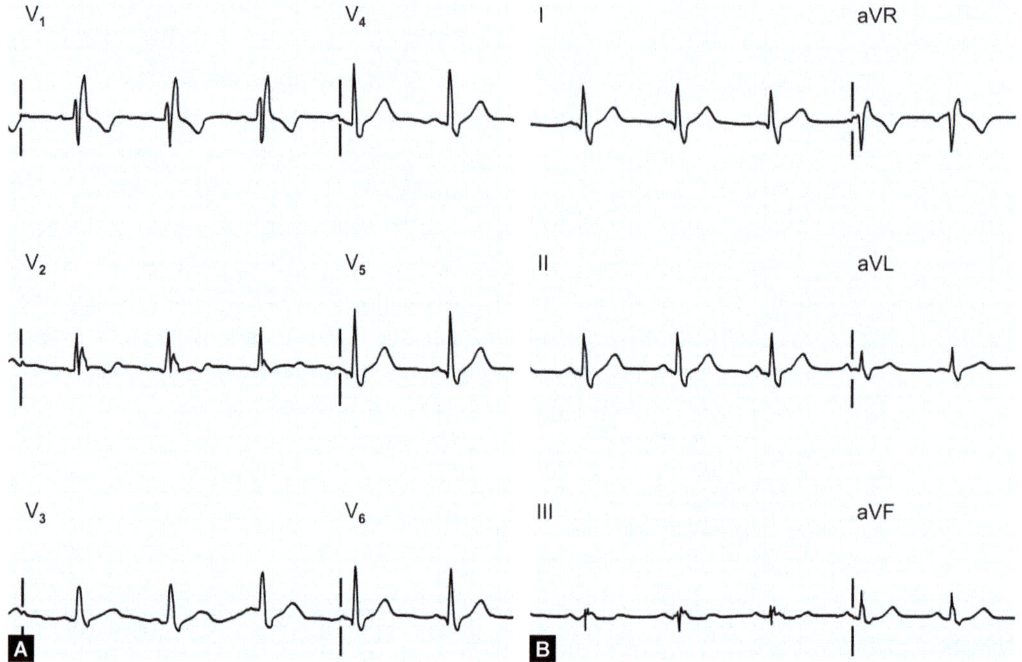

Figs. 2.7A and B: (A) QRS duration in V$_1$ greater than or equal to 0.12 second; RSR′ (M-shaped complex) in V$_1$; and wide, slurred S wave in leads I, V$_5$, and V$_6$ indicate right bundle branch block. (B) Limb leads; slurred, wide S wave in lead I, and the amplitude (length or duration) of the S wave is greater than the preceding R wave.

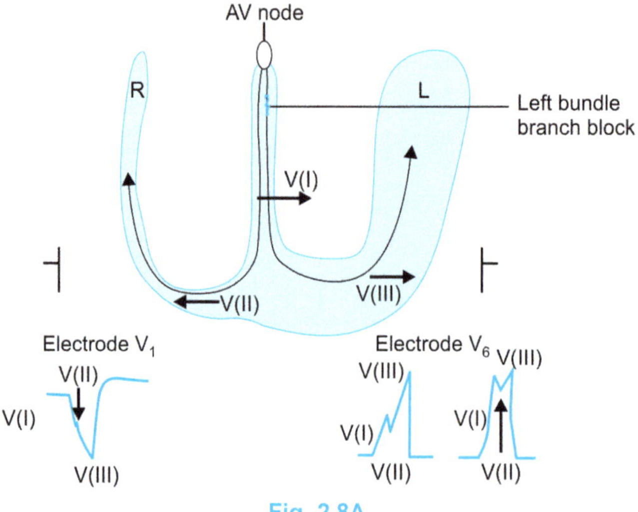

Fig. 2.8A

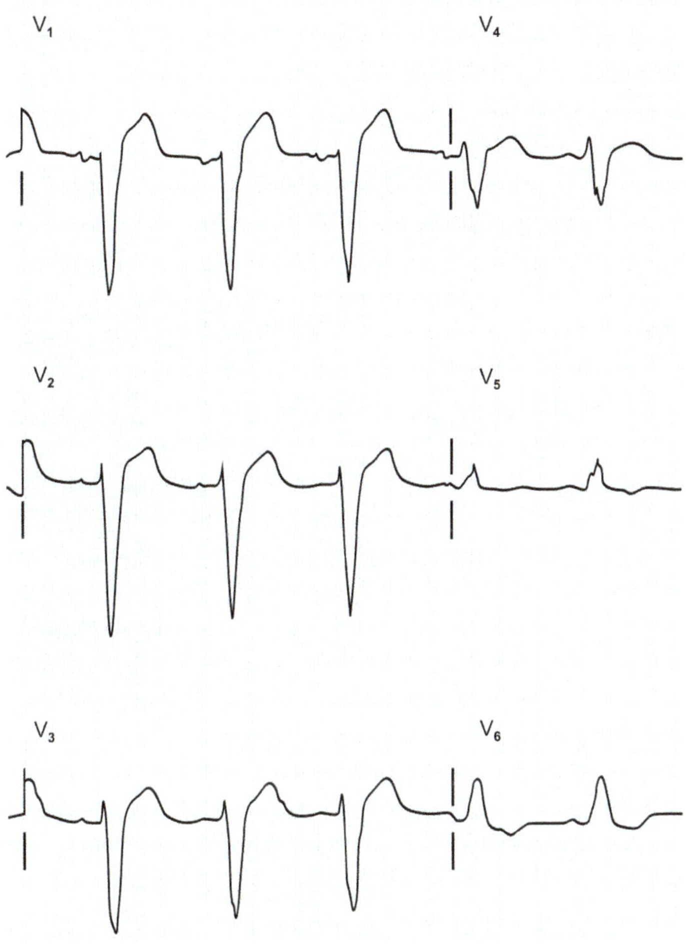

Fig. 2.8B

Figs. 2.8A and B: (A) The contribution of vectors I, II, and III, labeled V(I), V(II), and V(III), to the genesis of left bundle branch block; (B) QRS duration more than 0.12 second; small R waves in V_1 to V_3; and notched R wave in V_5 indicate left bundle branch block.
Source of Fig. 2.8A: Adapted with permission from Khan MG. On Call Cardiology, 3rd edition. Philadelphia: WB Saunders, Elsevier Science; 2006.

STEP 3: ASSESS FOR NONSPECIFIC INTRAVENTRICULAR CONDUCTION DELAY AND WOLFF-PARKINSON-WHITE SYNDROME (FIG. 2.9)

- If the QRS duration is prolonged more than or equal to 0.11 second and bundle branch block appears to be present but is atypical, consider WPW syndrome, particularly if there is a tall R wave in V_1 and V_2 (Table 2.3).
- Assess for a short PR interval less than or equal to 0.12 second and for a delta wave (Fig. 2.10).

The WPW syndrome may mimic an inferior MI (*see* Chapters 6 and 11 for discussion of WPW syndrome). If WPW syndrome, RBBB, or LBBB is not present, interpret as nonspecific IVCD and assess for the presence of electronic pacing (*see* Figs. 2.7, 2.8, 2.11).

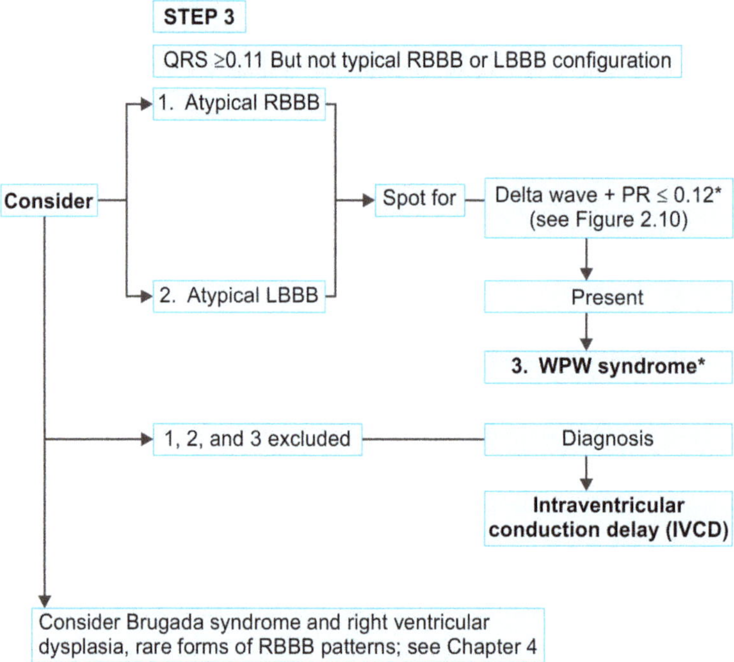

Fig. 2.9: Step-by-step method for accurate ECG interpretation. Step 3: assess for nonspecific intraventricular conduction delay and Wolff-Parkinson-White (WPW) syndrome (*see* Figs. 2.10 and 2.11). [See Chapter 4 for Brugada syndrome and right ventricular dysplasia, rare forms of right bundle branch block (RBBB) patterns, and Chapter 11 for WPW syndrome.]
* In ~ 20% the QRS is < 0.11 second; in ~23% the PR interval is 0.12 second or slightly longer.

TABLE 2.3: Causes of tall R waves in V_1 and V_2.

1. Thin chest wall or normal variant, age <20, early transition (*see* Fig. 2.2C)
2. Right bundle branch block (*see* Fig. 2.7)
   Note: Slurred S wave in leads I, V_5, and V_6
3. Right ventricular hypertrophy
   Note: No slurred S wave in leads I, V_5, and V_6
4. Wolff-Parkinson-White syndrome (*see* Fig. 2.10)
5. True posterior infarction
   Note: Associated inferior MI, no slurred S in V_5 and V_6, and T upright in V_1 and V_2
6. Hypertrophic cardiomyopathy
7. Duchenne muscular dystrophy
8. Low placement of leads V_1 and V_2
9. Dextroposition

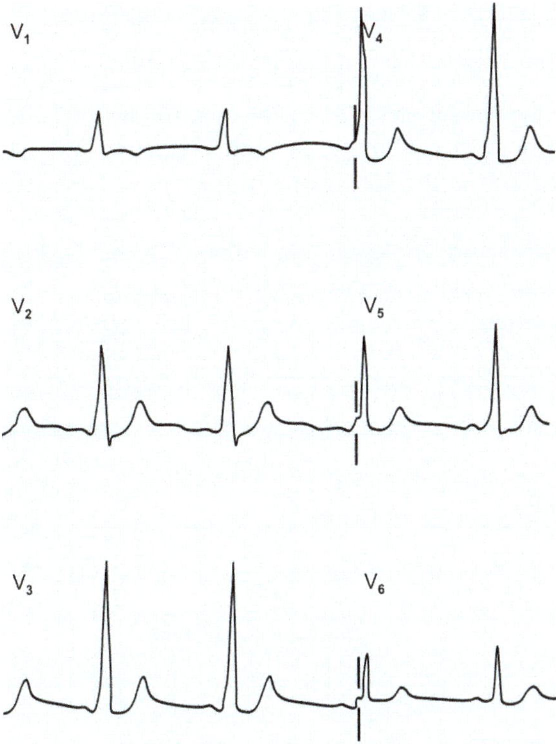

Fig. 2.10: Tall R waves in leads V₁ and V₂; QRS duration ≥0.11 second; and delta wave in V₃ through V₅ indicate Wolff-Parkinson-White syndrome.

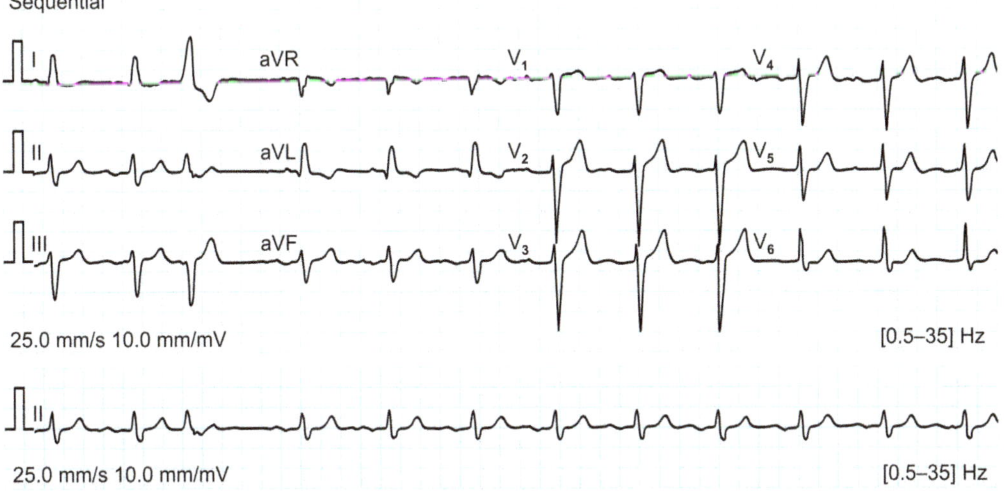

Fig. 2.11: Sinus rhythm 72/minute; ventricular premature beats; QRS duration 0.14 second, 140 ms: intraventricular conduction delay (IVCD). Abnormal ECG.

STEP 4: ASSESS FOR ST SEGMENT ELEVATION OR DEPRESSION (FIG. 2.12)

- Focus on the ST segment for elevation or depression (see Fig. 2.12). ST elevation more than or equal to 1 mm (0.1 mV) in two or more contiguous ECG leads in a patient with chest pain indicates STEMI. The diagnosis is strengthened if there is reciprocal depression (Figs. 2.13A to C).
- Figure 2.13A shows marked ST elevation in leads II, III, and aVF, with marked reciprocal depression in leads I and aVL, diagnostic of acute inferior MI.
- Figure 2.13B shows marked ST segment elevation in V_1 through V_5, caused by extensive acute anterior MI.
- Figure 2.13C shows the ECG of a patient with a subtotal occlusion of the left main coronary artery. Note the ST elevation in aVR is greater than the ST elevation in V_1, a recently identified marker of left main coronary disease. (See Chapter 5 for an in-depth discussion of Step 4: ST segment elevation.)

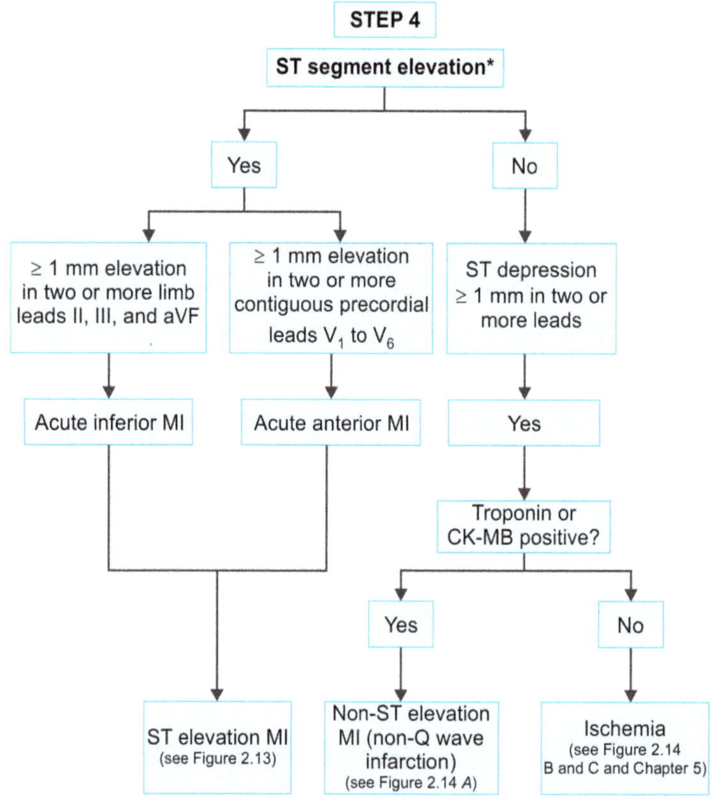

Fig. 2.12: Step-by-step method for accurate ECG interpretation. Step 4: assess for ST segment elevation or depression.
*Reciprocal depression increases probabilities of acute myocardial infarction (MI)

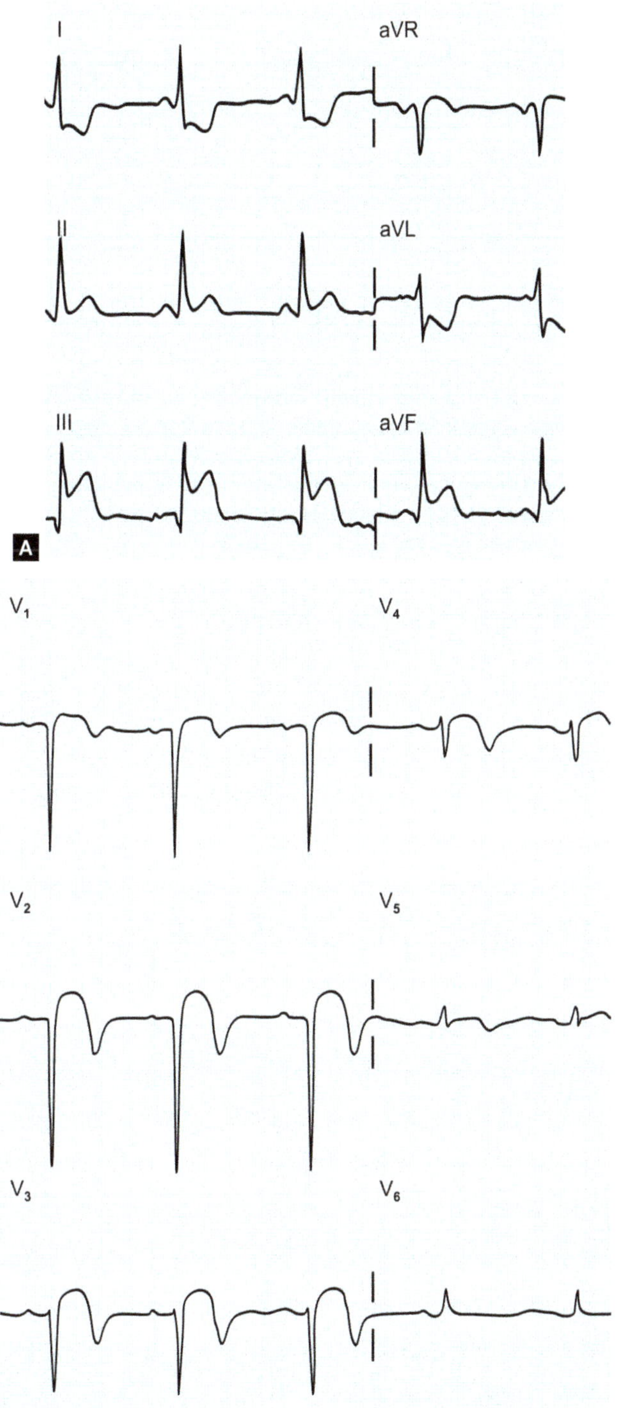

Figs. 2.13A and B

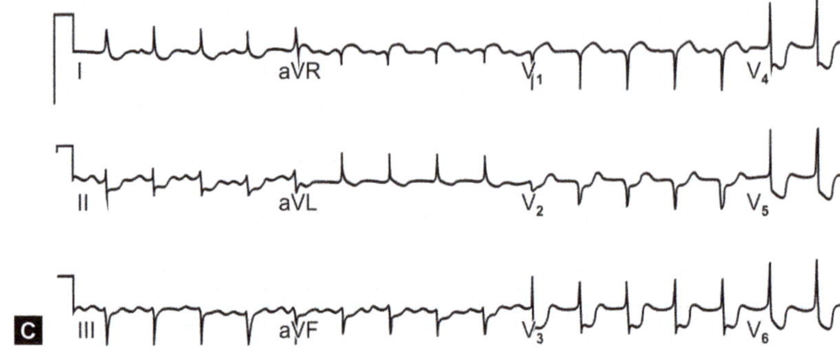

Fig. 2.13C

Figs. 2.13A to C: (A) Marked ST segment elevation in leads II, III, and aVF with reciprocal depression in leads I and aVL indicates acute inferior infarction. (B) Marked ST segment elevation in leads V_1 through V_5 indicates acute anterior infarction. (C) Electrocardiogram of a 79-year-old woman with an apparent acute subendocardial myocardial infarction attributed to subtotal occlusion of the left main coronary artery, associated with global hypokinesis and an estimated left ventricular ejection fraction of 10%. ST segment is depressed in leads I, II, III, aVL, aVF, and V_2 through V_6. Apparent "reciprocal" ST segment elevation is seen in leads aVR and V_1.

Source: Adapted with permission from Surawicz B, Knilans TK. Chou's Electrocardiography in Clinical Practice, 5th edition. Philadelphia: WB Saunders, Elsevier Science; 2001.

- Figure 2.14A shows features of non-ST elevation MI (non-Q wave MI).
- Figures 2.14B and C illustrate ECG features diagnostic of myocardial ischemia.

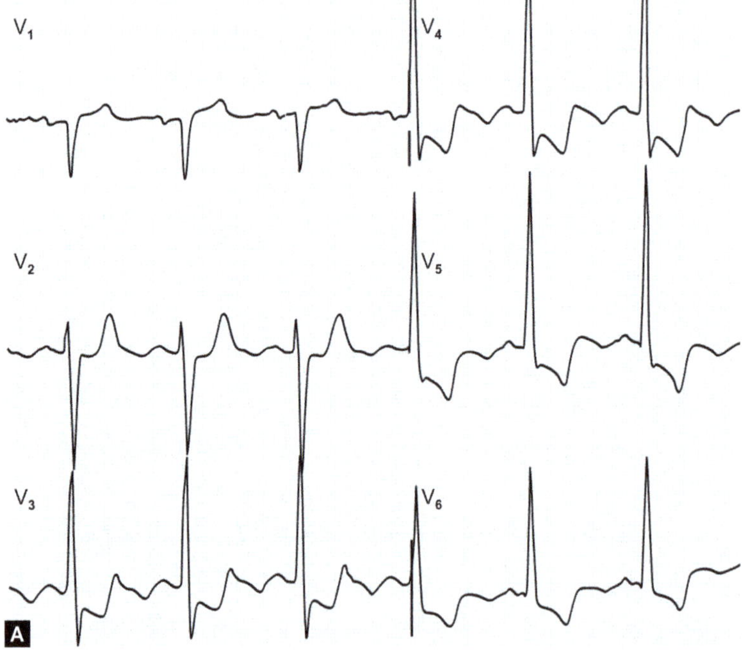

Fig. 2.14A

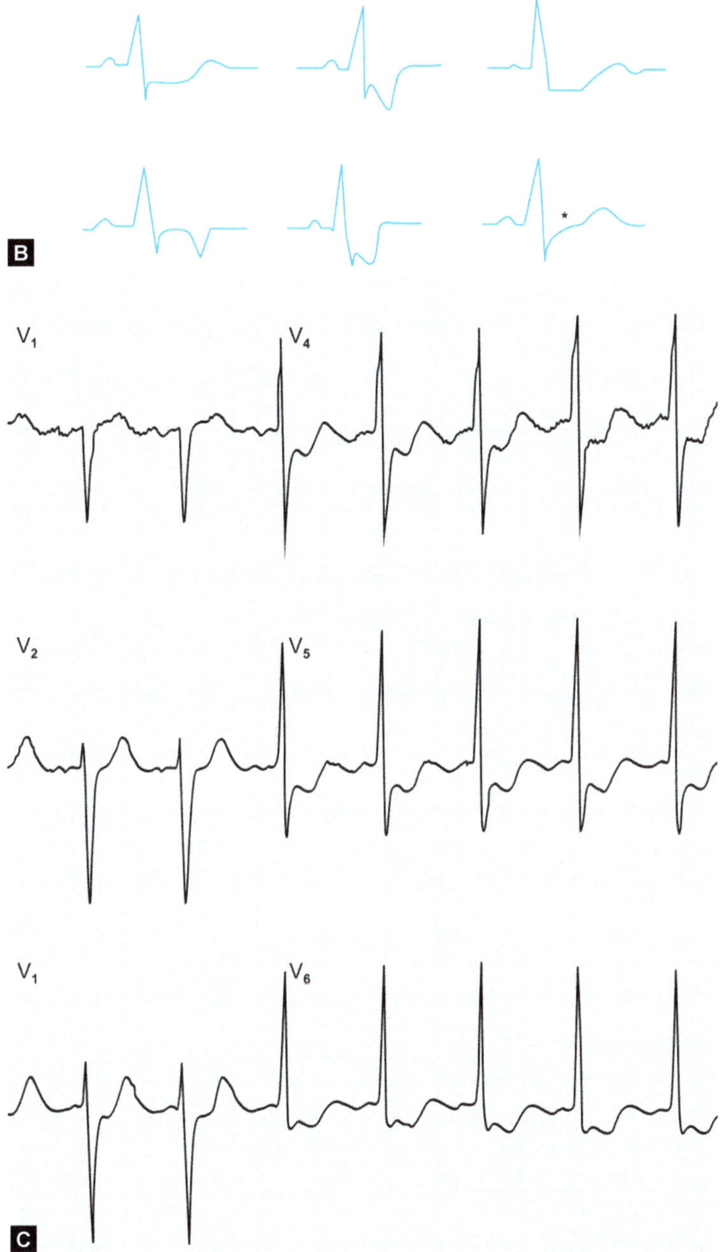

Figs. 2.14B and C

Figs. 2.14A to C: (A) Marked ST segment depression and elevated creatine kinase (CK) and CK-MB indicate non-Q wave myocardial infarction. (B) ECG patterns of myocardial ischemia. (C) Leads V₄ through V₆ show ST segment depression; V₄ through V₆ are in keeping with myocardial ischemia from a patient known to have unstable angina.

*Upsloping ST depression is nonspecific; commonly seen with tachycardia.

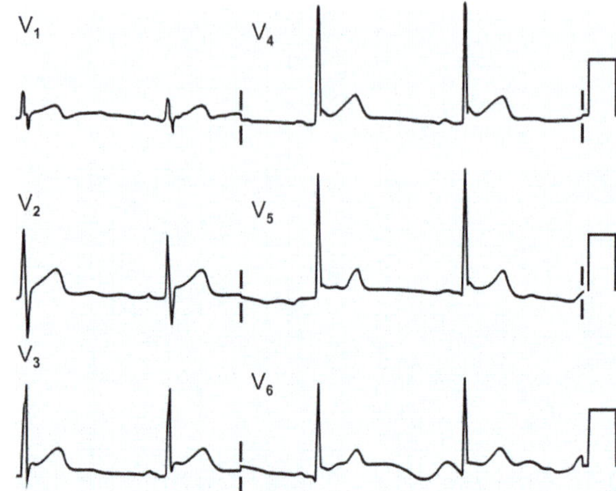

Fig. 2.15: ST elevation with typical fishhook appearance in the V leads is a normal variant.

- Elevation of the ST segment may occur as a normal variant (Fig. 2.15). See Chapters 5 and 6 for further discussion of ST segment abnormalities and MI.

Note: This text advises scrutiny of the ST segment before assessment of T waves, electrical axis, QT interval, and hypertrophy because the diagnosis of acute MI or ischemia is vital and depends on careful assessment of the ST segment.

Exclude other causes of ST elevation:

- *Normal variant:* 1- to 2-mm ST segment elevation, mainly in leads V_2 through V_4, nonconvex, and with fishhook appearance. Common in African Americans: even 4-mm ST segment elevation (see Fig. 2.15 and sections on acute myocardial infarction in Chapters 5 and 6).
- *Coronary artery spasm:* ST returns to normal with nitroglycerin or with pain relief.
- *Left bundle branch block:* QRS more than 0.12 second and typical configuration (see Fig. 2.8B, and Chapter 4).
- Left ventricular aneurysm and known old infarct with old Q waves (see Chapter 6).

STEP 5: ASSESS FOR PATHOLOGIC Q WAVES (THAT IS, LOSS OF R WAVES) (FIG. 2.16)

- Assess for the loss of R waves—pathologic Q waves—in leads I, II, III, aVL, and aVF (*see* Figs. 2.17A and B, and Chapter 6 for detailed discussion).
- Assess for R wave progression in V_2 through V_4. Figure 2.17C illustrates the variation in the normal QRS configuration that occurs with rotation. The R wave amplitude should measure from 1 mm to at least 20 mm in V_3 and V_4 (*see* Table 2.1). Loss of R waves in V_1 through V_4 with ST segment elevation indicates acute anterior MI (Fig. 2.18A).

- Loss of R wave in V_1 through V_3 with the ST segment isoelectric and the T wave inverted may be interpreted as anteroseptal MI age indeterminate (i.e. infarction in the recent or distant past) (Fig. 2.18B). Features of old anterior MI are shown in Figures 2.18C and D and lateral infarction is shown in Figure 2.19.

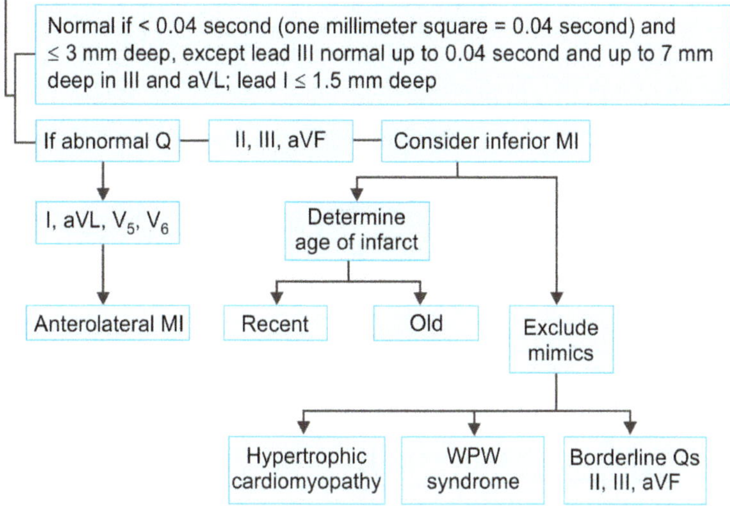

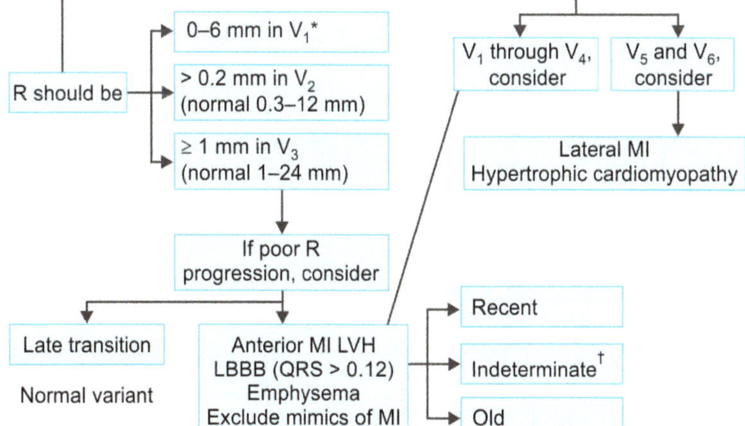

Fig. 2.16: Step-by-step method for accurate ECG interpretation. Step 5: assess for pathologic Q waves (i.e. loss of R waves).
Age >30; see chapter 6 and Table 2.1 for exceptions and normal parameters.
†Compare old ECGs.

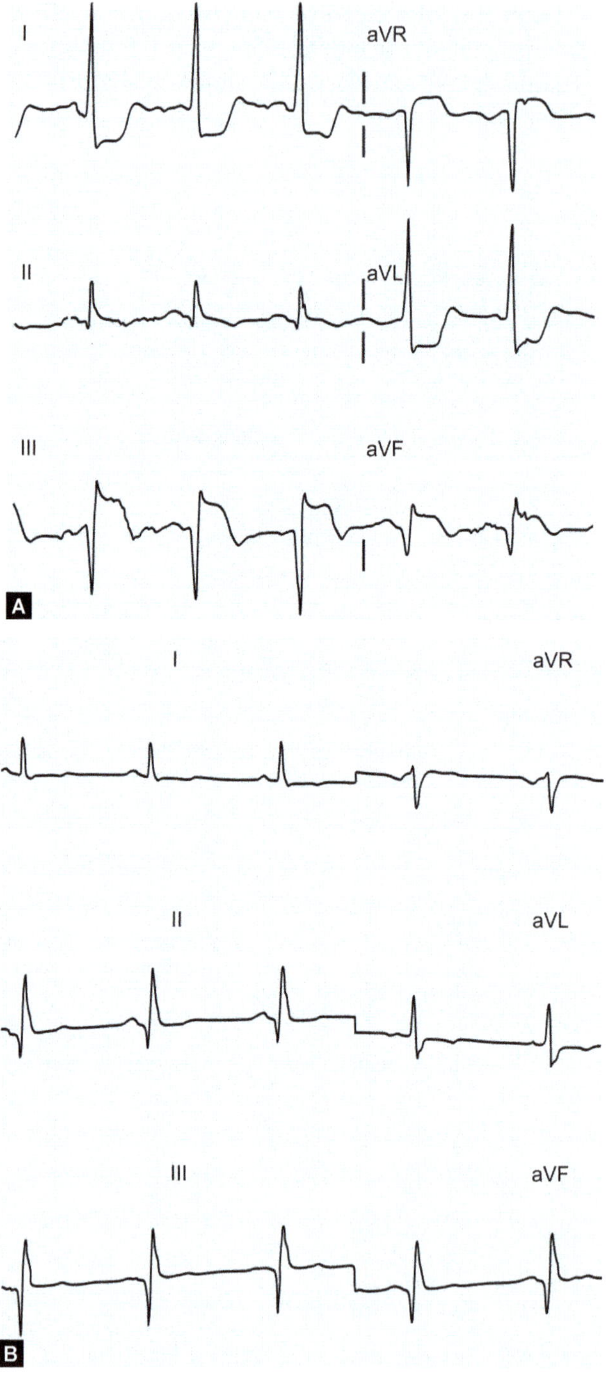

Figs. 2.17A and B

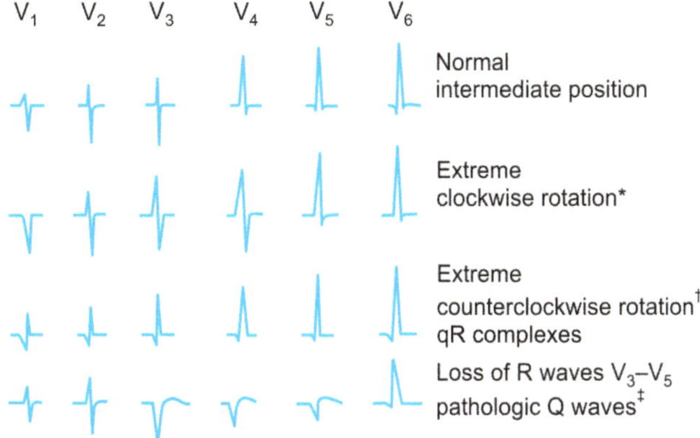

Fig. 2.17C

Figs. 2.17A to C: (A) Loss of R wave in leads III and aVF (i.e. pathologic Q waves associated with marked ST segment elevation in leads III and aVF) and minimal elevation in lead II and reciprocal depression in leads I and aVL indicate typical acute Q wave inferior infarction; (B) Wide, deep pathologic Q waves in leads II, III, and aVF and isoelectric ST segment indicate old inferior myocardial infarction; (C) Variation in QRS configuration caused by rotation.

*With clockwise rotation, the V_1 electrode, like aVR, faces the cavity of the heart and records a QS complex; no initial q in lead V_6.

†qR complexes, q < 0.04 second, <3 mm deep, therefore not pathologic Q waves

‡Loss of R wave V_3 to V_5 pathologic Q waves: signifies anterior myocardial infarction.

Source: Adapted with permission from Khan MG. On Call Cardiology, 3rd edition. Philadelphia: WB Saunders, Elsevier Science; 2006.

Poor R wave progression in V_2 through V_4 may be caused by the following:

- Improper lead placement.
- Late transition (Fig. 2.20).
- Anteroseptal or anteroapical MI.
- Left ventricular hypertrophy (*see* Chapter 7).
- Severe chronic obstructive pulmonary disease, particularly emphysema—emphysema may cause QS complexes in leads V_1 through V_4, which may mimic MI; a repeat ECG with recording electrodes placed one intercostal space below the routine locations should cause R waves to be observed in leads V_2 through V_4 (*see* Chapter 6).
- Hypertrophic cardiomyopathy.
- Left bundle branch block (Fig. 2.8B).

In women, albeit rarely, the R wave in V_2 or V_3 may be less than 1 mm tall; this may cause an erroneous diagnosis of anteroseptal infarction.

In summary: An abnormal, pathologic Q wave is defined in adults as one that has a duration of more than 40 ms, but the definition does not apply to leads aVR and V_1, which may normally lack the initial R wave. In addition, in leads III, aVF, and aVL, the initial R wave may be absent; the resultant QS or QR pattern represents a normal variant. A QS pattern is disturbing to students and clinicians. The student is warned: Sound knowledge of normal variants and features of normal ECG deflections that look abnormal but are indeed normal must be mastered by the competent interpreter of ECGs. A QS is often observed in lead aVL in thin subjects with a vertical heart. A QS in lead III is common in individuals with a horizontal heart position, some of whom are obese. See Chapter 6 for an in-depth discussion of Step 5: Q wave abnormalities.

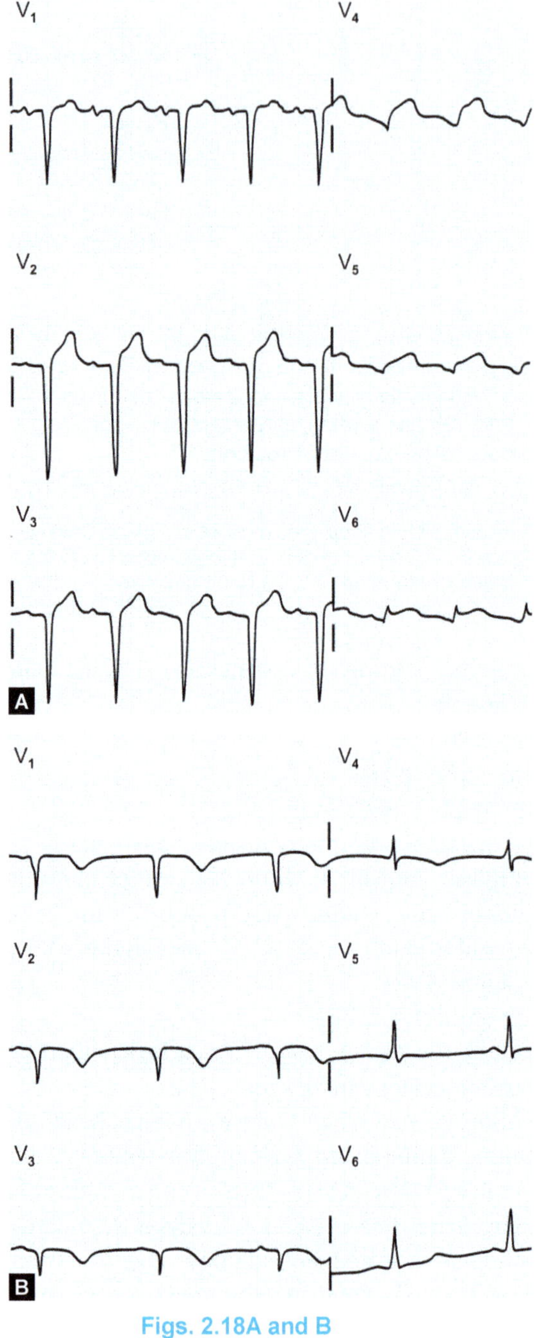

Figs. 2.18A and B

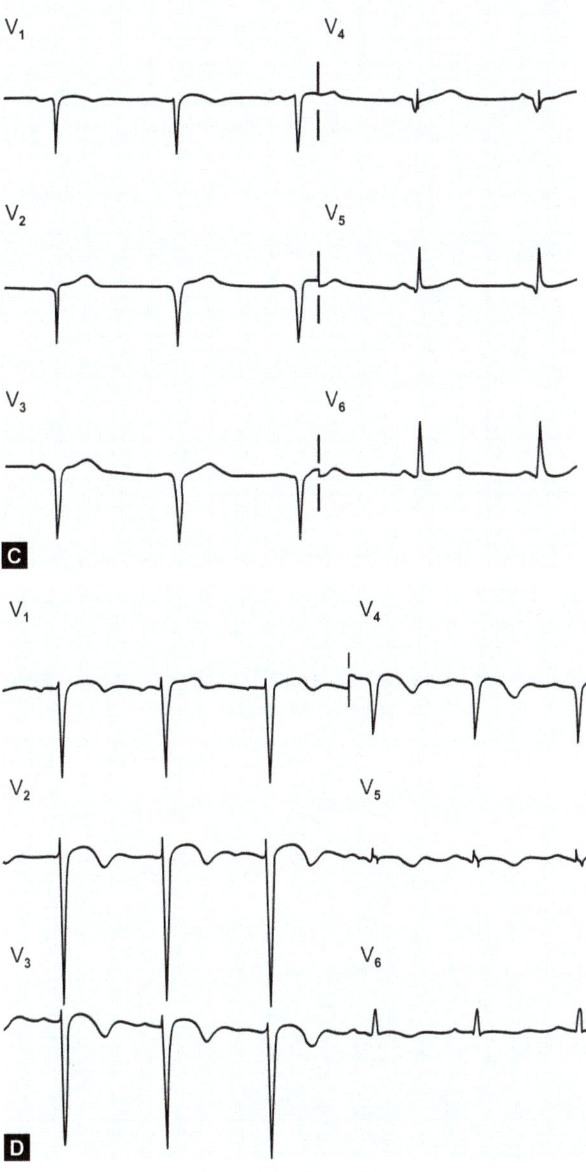

Fig. 2.18C and D

Figs. 2.18A to D: (A) Loss of R waves in V_2 through V_5 (i.e. pathologic Q waves associated with abnormal ST segment elevation) indicates acute anterior infarction; (B) Loss of R wave in V_1 through V_3 (i.e. pathologic Q waves associated with an isoelectric ST segment) and T wave inversion indicate anteroseptal infarction, age indeterminate, infarction occurring approximately 1–12 months before the recording of this tracing; comparison with previous ECGs and clinical history required to determine the age of infarction; (C) Loss of R waves in V_2 through V_5 (i.e. pathologic Q waves in V_2 through V_4 not associated with acute ST segment changes) indicates old anterior infarction; (D) Loss of R waves in V_4 and V_5 indicates anterior myocardial infarction, age indeterminate.

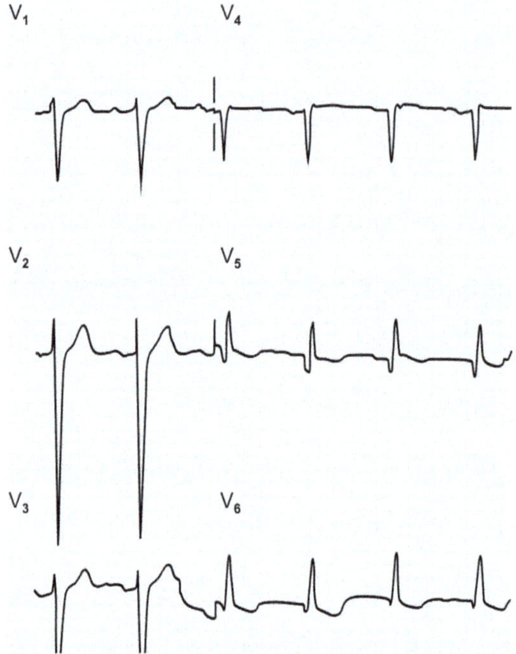

Fig. 2.19: Pathologic Q waves in V₄ through V₆ and ST segment in keeping with an old anterolateral infarct; clinical correlation necessary to confirm the presence of an old infarction.

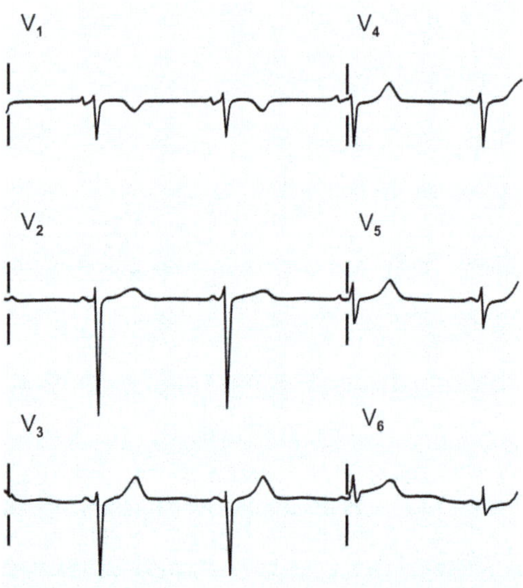

Fig. 2.20: Poor R wave progression in leads V₂ through V₅. *Note*: The negative QRS complex in V₅ is caused by late transition and not by other causes of poor R wave progression such as anterior infarction. ECG with normal limits.

STEP 6: ASSESS P WAVES (FIG. 2.21)

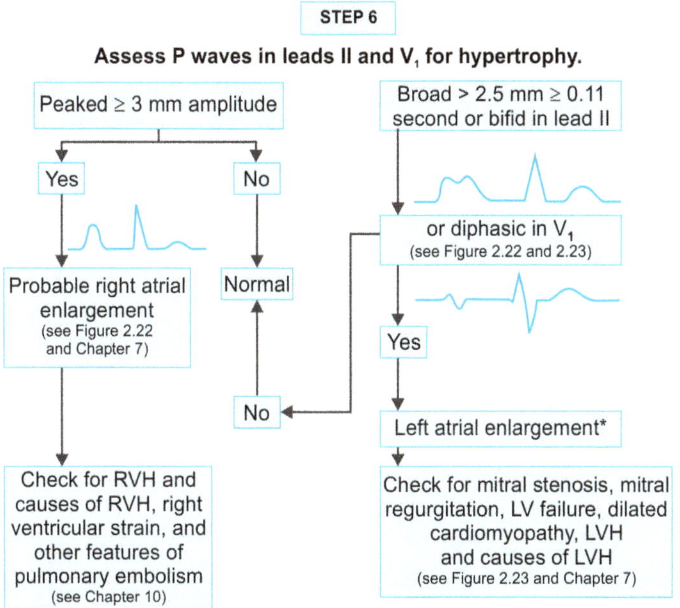

Fig. 2.21: Step-by-step method for accurate ECG interpretation. Step 6: assess P waves.
*Left atrial abnormality: enlargement, hypertrophy, or increased atrial volume or pressure.

- Assess the P waves for abnormalities including atrial hypertrophy (Figs. 2.22 and 2.23).

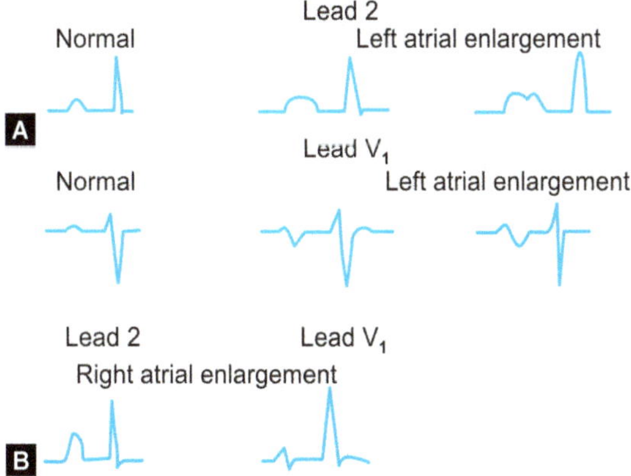

Figs. 2.22A and B: (A) Left atrial enlargement: P wave duration greater than three small squares (0.12 second) in lead 2; in lead V₁ the negative component of the P wave occupies at least one small box: 1 mm × 0.04 second = P terminal force more than or equal to −0.04 mm s; (B) Right atrial enlargement: lead 2 shows P amplitude more than 3 mm; in V₁, the first half of the P wave is positive and more than 1 mm wide (see Figs. 2.23, 7.2, and 7.3).
Source: Adapted with permission from Khan MG. On Call Cardiology, 3rd edition. Philadelphia: WB Saunders, Elsevier Science; 2006.

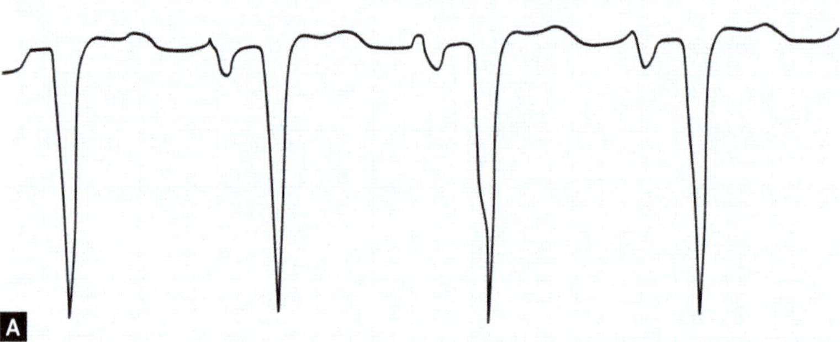

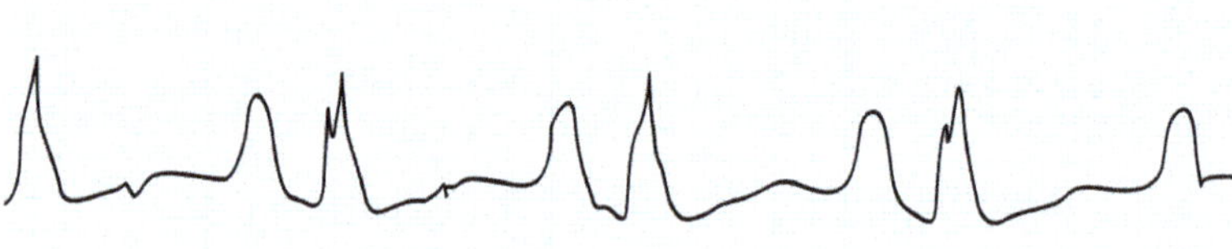

Figs. 2.23A and B: Lead V_1 shows right and left atrial hypertrophy. Lead II shows peaked P waves caused by right atrial enlargement.

STEP 7: ASSESS FOR LEFT AND RIGHT VENTRICULAR HYPERTROPHY (FIG. 2.24)

- Assess for LVH (*see* Figs. 2.24 and 2.25, and Chapter 7) and RVH (*see* Figs. 2.26A and B, and Chapter 7 for further details).
- Criteria for LVH and RVH are not applicable if bundle branch block is present. Thus, it is essential to exclude LBBB and RBBB early in the interpretive sequences as delineated previously in Steps 2 and 3.

STEP-7

A. Assess for left ventricular hypertrophy.[*]

1. S wave in V_1 + R wave in V_5 or V_6 >35 mm = LVH ≈ 90% specificity; sensitivity <40%
2. R wave in aVL + S wave in men ≥ 24 mm and in women ≥18 mm = LVH ≈90% specificity; sensitivity <40%
3. Specificity of (1) or (2) increased to ≈ 98% in presence of:
   i.   Left atrial enlargement *or*
   ii. ST segment depression and T wave inversion (strain pattern) in V_5 or V_6 (see Figs. 2.23 and 2.25)

B. Assess for right ventricular hypertrophy.

1. R wave in V_1 ≥ 7 mm[†]
2. S wave in V_5 or V_6 ≥ 7 mm
3. R/S ratio in V_1 ≥ 1
4. R/S ratio in V_5 or V_6 ≤ 1
5. Right axis deviation   ≥ +110°
   Any two of above = RVH likely (see Fig. 2.26)
6. Specificity increased if ST depression and T wave inversion in V_1 to V_3 or right atrial hypertrophy (see Figs. 2.26)

Fig. 2.24: Step-by-step method for accurate ECG interpretation. Step 7: assess for left ventricular hypertrophy (LVH) and right ventricular hypertrophy (RVH) (not applicable if QRS duration ≥0.12 second or in presence of LBBB or RBBB).
*Age >30; ≥40 mm, age 20–30.
†Age >30; see Table 2.1.

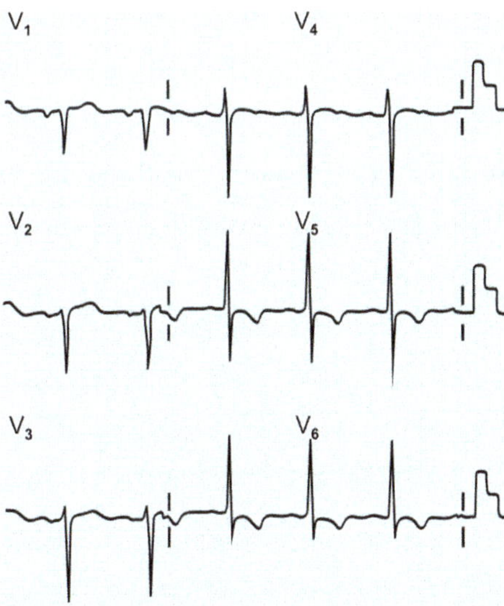

Fig. 2.25: Note that the standardization at half voltage in V_1 through V_6 is markedly increased; ST-T strain pattern in V_5 and V_6 and left atrial enlargement are typical features of left ventricular hypertrophy.

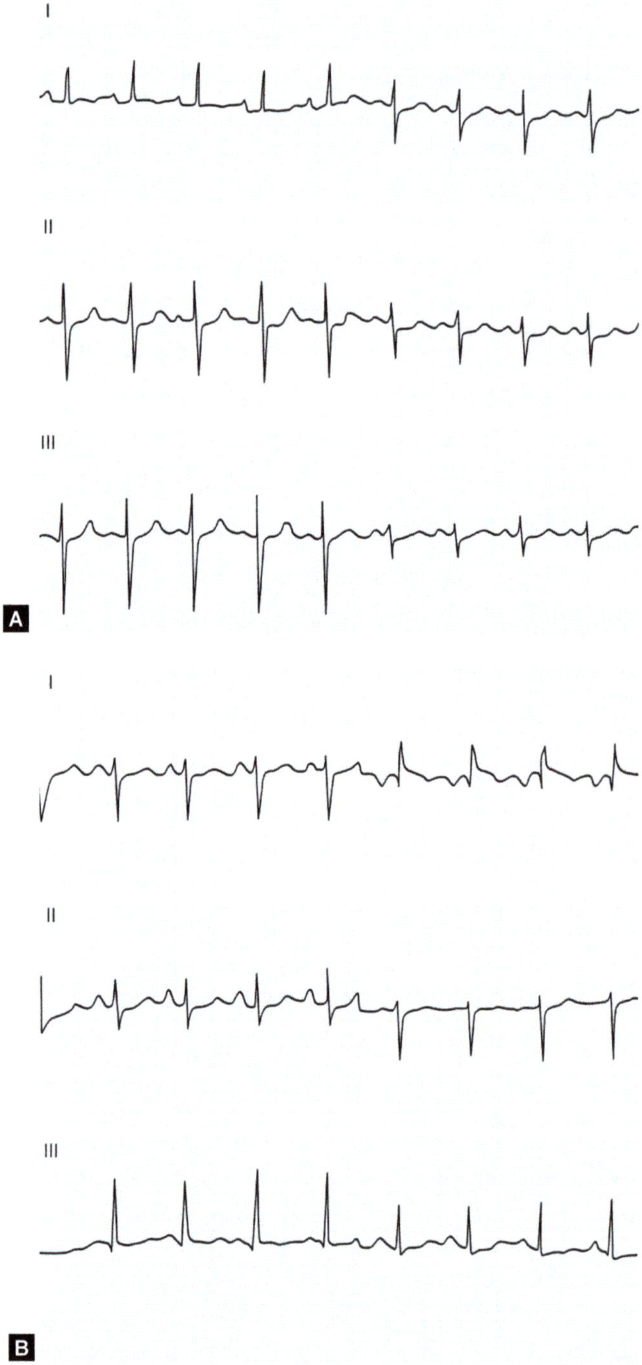

Figs. 2.26A and B: (A) Leads V_1 through V_6: A tall R wave in V_1, R/S ratio in V_1 >1, and R/S ratio in V_5 or V_6 <1 are features of right ventricular hypertrophy; (B) Limb leads: right axis deviation +140°, peaked P wave in lead II, and right atrial enlargement are all in keeping with right ventricular hypertrophy.

STEP 8: ASSESS T WAVES (FIGS. 2.27A AND B)

- Assess the pattern of T wave changes (*see* Figs. 2.27A and B). T wave changes are usually nonspecific (Fig. 2.28). T wave inversion associated with ST segment depression or elevation indicates myocardial ischemia (Fig. 2.29). See Chapter 8 for further information on T wave abnormalities.

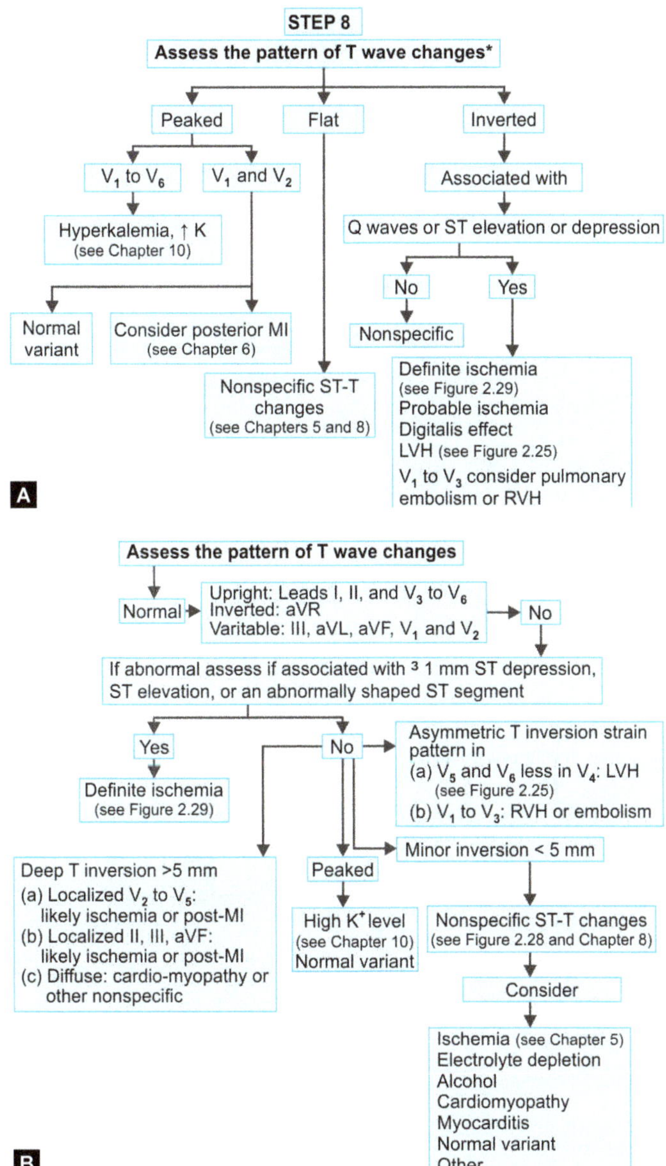

Figs. 2.27A and B: Step-by-step method for accurate ECG interpretation. (A) Step 8: assess T wave changes; (B) Step 8: Alternative approach for the assessment of T wave changes.

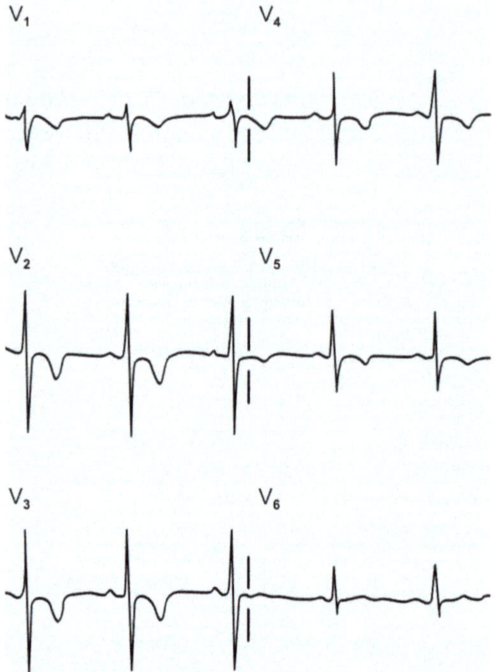

Fig. 2.28: T wave inversion in V$_2$ through V$_5$ not associated with ST segment depression or elevation; nonspecific ST-T wave changes; cannot exclude ischemia, but the tracing is not diagnostic. Abnormal ECG.

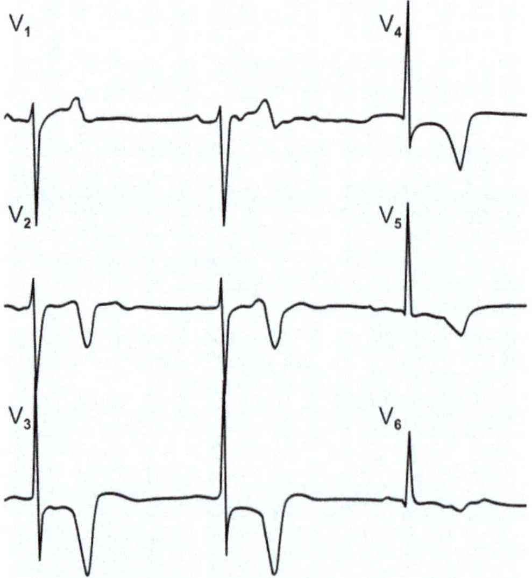

Fig. 2.29: The deep T wave inversion in V$_2$ through V$_5$, which is associated with an abnormal ST segment that is hitched up in V$_2$ and abnormally shaped in V$_3$ and V$_4$, is in keeping with myocardial ischemia and likely left anterior descending artery obstruction.

STEP 9: ASSESS ELECTRICAL AXIS (FIGS. 2.30A AND B)

Assess the electrical axis (*see* Figs. 2.30A and B, and Table 2.4). using two simple clues:

1.   If leads I and aVF are upright, the axis is normal.

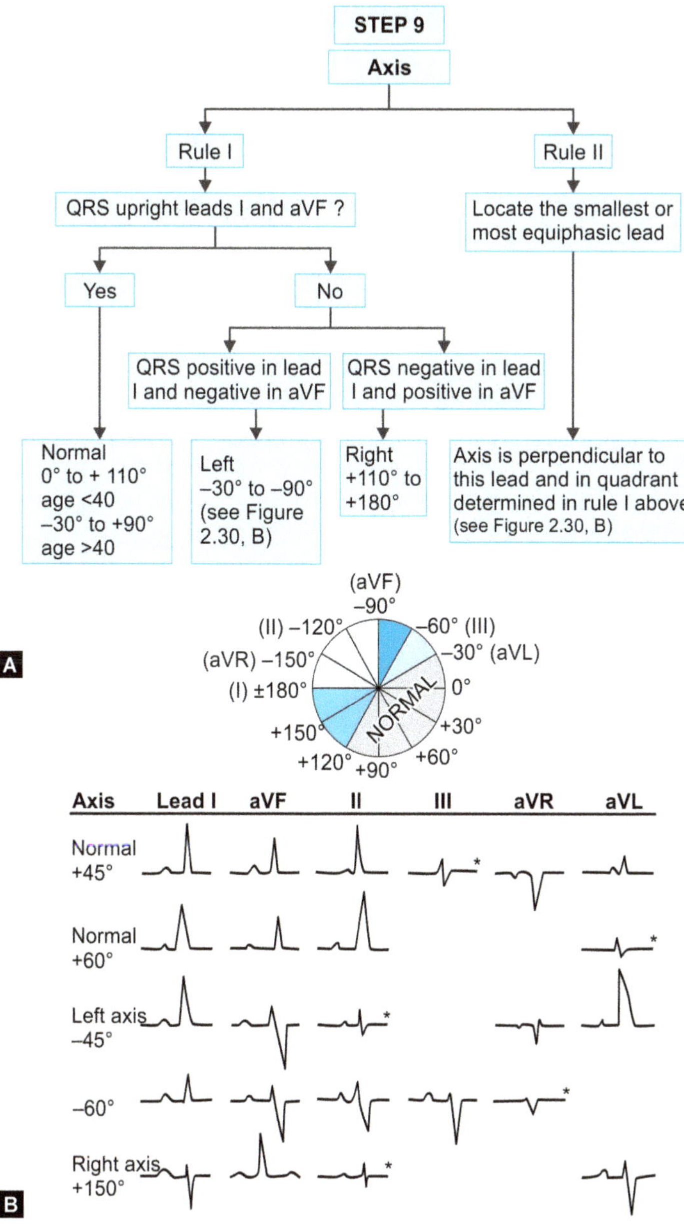

Figs. 2.30A and B: (A) Step-by-step method for accurate ECG interpretation. Step 9: assess the electrical axis. Leads are indicated in parentheses. (B) The axis is perpendicular to the lead with the most equiphasic or smallest QRS deflection.

*Most equiphasic lead.

The axis is perpendicular to the lead with the most equiphasic or smallest QRS deflection (*see* Fig. 2.30B). Figure 2.31 shows left-axis deviation and the commonly associated left anterior fascicular block (*see* Chapter 9).

TABLE 2.4: Electrical axis.

Most equiphasic lead	*Lead perpendicular**	*Axis*
		Leads I and aVF positive = normal axis
III	aVR	Normal = +30°
aVL	II	Normal = +60°
		Lead I positive and aVF negative = left axis
II	aVL (QRS positive)	Left = −30°
aVR	III (QRS negative)	Left = −60°
I	aVF (QRS negative)	Left = −90°
		Lead I negative and aVF positive = right axis
aVR	III (QRS positive)	Right = +120°
II	aVL (QRS negative)	Right = +150°

*Lead perpendicular (at right angles) to the most equiphasic (isoelectric) lead usually has the tallest R or deepest S wave.

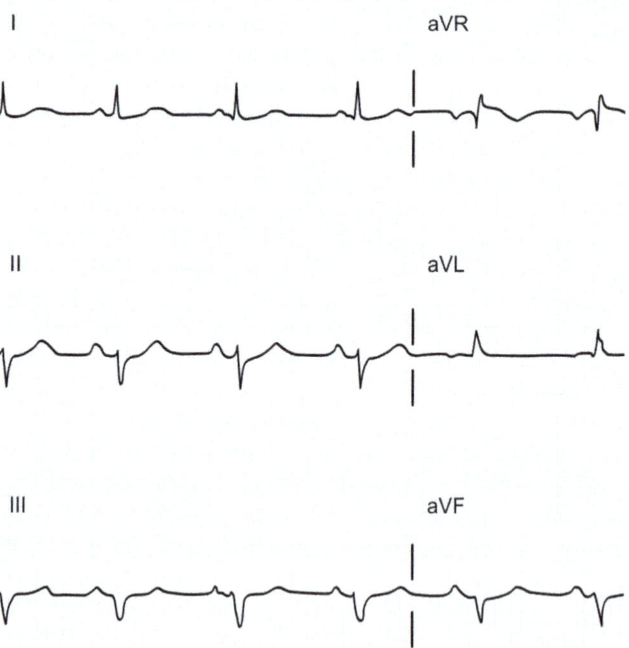

Fig. 2.31: Lead aVR is the most equiphasic: the lead perpendicular to aVR is lead III, indicating a left axis of −60°. There is a small normal Q wave in lead I and a small R wave in lead III in keeping with left anterior fascicular block (hemiblock). Borderline ECG.

STEP 10: ASSESS FOR MISCELLANEOUS CONDITIONS (FIG. 2.32)

Perform a rapid screen for miscellaneous conditions. Chapter 10 gives details and relevant ECGs.

- *Artificial pacemakers:* If electronic pacing is confirmed, usually no other diagnosis can be made from the ECG (*see* Chapter 10).
- *Prolonged QT syndrome:* See normal QT parameters listed in Table 2.5. No complicated formula is required for assessment of the QT intervals (see Chapter 10 for further details).

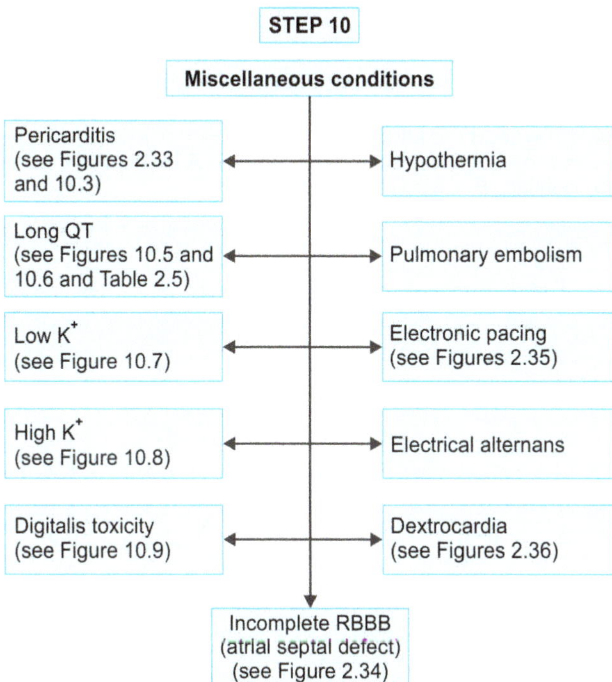

Fig. 2.32: Step-by-step method for accurate ECG interpretation. Step 10: assess for miscellaneous conditions (*see* Chapter 10)

TABLE 2.5: QT intervals.*		
Clinically useful approximation of upper limit of QT interval(s)		
Heart rate (bpm)	Male	Female
45–65	< 0.47	< 0.48
66–100	< 0.41	< 0.43
>100	< 0.36	< 0.37

*ECG paper speed 25 mm/s. No complicated formula required.

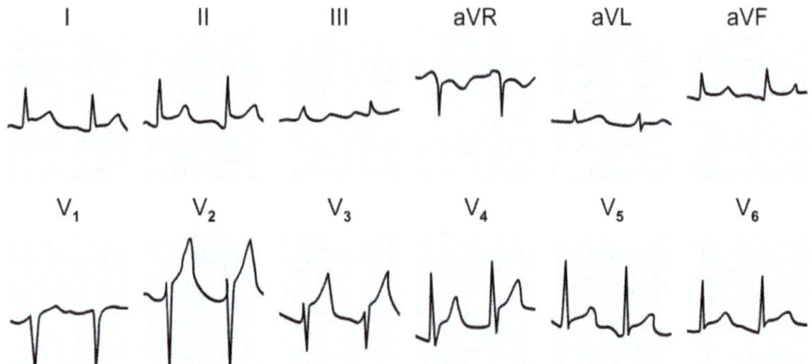

Fig. 2.33: Stage 1 electrocardiographic changes from patient with acute pericarditis. Diffuse ST segment elevation, which is concave upward, is present in all leads except aVR and V_1. Depression of the PR segment, an electrocardiographic abnormality that is common in patients with acute pericarditis, is not evident because of the short PR interval.
Source: Adapted with permission from Braunwald E. Heart Disease: A Textbook of Cardiovascular Medicine, 5th edition. Philadelphia: WB Saunders, Elsevier Science; 1997.

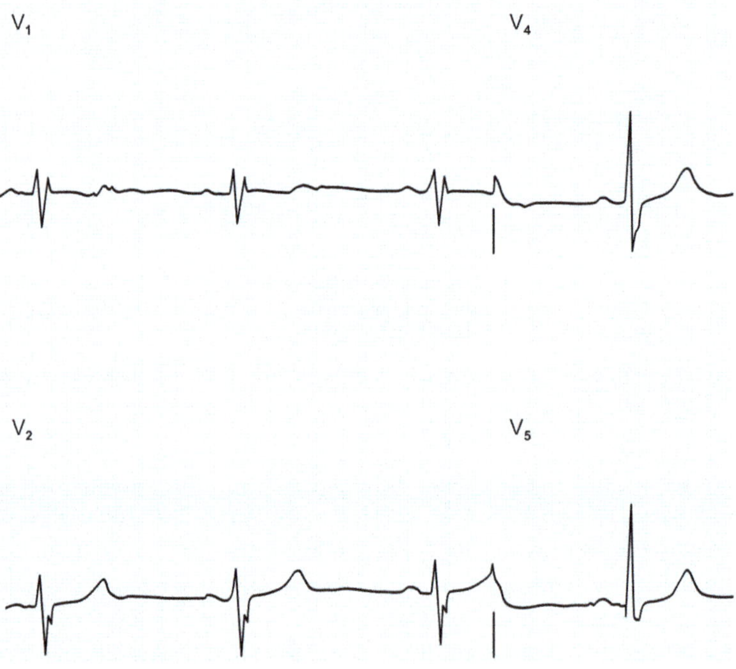

Fig. 2.34: V leads of a 39-year-old woman who had a large atrial septal defect repaired 5 years earlier. Note the RSr' in lead V_1 and a wide, slurred S wave in V_5; the QRS duration is 0.1 second: Incomplete right bundle branch block.

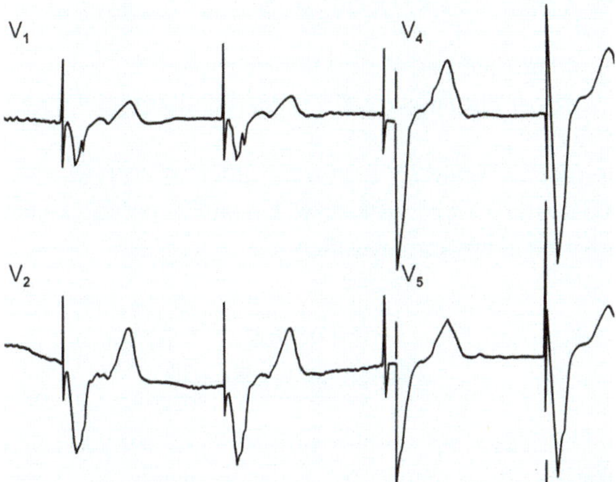

Fig. 2.35: ECG showing electronic pacing and ventricular capture; rate is 60 beats/minute. No further analysis is possible because of pacemaker rhythm.

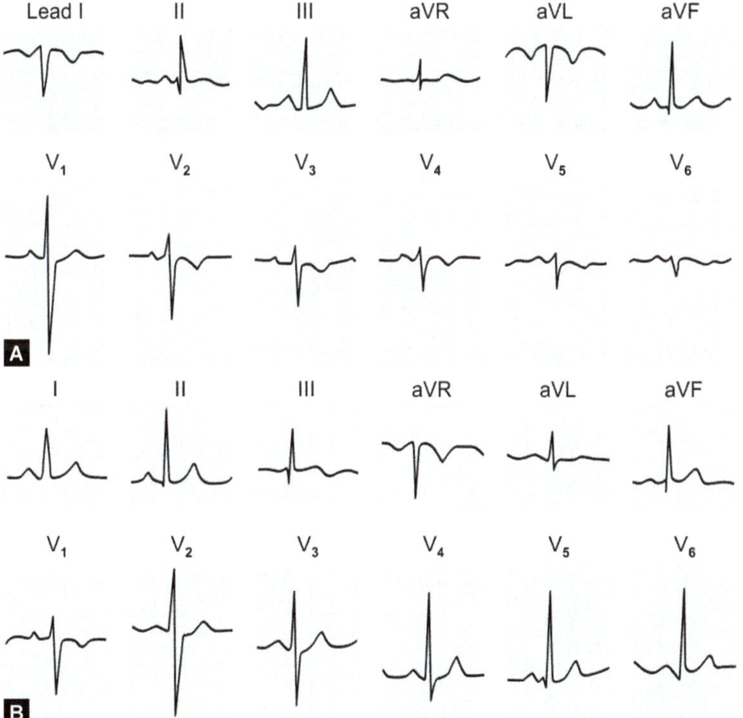

Figs. 2.36A and B: Mirror-image dextrocardia with situs inversus. The patient is a 15-year-old girl. There is no evidence of organic heart disease. (A) Tracing recorded with conventional electrode placement; (B) Tracing obtained with the left and right arm electrodes reversed. The precordial lead electrodes also were located in the respective mirror-image positions on the chest. The tracing is within normal limits.
Source: Adapted with permission from Chou TC. Electrocardiography in Clinical Practice, 4th edition. Philadelphia: WB Saunders, Elsevier Science; 1996.

STEP 11: ASSESS ARRHYTHMIAS (FIGS. 2.37A AND B)

Tachyarrhythmias should be analyzed as the following:

- *Narrow complex tachycardia:* Figure 2.37A gives the differential diagnosis of narrow QRS complex tachycardia.
- *Wide complex tachycardia:* Figure 2.37B gives the differential diagnosis of wide QRS complex tachycardia. See Chapter 11 for relevant ECGs and detailed discussion of arrhythmia diagnosis including that of bradyarrhythmias.

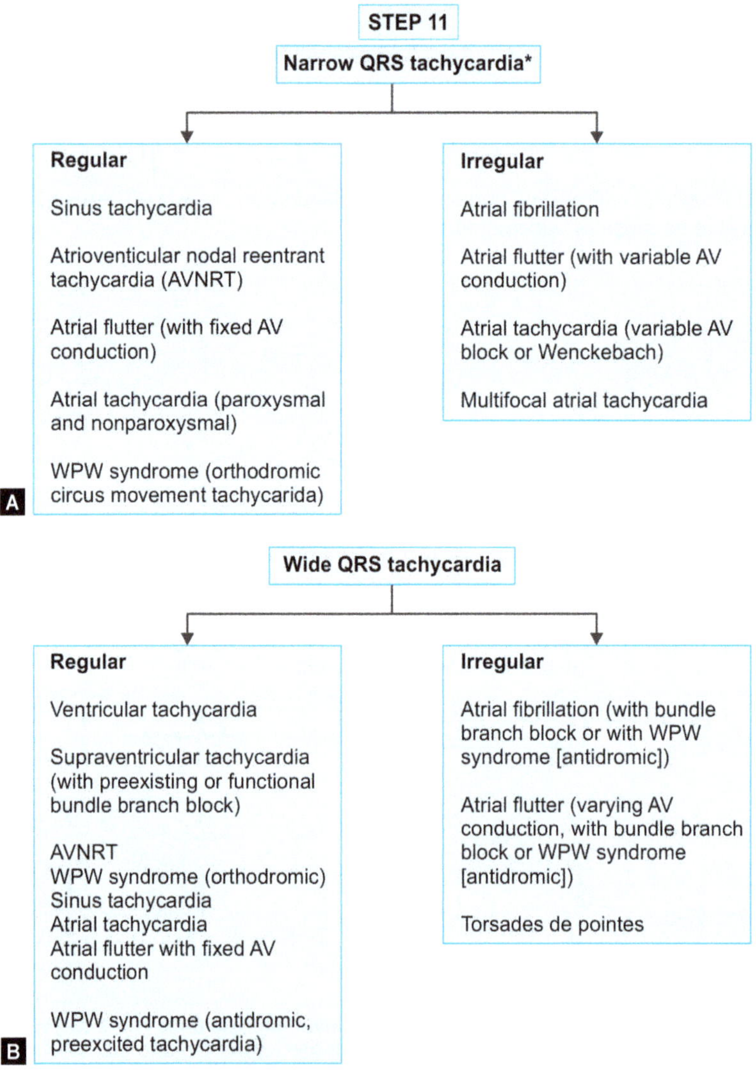

Figs. 2.37A and B: Step-by-step method for accurate ECG interpretation. Step 11: assess arrhythmias: (A) Differential diagnosis of narrow QRS tachycardia and (B) Wide QRS tachycardia.
*See Chapter 11.

ELECTROCARDIOGRAM TECHNIQUE

- Ensure the standardization is 1 mV displayed as a 10-mm deflection (10 small squares in amplitude).
- Always record the ECG at a standard paper speed of 25 mm/s.
- Remember that artifacts such as baseline drift are often caused by loose or improperly installed sensors.
- Most ECG machines have two modes of operation: (1) automatic or (2) manual. Familiarize yourself with the procedure in the ECG department of your hospital so that you can do the ECG, if called, when there is no technician or nurse available to do the procedure.
- Attach the electrodes (bulb suction cup or flat sensors) on a smooth, fleshy part of the lower arm or forearm and on the fleshy parts of the lower leg.
- Attach the chest lead sensors as indicated in Figure 2.38 (bulb sensor suction cups or flat sensors).

Ensure that electrodes are properly placed. Incorrect lead placement can lead to serious errors with interpretation (Figs. 2.39A and B).

Untrained technicians often place leads V_5 and V_6 too anteriorly; this may not give a true recording of the left ventricular muscle mass. The leads must be placed in the anterior and midaxillary line (*see* Fig. 2.38). Incorrect placement of V_2 and V_3 may render a false interpretation of old anteroseptal MI. Thus, much care is needed in placing the chest leads. Feel for the bony.

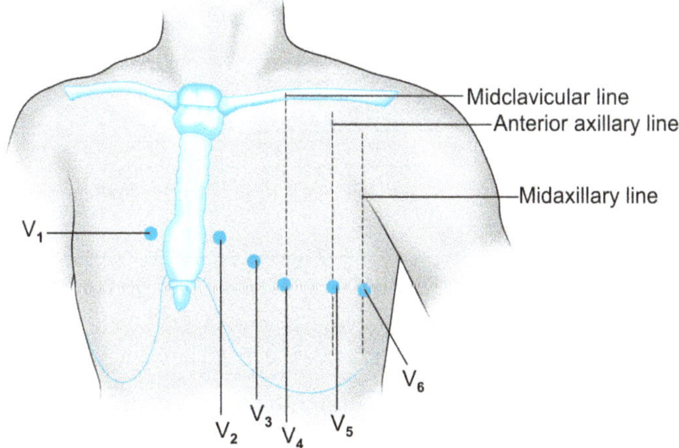

V_1 = 4th interspace at the right margin of the sternum
V_2 = 4th interspace at the left margin of the sternum
V_3 = Midway between position for V_2 and V_4
V_4 = 5th interspace at junction of left midclavicular line (apex)
V_5 = At horizontal level of position V_4 at left anterior axillary line
V_6 = Same horizontal line as for position V_4 but in the midaxillary line

Fig. 2.38: Chest leads placement. V_1, 4th interspace at the right margin of the sternum; V_2, 4th interspace at the left margin of the sternum; V_3, midway between positions for V_2 and V_4; V_4, 5th interspace at junction of left midclavicular line (apex); V_5, at horizontal level of position V_4 at left anterior axillary line; V_6, same horizontal line as for position V_4 but in the midaxillary line.

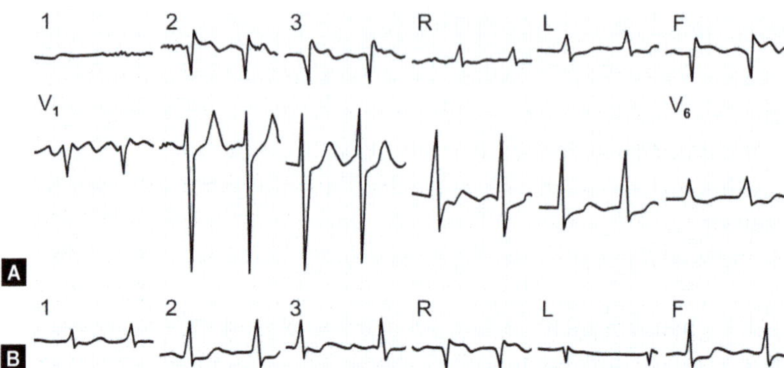

Figs. 2.39A and B: (A) Atrial fibrillation and pseudoinferior infarction resulting from electrode misplacement. With Q waves and ST elevation in leads 2, 3, and aVF and with reciprocal depression of the ST segment in aVL and chest leads, this tracing suggests acute inferior infarction. However, lead 1, with virtually no deflections, is the tip-off: The two arm electrodes are on the two legs (and the leg electrodes are on the arms); (B) Limb leads with the electrodes attached correctly.
Source: Adapted with permission from Marriott HJ. *Practical Electrocardiography*, 8th edition. Baltimore: Williams & Wilkins; 1988.

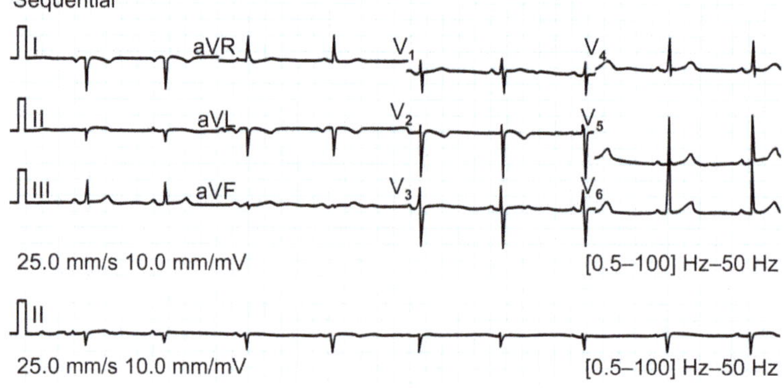

Fig. 2.40: Arm electrodes interchanged. Otherwise ECG within normal limits.

Small changes in electrode position can cause significant changes in the record obtained with these leads.

The most common error is the reversal of the left and right arm leads. The ECG records the following: the P wave is negative in lead I and upright in aVR; lead I is a mirror image of I, and therefore the entire complex that is usually positive becomes negative; there is reversal of lead aVR and aVL (aVR is aVL: aVL shows a negative P wave and a relatively negative complex because it is aVR); and there is reversal of leads II and III (lead II is III and lead III is II). Figure 2.40 shows the effect of the reversal of the arm leads. The P, QRS, and T waves are inverted in leads I and aVL; the precordial (V) leads remain normal, however, and thus rule out dextrocardia, in which the limb leads are similar but there is loss of R waves or poor R wave progression from V_2 through V_6 (*see* Figs. 2.36A and B).

P Wave Abnormalities

INTRODUCTION

The P wave represents the spread of the electrical impulse through both atria (*see* Fig. 1.8). The electrical impulse begins in the sinoatrial node (SA) node and depolarizes the right atrium and then the left atrium. Thus, the first part of the P wave reflects right atrial activity, and the late portion of the P wave represents electrical potential generated by the left atrium.

FEATURES OF THE NORMAL P WAVE

The following are some features of the normal P wave:
- It should be upright in leads I and II, as well as in the precordial leads V_3 through V_6 (Figs. 3.1 and 3.2).
- It is always inverted in aVR.
- It is usually upright in aVF and V_3, but occasionally a diphasic or flat P wave may be seen.
- It is variable in leads III, aVL, V_1, and V_2: upright, inverted, or diphasic. (A P or T wave that is partly above the baseline and partly below it is referred to as diphasic.)

FEATURES OF ABNORMAL P WAVES (SEE FIGS. 2.21 AND 2.22)

- Inverted in II, III, and aVF and upright in aVR: diagnostic of an atrioventricular (AV) junctional (*see* Fig. 3.2) or ectopic atrial rhythm. When there is abnormal propagation of the electrical impulse through the atria, the polarity or axis of the P wave is abnormal.

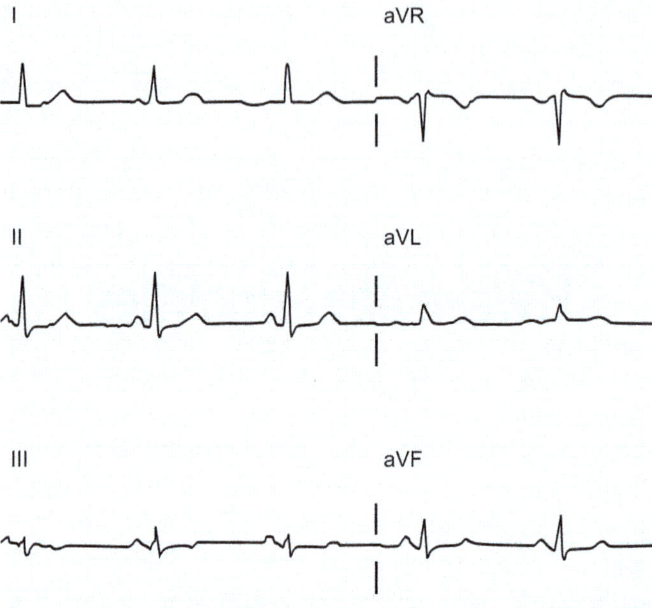

Fig. 3.1A: Limb leads of a normal tracing. Normal upright P waves are seen in lead I but are best seen in lead II, are inverted in aVR, and usually are variable in aVL and lead III.

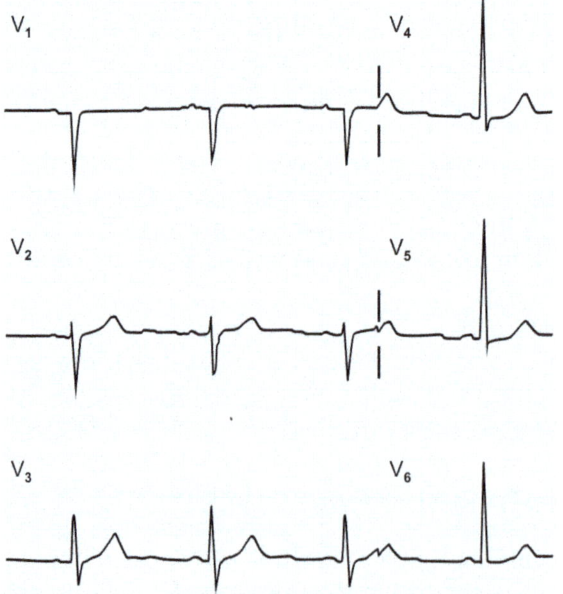

Fig. 3.1B: Same tracing as in (3.1A) showing normal upright P waves in leads V_3 through V_6.

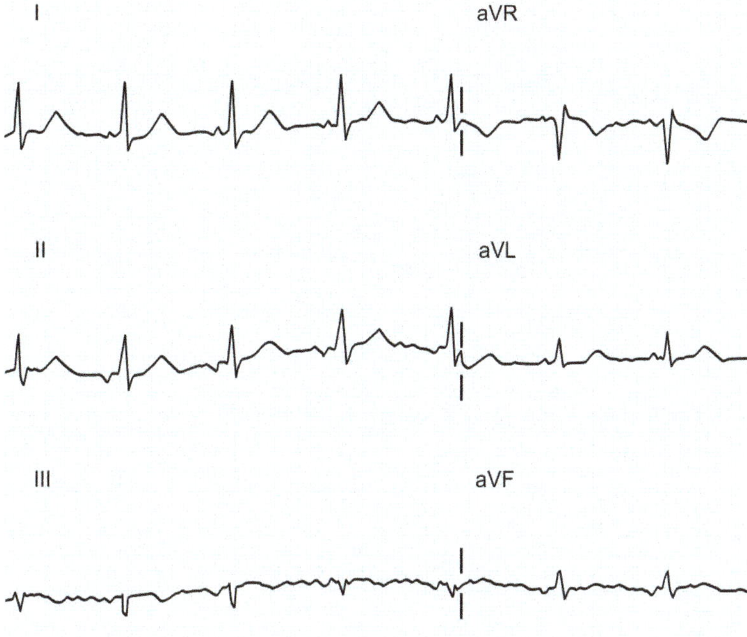

Fig. 3.2: P wave is inverted in leads II, III, and aVF and is upright in aVR, indicating junctional rhythm.

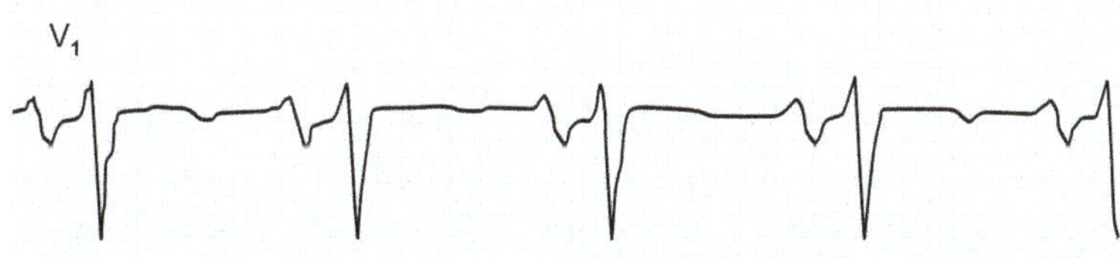

Fig. 3.3: The second half of the P wave in V₁ is dominantly negative and wide, indicating left atrial enlargement.

- Inverted in lead I and upright in aVR, with lead I being the mirror image of I: caused by reversed arm leads or dextrocardia, but in true dextrocardia there is a loss of R wave in V_4 through V_6 (*see* Figs. 2.36 and 2.40).
- Duration more than or equal to 0.12 second (three small squares). Most prominent in leads II, III, and aVF; caused by left atrial enlargement (*see* Figs. 2.21 and 2.40). P waves are seen best in leads II and V_1; thus, these leads should be used for rhythm strips and arrhythmia detection.

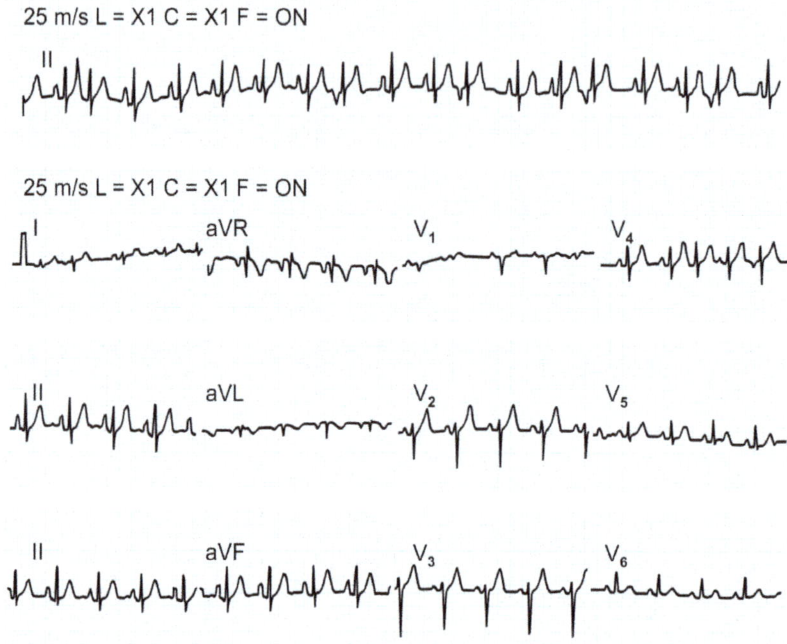

Fig. 3.4: Tall pointed P waves, high amplitude (>2.5 mm), particularly in leads II, III and aVF. Note the P wave is much taller in lead III than in lead I; typical features of right atrial hypertrophy (enlargement).

- *Notching of a wide P wave in lead II, III, or aVF*: A distance between peaks more than 0.04 second usually indicates left atrial enlargement (*see* Fig. 2.22).
- *Diphasic in V_1*: The second half of the P wave is dominantly negative and wide (*see* Figs. 2.22, 2.23, and 3.3). The depth of the inversion multiplied by the width represents the P terminal force; if it is more than or equal to −0.04 mm (i.e. a negative amplitude of 1 mm with duration of 0.04 second), consider left atrial enlargement (*see* Figs. 2.22, 2.23, and 3.3). In V_1, the negative deflection is normally less than 1 mm.
- *Large diphasic in V_1*: If the first half of the P wave is positive more than or equal to 1.5 mm and the second half is negative more than or equal to 1 mm and wide, consider biatrial enlargement (*see* Fig. 2.23).
- *High amplitude, peaking (see Figs. 2.22 and 2.23)*: Tall, pointed P waves, taller in lead III than in lead I; high amplitude (≥2.5 mm), particularly in lead II, III, or aVF, indicates right atrial enlargement (Fig. 3.4). Consider the presence of right ventricular hypertrophy (RVH), cor pulmonale, pulmonary hypertension, or pulmonary and tricuspid stenosis (Figs. 3.5A to C).
- *Absent P waves*: consider SA block and AV junctional rhythms. If the rhythm is irregular, consider atrial fibrillation (*see* Chapter 11).

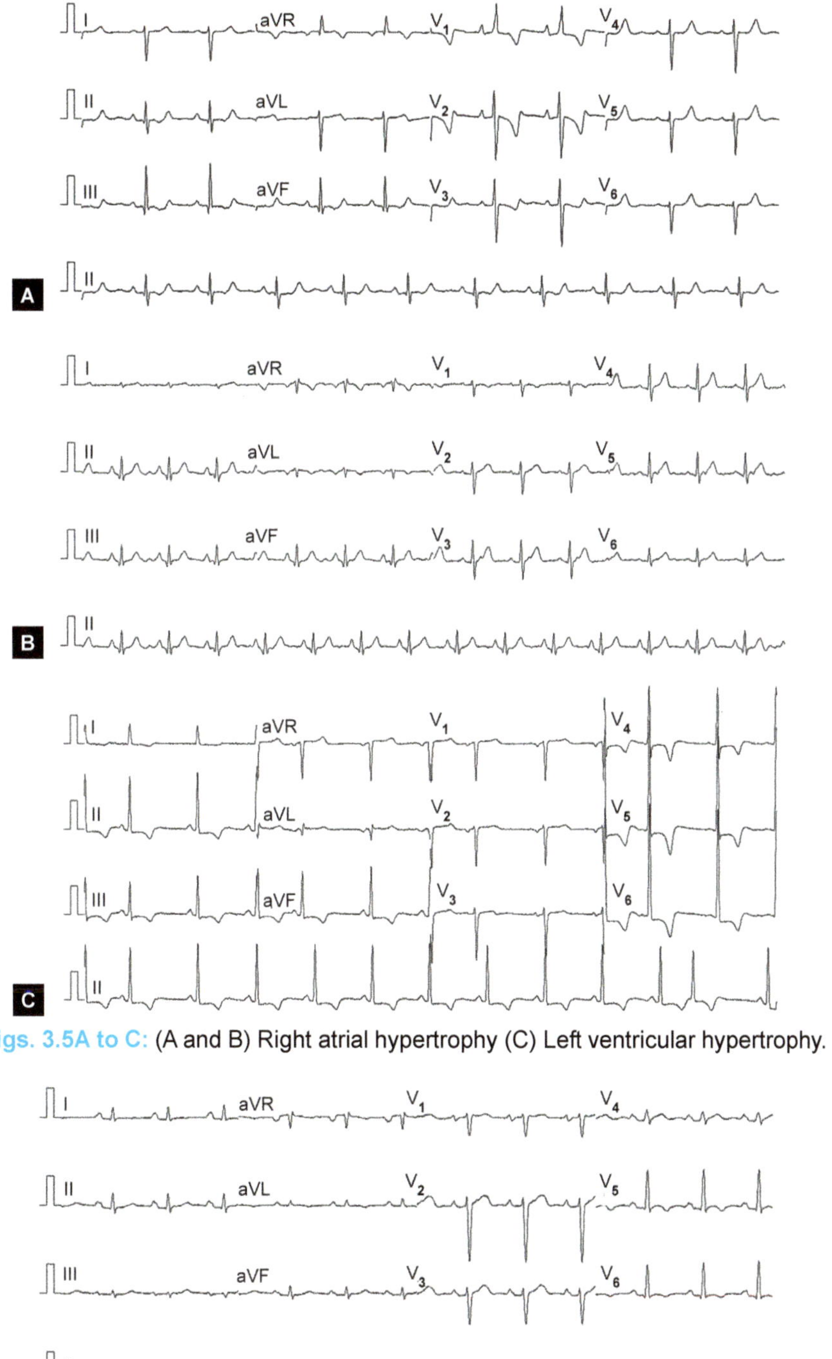

Figs. 3.5A to C: (A and B) Right atrial hypertrophy (C) Left ventricular hypertrophy.

Fig. 3.6: Left atrial hypertrophy (LAH)—sinus rhythm. S-T, T wave changes/nonspecific (abnormal ECG of a male patient aged 44 years old, QRS 114 ms).

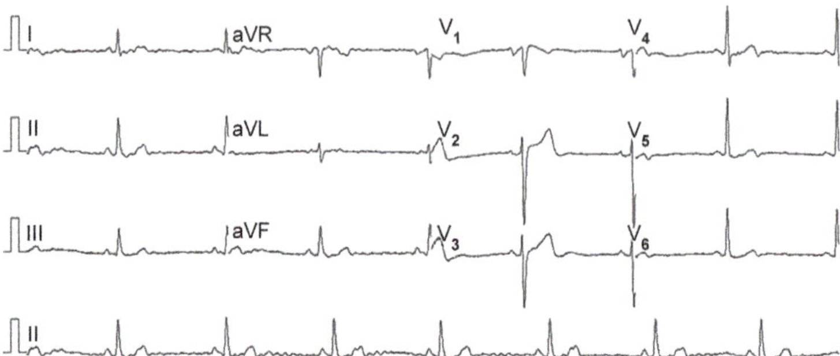

Fig. 3.7: Left atrial hypertrophy. Note best seen in V_1; thus, I advise looking at lead V_1 early in interpretation sequence as to see sinus rhythm, atrial fibrillation or hypertrophy or AV block all can be seen in V_1.

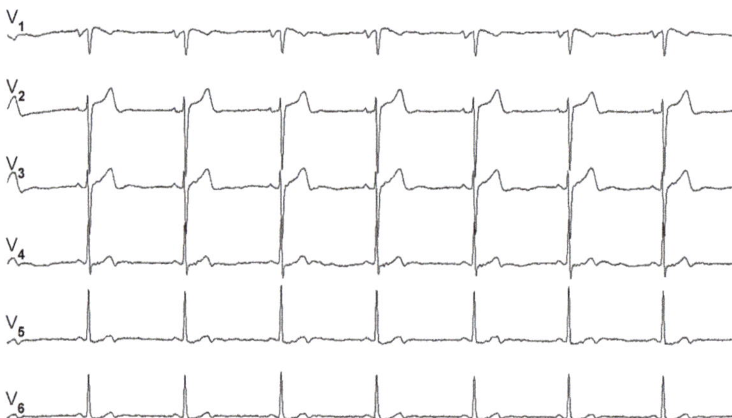

Fig. 3.8: Sinus bradycardia—left atrial hypertrophy. Mild left ventricular hypertrophy (LVH); clinical correlation required.

- *Different morphologies*: At least three different P wave morphologies in the same lead: consider multifocal atrial tachycardia (*see* Chapter 11). Other examples of P wave abnormalities are given in Figures 3.6 to 3.8.

Bundle Branch Block

RIGHT BUNDLE BRANCH BLOCK

Diagnostic Criteria

- Wide QRS more than or equal to 0.12 second.
- A secondary R wave (R′) in V_1 or V_2 (i.e. an rSR′, rsR′, or rsr′ complex that often is M-shaped). The secondary R wave (R′) is usually taller than the initial R wave (Figs. 4.1, 4.2A, and 2.7A).
- A wide, slurred S wave in leads V_5, V_6, and I with duration more than 40 ms; the S wave is longer in duration (length) than the preceding R wave in leads V_6 and I (*see* Figs. 2.7A, B and 4.2).
- The axis may be normal, right, or left. If left axis is present, consider left anterior fascicular block (hemiblock) (*see* Chapter 9).

Genesis of the QRS in Right Bundle Branch Block

The typical M-shaped complex in V_1 or V_2 is derived from an alteration of the normal vector forces (*see* Fig. 4.1).

- The initial impulse depolarizes the septum normally from left to right. With right bundle branch block (RBBB), vector I remains intact; the electrical current traveling toward the electrode V_1 positioned over the right ventricle registers an initial small R wave in leads V_1 and V_2 (*see* Fig. 4.1). Because the right bundle branch does not conduct the electrical impulse, vector II is directed leftward only, activates the left ventricle, and records an S wave in V_1 and

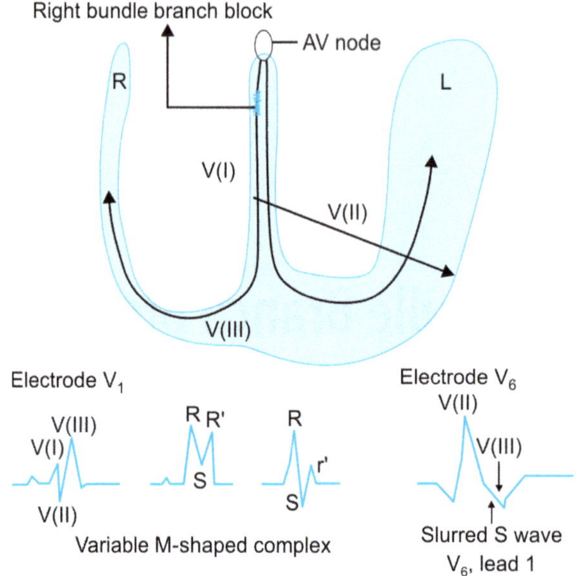

Fig. 4.1: Genesis of the QRS complex in right bundle branch block.
Source: Adapted with permission from Khan MG. On Call Cardiology, 3rd edition. Philadelphia: WB Saunders, Elsevier Science; 2006.

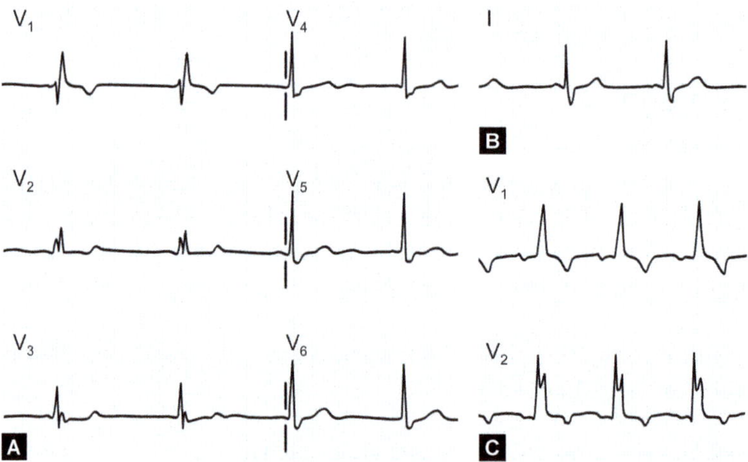

Figs. 4.2A to C: (A) An rSR′ in V_1; M-shaped complex in V_1 and V_2; QRS duration ≥0.12 second; and wide, slurred S waves in V_5 and V_6 indicate right bundle branch block. (B) Same patient as in (A). Lead I, wide, slurred S wave indicates RBBB. (C) Right bundle branch block.

V_2. Right ventricular activation occurs later (i.e. unopposed by left ventricular activation); the resultant force, vector III, causes a large R, termed R′ in V_1 or V_2. Thus, the rsR′ or rSR′ complex depicts an M shape. The deflection R′ is usually greater than the amplitude of the small R produced by vector I septal depolarization.

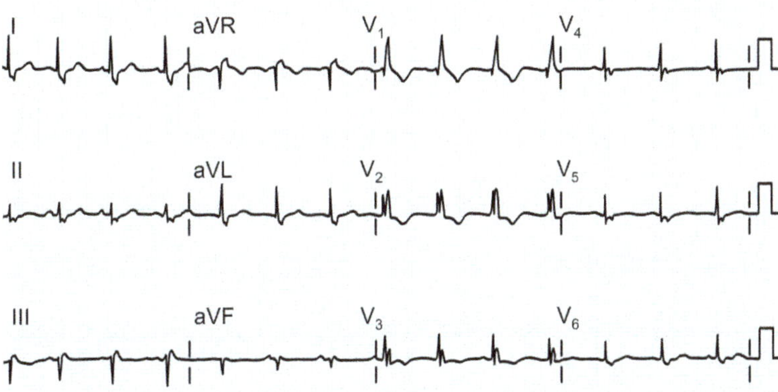

Fig. 4.2D: Typical right bundle branch block: QRS, 0.14 second; rsR′ in V₁; M-shaped complex in lead V₂; and a slurred S wave in V₅ and V₆. The S wave in lead I and V₆ is longer in duration (length) than the preceding R wave.

- The unopposed late depolarization of the right ventricle, which causes the R′ in V_1 or V_2, is recorded as a wide, slurred S wave in leads V_5, V_6, and I, the electrodes overlying the left ventricle (*see* 4.1 and 4.2).
- Because of delayed right ventricular activation, the QRS duration is increased to 0.12 second or more. Figure 4.2D shows typical features of RBBB.
- *Brugada syndrome* is a special form of incomplete or complete RBBB pattern. Although the condition is rare, it is a common cause of idiopathic ventricular fibrillation and sudden cardiac death in young adults, particularly of Asian origin, and notably in individuals without evidence of structural heart disease. Attention must be given to any condition that causes sudden death, particularly in young individuals. The typical electrocardiogram (ECG) features are illustrated in Figure 4.3. Note the RBBB pattern and persistent ST segment elevation in V_1, V_2, and V_3 that has a typical pattern: coved or saddleback-shaped, a marker for sudden death in individuals without demonstrable structural heart disease. Note that this is an atypical incomplete or complete RBBB pattern, because there are usually no widened S waves in V_5 and V_6 of true RBBB: the S wave in V_6 or lead I in RBBB is longer in duration than the preceding R wave. The ST segment elevation appears to be caused by an early high take-off (J wave) and mimics RBBB.
- Arrhythmogenic right ventricular dysplasia, another rare condition that shows an atypical RBBB pattern, is a marker for sudden cardiac death in younger individuals. With this condition, there is structural heart disease caused by a type of cardiomyopathy that involves the right ventricle and the left ventricle at a later stage. Fatty and fibro-fatty degeneration occurs in the right ventricular inflow and outflow tracts and in the apex. Either incomplete or complete RBBB is observed. In approximately 40% of cases, a characteristic terminal notch is observed in the QRS of V_1 and V_2 (termed an epsilon wave) that is a result of slowed intraventricular conduction. Another feature is T wave inversion in V_1, V_2, and V_3. The echocardiogram may show an abnormal right ventricle as the disease progresses.

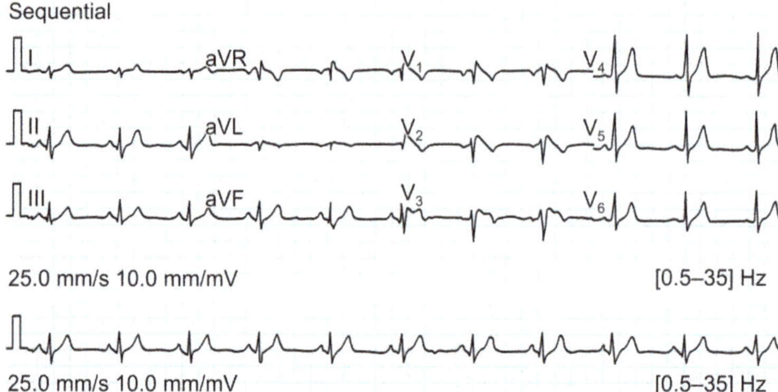

Fig. 4.3: Typical features of Brugada syndrome. Atypical, incomplete right bundle branch block (RBBB) with a curious (odd shape) ST segment elevation/deformity in V_1 to V_3, described as the coved (in V_1, V_2) and saddleback patterns (V_3). Note there is no widened S wave in V_5 or in V_6, as seen in true incomplete or complete RBBB. Thus, if you recognize an atypical RBBB, think of Brugada syndrome and reassess for the characteristic features of this rare but important diagnosis. ECG from a 40-year-old man with episodes of syncope/collapse. No recurrence of syncope over 3 years following ICD.

Causes of Right Bundle Branch Block

- A normal finding in adults of all ages.
- Coronary artery disease (CAD) and hypertensive and rheumatic heart disease.
- Congenital heart disease, often associated with ventricular septal defect (VSD) and tetralogy of Fallot. With secundum atrial septal defect (ASD), more than 90% of individuals have incomplete RBBB.
- Coarctation of the aorta.
- Pericarditis and myocarditis including Chagas disease.
- Pulmonary embolism and cor pulmonale.
- Cardiomyopathy.
- Brugada syndrome and right ventricular dysplasia (atypical RBBB pattern).

Incomplete Right Bundle Branch Block

Diagnostic Criteria

- The presence of an rSR′ (i.e. RBBB pattern) in V_1 or V_2 and an S wave in leads I and V_6 should be confirmed.
- The QRS duration should be 0.08–0.11 second.

Causes of Incomplete Right Bundle Branch Block

- Incomplete RBBB is a common ECG finding in normal individuals.
- More than 90% of patients with a secundum ASD show incomplete RBBB (*see* Figs. 2.34 and 4.3).

- Wolff-Parkinson-White (WPW) syndrome may mimic incomplete RBBB.
- Brugada syndrome and right ventricular dysplasia.

RSr′ Variant

More than 5% of individuals without heart disease show an RSr′ in V_1 or V_2. If the QRS duration is more than or equal to 0.08 second and there is an S wave in V_5 or V_6 (*see* Fig. 4.3), the diagnosis of incomplete RBBB should be made. The diagnosis is strengthened if there is a slurred S wave in I, V_5, or V_6.

- If a slurred S wave is absent in leads I, V_5, or V_6 with QRS duration less than 0.08 second, the ECG is interpreted as an rSR′, RSR′, or RSr′ variant, borderline ECG. An R′ less than 6 mm with an R′/S ratio less than 1 suggests normality.

Causes of rSR′, RSR′, and RSr′ in V_1 or V_2: QRS Duration ≤0.11 Second

- Idiopathic; a normal finding in 5% of individuals without heart disease.
- Incomplete RBBB.
- Straight back syndrome or pectus excavatum.
- Atrial septal defect.
- Rarely, VSD and coarctation of the aorta.
- Mitral stenosis and other acquired heart diseases.
- Right ventricular hypertrophy.
- Right ventricular volume overload.
- Cor pulmonale or pulmonary embolism.
- WPW syndrome (may mimic incomplete RBBB).
- Atrioventricular nodal reentrant tachycardia (*see* Chapter 11).
- Muscular dystrophy.
- Late activation of the outflow tract of the right ventricle, the crista supraventricularis (may cause r′ wave in V_1).
- Incorrect placement of the V_1 electrode.

The RSr′ may appear if V_1 is placed in the third interspace and may disappear with the electrode in the fifth interspace, or incomplete RBBB may be recorded. The appearance at a higher intercostal space may be the only abnormality in some patients with a secundum ASD (*see* Figs. 2.34).

Right Bundle Branch Block and Myocardial Infarction

- With acute anterior myocardial infarction (MI), pathologic Q waves occur in V_1, V_2, V_3, or V_4. A Q wave in V_1 and V_2 is not sufficient evidence for the diagnosis of MI.
- Consider inferior MI only if pathologic Q waves are present in leads II, III, and aVF. Q waves in leads III and aVF are not diagnostic.
- The right bundle branch and the septum are supplied blood by the same artery; thus, anteroseptal infarction commonly is associated with RBBB. In anteroseptal MI, the initial septal force, vector I, is lost. Thus, a loss of the initial r wave occurs in V_1 with resultant q or Q wave in V_1, V_2. In addition, the normal small q wave in V_6 disappears.

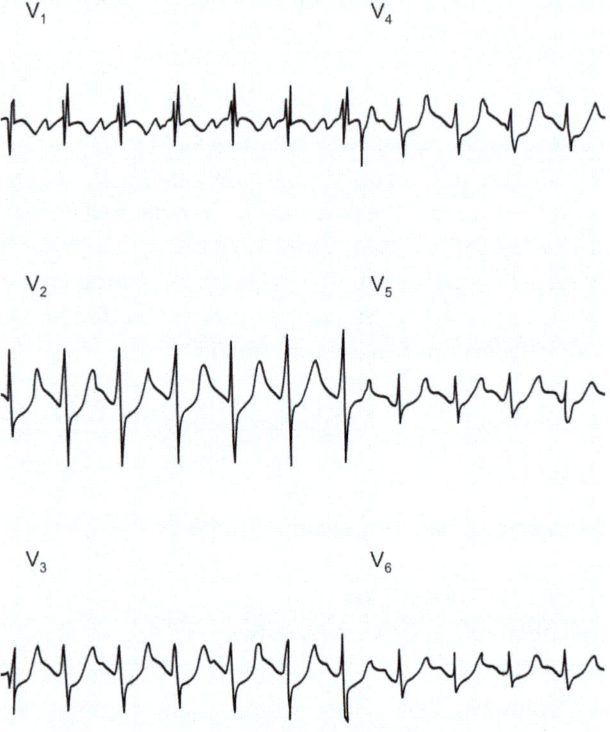

Fig. 4.4: Sinus tachycardia, rate 147 beats/minute. QRS duration 0.10 second and rSR′ in V_1 indicates incomplete right bundle branch block.

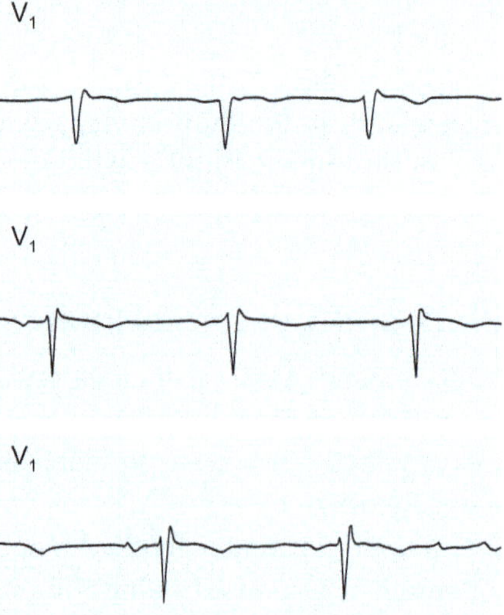

Fig. 4.5: RSr′ and rSR′ in V_1; recorded in different intercostal spaces.

LEFT BUNDLE BRANCH BLOCK

Diagnostic Criteria

- QRS duration more than or equal to 0.12 second.
- A broad monophasic R wave that is often notched or slurred in lead I, aVL, V_5, or V_6 (Figs. 4.6 to 4.8 and Fig. 2.8B).
- Late intrinsicoid deflection in leads I, V_5, and V_6 greater than 0.05 second.
- Leads V_1 and V_2 reveal QS or rS pattern with poor R wave progression in V_2 and V_3 (*see* Figs. 4.6 to 4.8). Figure 4.9A shows notching of lead I. Figure 4.9B shows all the typical features of left bundle branch block (LBBB).
- A presumptive diagnosis of incomplete LBBB may be made if the QRS duration is 0.10–0.11 second with notching of the R wave in V_5 or V_6.

Genesis of the QRS Complex in Left Bundle Branch Block

- Depolarization of the left ventricle is delayed, and the QRS duration is prolonged to more than or equal to 0.12 second.
- The septum and left ventricle are activated by the electrical impulse from the right bundle.
- The normal direction of septal activation from left to right is reversed.
- Vector I flows from right to left through the lower septum rather than from left to right. Thus, an electrode over the left ventricle records an R wave in V_5, V_6, and I and a QS or rS in V_1 (*see* Figs. 4.6, 4.7, and Fig. 2.8B).
- Vector II travels from left to right through the right ventricular mass and may cause a slur or notch in the R wave of leads I, aVL, V_5, and V_6 [marked V(II) in Fig. 4.6]. The notched R and R′ may result in an M-shaped complex in lead I, V_4, V_5, or V_6 (*see* Figs. 4.6 to 4.9).
- Vector III travels right to left and causes an R′ in V_6 [marked V(III) in Fig. 4.6].

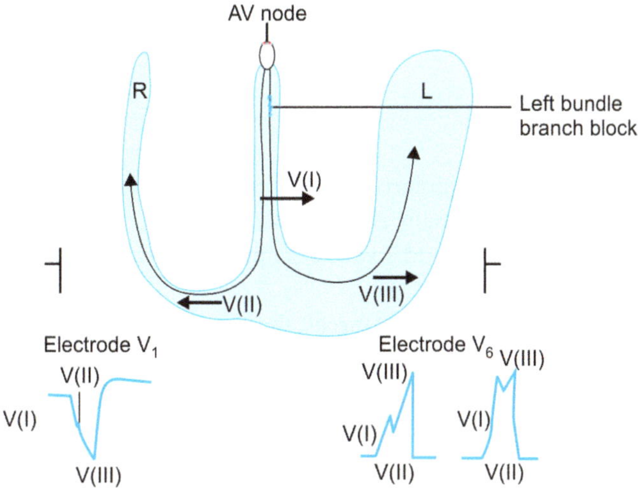

Fig. 4.6: Genesis of the QRS complex in left bundle branch block.

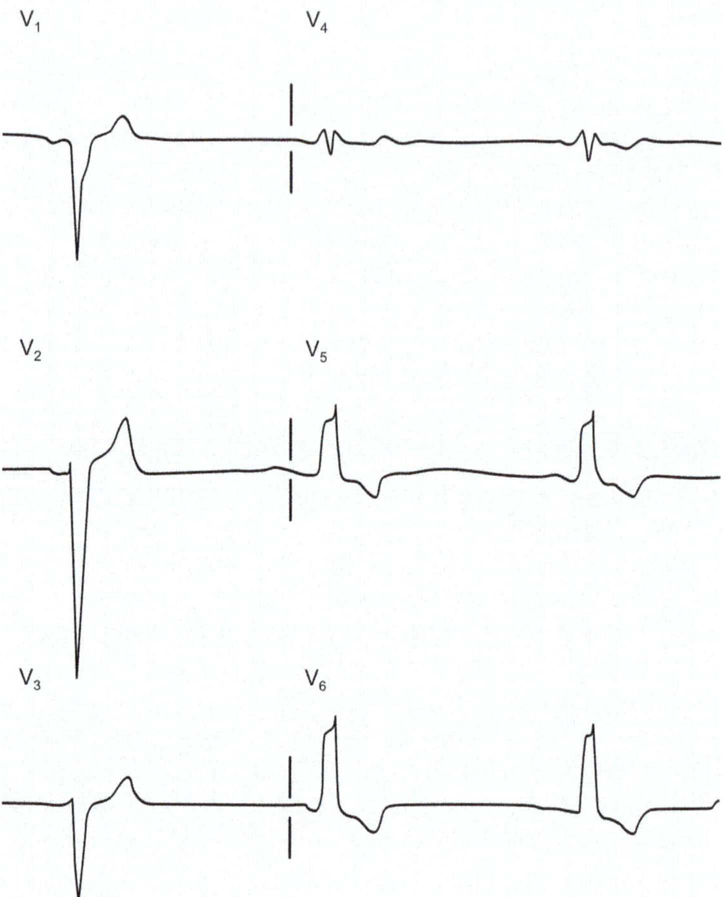

Fig. 4.7: Sinus bradycardia, 40 beats/minute; QRS duration >0.12 second. Note the broad, monophasic R wave, notched in V_5 and V_6, and poor R wave progression in V_2 and V_3, typical features of left bundle branch block.

- The marked derangement in depolarization of the left ventricle causes the ST segment in leads V_1 through V_4 to be abnormally elevated (*see* Fig. 4.8).
- The direction of the ST segment and T waves is opposite the direction of the terminal QRS (*see* Figs. 4.6 to 4.8).
- Because LBBB deranges normal vector forces, the diagnosis of left ventricular hypertrophy (LVH) cannot be made in the presence of LBBB. ST elevation, poor R wave progression in V_1 through V_3, and increased voltage are common features of LBBB and do not indicate LVH, myocardial injury, or MI (*see* Figs. 4.7, 4.8, and Fig. 2.8B and Chapter 6).

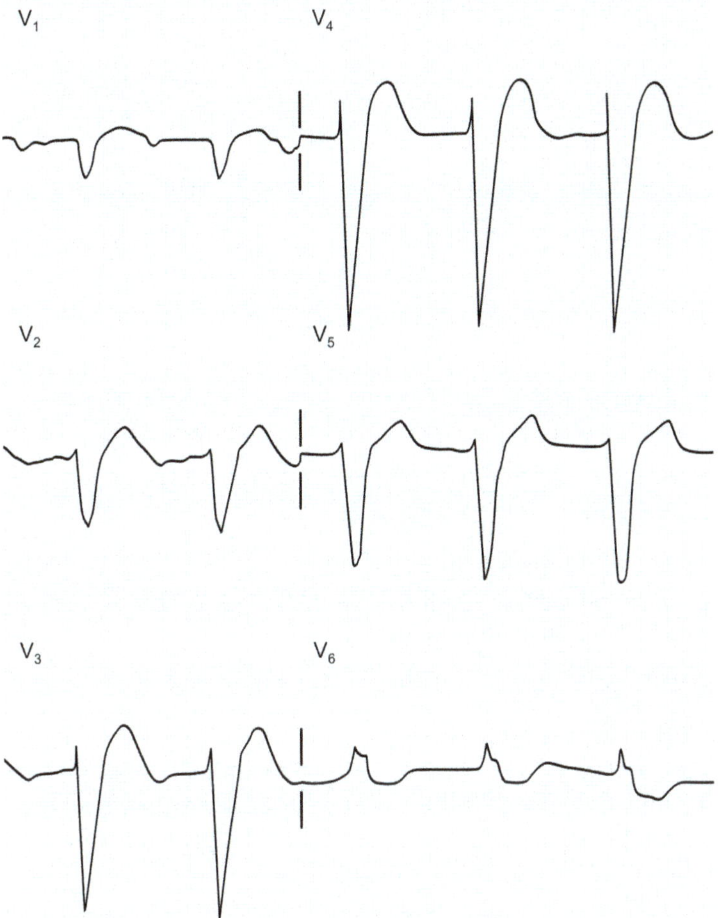

Fig. 4.8: QRS duration ≥0.12 second; poor R wave progression; and notched R wave in V_6. Note ST segment elevation in V_1 through V_5, typical of left bundle branch block that mimics anterior myocardial infarction.

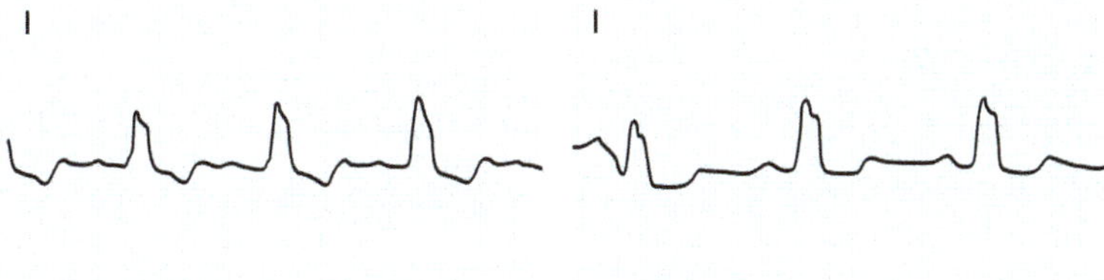

Fig. 4.9A

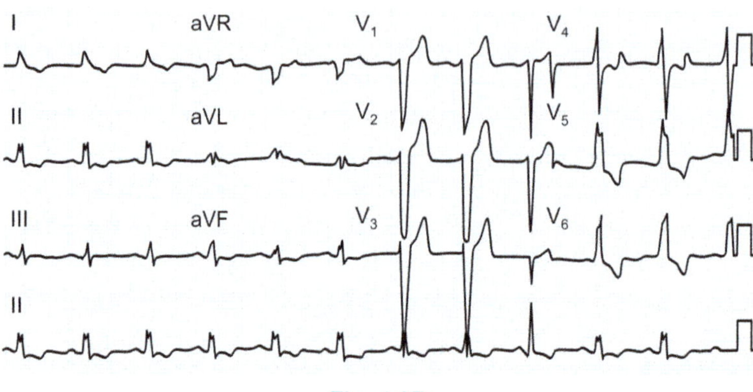

Fig. 4.9B

Figs. 4.9A and B: (A) Notching in lead I indicates left bundle branch block (two patients); (B) All of the typical electrocardiographic features of LBBB. Note the absence of normal Q waves in V_5 and V_6.

Causes of Left Bundle Branch Block

- Cardiomyopathies and degenerative diseases.
- Coronary artery disease; patients with CAD and LBBB have a high incidence of left ventricular dysfunction and congestive heart failure.
- Hypertensive heart disease.
- Advanced valvular heart disease.
- Congenital heart disease.
- Idiopathic in patients with structurally normal hearts. Although LBBB usually occurs in patients with underlying heart disease, the condition may occasionally occur in individuals with structurally normal hearts. These individuals fall primarily into a category of young, healthy adults with idiopathic LBBB or older subjects with primary disease of the conducting system. New LBBB that develops at age 45 or later is likely caused by a significant disease process. In the Framingham study, 55 individuals developed new LBBB at an average age of 62, and coronary heart disease was evident in 89% of these; 50% died within 10 years of onset of LBBB.

Nonspecific Intraventricular Conduction Delay

Diagnostic Criteria

- QRS duration more than 0.11 with QRS morphology that does not satisfy the criteria for either RBBB or LBBB.
- Figure 4.10 illustrates steps to consider before making the diagnosis of nonspecific intraventricular conduction delay (IVCD). Notching of a QRS complex with a QRS duration less than 0.11 should not be classified as nonspecific IVCD.

Causes of Intraventricular Conduction Delay

- Coronary heart disease.

QRS ≥ 0.11 second but not typical RBBB or LBBB configuration

Assess for

1. Atypical RBBB or LBBB → **Spot for** → Delta wave + PR ≤0.12
   (Figure 11.27)

Present

WPW syndrome*

2. Atypical RBBB but WPW excluded and no slurred S wave in V_5 and V_6
   (therefore not true RBBB)

Spot for ST elevation in V_1 and V_2
(Coved or saddleback)

Present

Brugada syndrome↑(Figure 4.3)

3. Atypical RBBB 1 and 2
   Excluded → **Spot for** A terminal notch
   in the QRS **(Epsilon wave)**
   + T ↓ $V_1 V_3$

Present

Right ventricular dysplasia

4. 1 to 3 excluded → Diagnosis

IVCD

* = In=20%, the QRS is <0.11 second
↑ = QRS duration may be 0.10 to 0.12 second

Fig. 4.10: Before making the diagnosis of nonspecific intraventricular conduction delay (IVCD), consider steps 1, 2, and 3.

- Hypertensive heart disease.
- Severe valvular heart disease.
- Congenital heart disease.
- Cardiomyopathies.
- Heart failure (all causes).
- Antiarrhythmic agents.
- Tricyclic antidepressants.

Further examples of RBBB are shown in Figures 4.11 to 4.13; and Figure 4.14 shows incomplete RBBB. QRS must be more than 90 ms and less than 120 ms.

Further examples of LBBB are shown in Figures 4.15 and 4.16.

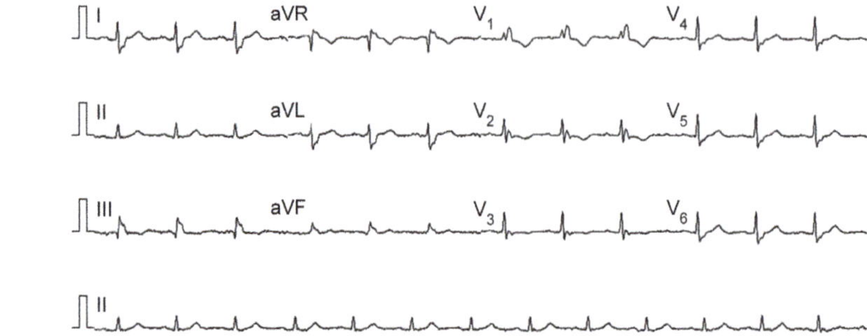

Fig. 4.11: Sinus rhythm—right axis deviation—right bundle branch block. QRS = 150 ms; notched R in V_1; RSR' in V_2; S >30 ms in I, V_5, and V_6.

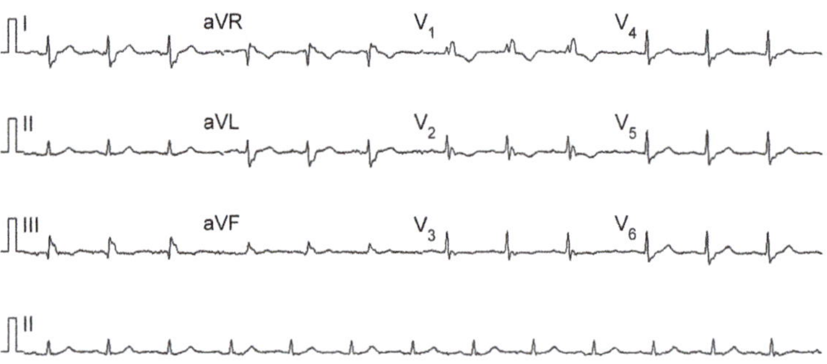

Fig. 4.12: Sinus rhythm; right bundle branch block (RBBB). QRS = 150 ms; notched R in V_1.

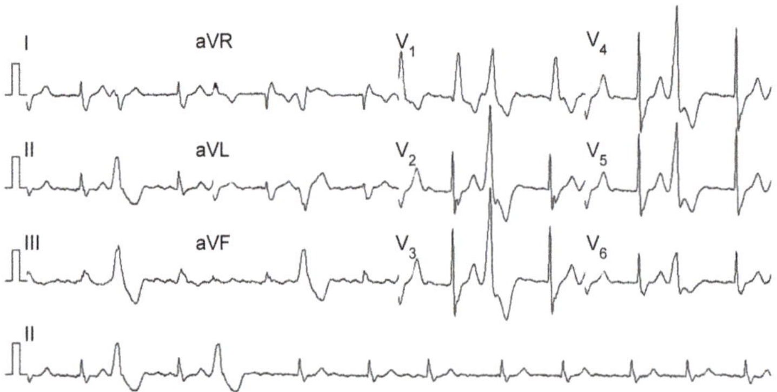

Fig. 4.13: Right bundle branch block (RBBB), also ventricular premature beats (VPBs) and atrial fibrillation; RSR' in V_2, V_5, V_6, lead I slurred S >30 ms.

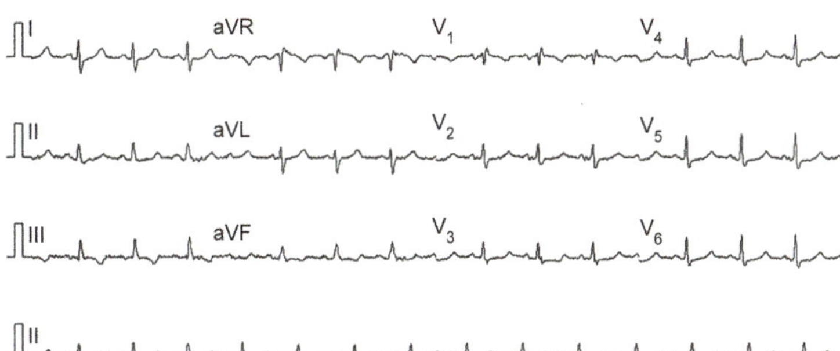

Fig. 4.14: Incomplete RBBB: RSR1 in V_1; the end of the S wave in V_6 is slightly slurred resembling complete RBBB but the QRS duration is less than 120 ms; the QRS should be more than 90–120 to entertain the diagnosis of incomplete RBBB.

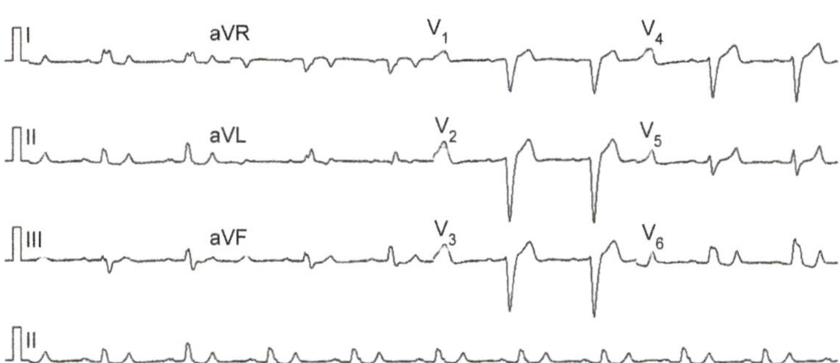

Fig. 4.15: Wide QRS notching in I, aVL, V_6; poor R wave progression V_1-V_3; typical pattern for left bundle branch block.

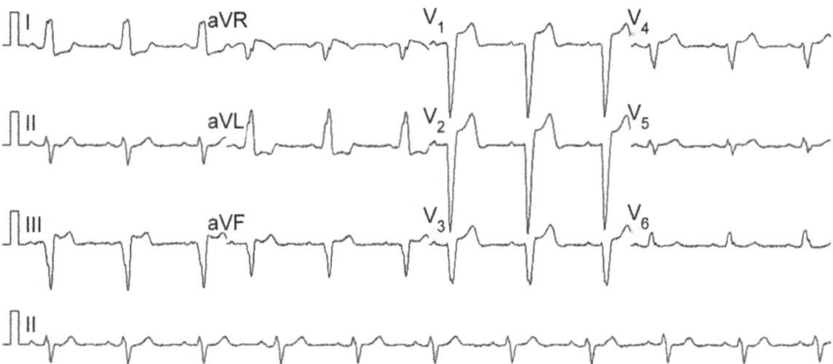

Fig. 4.16: Left bundle branch block loss of R or minute r V_1, V_3 may be mistaken for anteroseptal MI.

ST Segment Abnormalities

INTRODUCTION

The ST segment begins after the final deflection of the QRS complex and ends at the ascending limb of the T wave (*see* Fig. 2.1).

WHY EMPHASIZE THE ST SEGMENT?

Because important cardiac electrocardiogram (ECG) diagnoses are made from observation of abnormalities of the ST segment, the interpreter should rapidly focus on the ST segment. This assessment is Step 4 in the method for accurate ECG interpretation (Fig. 5.1). This step is carried out before the assessment for loss of R waves or for the presence of pathologic Q waves, T wave abnormalities, hypertrophy, and axis determination. The diagnosis of acute myocardial infarction (MI), ischemia, and pericarditis depends on careful scrutiny of the ST segment.

STEP 4

Assess the ST segment for the following:
- Elevation
- Depression
- Nonspecific changes.

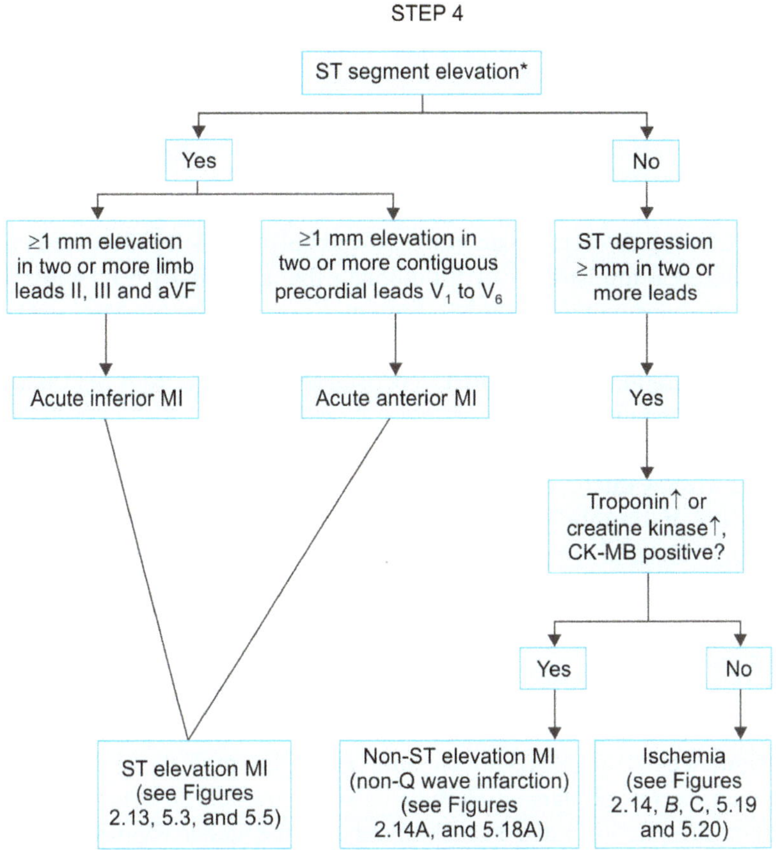

Fig. 5.1: Step-by-step method for accurate ECG interpretation. Step 4: assess for ST segment elevation or depression.
*Reciprocal depression increases probabilities of acute myocardial infarction (MI)

The PR segment is usually used to assess the degree of ST segment elevation or depression. The commencement of the ST segment is usually located at the same horizontal level as the T-P (the isoelectric interval, *see* Fig. 2.1).

Abnormal ST elevation can be caused by the following:

- Acute MI
- Coronary artery spasm
- Acute pericarditis
- Left ventricular (LV) aneurysm
- Left bundle branch block (LBBB)
- Left ventricular hypertrophy (LVH)

Exclude other causes of ST elevation:

- *Normal variant:* 1- to 2-mm ST elevation, mainly in leads V_2 through V_4, nonconvex, and with fishhook appearance. Common in African Americans: even 4-mm ST elevation (*see* Fig. 2.15).

- *Coronary artery spasm:* ST returns to normal with nitroglycerin or pain relief.
- *Left bundle branch block:* QRS more than or equal to 0.12 second and typical configuration (*see* Fig. 2.8B and Chapter 4).
- *Left ventricular aneurysm:* Known old infarction with old Q waves (*see* Chapter 6).

ST ELEVATION MYOCARDIAL INFARCTION

The early diagnosis of acute MI is paramount to successful percutaneous coronary intervention (PCI) or for the timely administration of thrombolytic therapy. This early diagnosis depends on the observation of abnormalities of the ST segment and not on the presence of Q waves or on the results of cardiac enzymes. Reliance on the presence of pathologic Q waves stems from the proven electrocardiographic principles that were used appropriately from 1930 to the late 1980s.

- ST segment depression = ischemia
- ST segment elevation = injury current
- Q waves = necrosis = infarction.

With the advent of thrombolytic therapy and PCI, it became necessary to diagnose acute MI within 1 hour of onset of symptoms, and the diagnosis has to be made without reliance on the presence of abnormal Q waves. Most patients with chest pain and abnormal ST segment elevation in two or more contiguous leads develop Q waves from 4 hours to 24 hours after the onset of symptoms.

Currently, two descriptive terms are used and recognized internationally:

1. ST elevation MI (STEMI)
2. Non-ST segment elevation MI (probable non-Q wave infarction).

The acute-injury current of infarction elevates the ST segment and deforms its shape. ST segment elevation patterns of infarction and a normal variant are illustrated in Figures 5.2A and B.

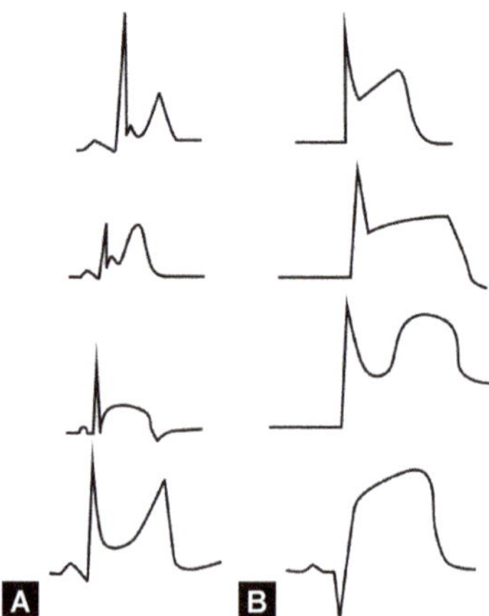

Figs. 5.2A and B: (A) ST segment elevation, pattern of normal variant. Note fishhook appearance; the ST segment usually retains the normal concave shape; the T waves are often prominent and peaked. (B) Abnormal ST elevation caused by acute myocardial infarction.
Source: Adapted with permission from Khan MG. On Call Cardiology, 3rd edition. Philadelphia: WB Saunders, Elsevier Science; 2006.

Diagnostic Criteria

Diagnostic criteria for STEMI (probable Q wave infarction) are as follows:
- Abnormal ST elevation of more than or equal to 1 mm in two or more contiguous limb leads.
- Elevation in leads II, III, and aVF indicates inferior infarction (Figs. 5.3, 5.4, and Fig. 2.13A). ST elevation in leads I, aVL, V_5, and V_6 indicates anterolateral infarction (*see* Fig. 2.18A).
- Abnormal ST elevation of more than or equal to 1 mm in two or more contiguous precordial leads indicates anterior infarction (*see* Fig. 5.1). ST elevation in V_1 through V_3 indicates anteroseptal infarction or anteroapical MI. Recent studies indicated that the area of necrosis is more likely to be anteroapical rather than anteroseptal (Fig. 5.5). Elevation in V_3 through V_6 (may involve V_2 and V_1) indicates anterior infarction (Fig. 5.6 and Fig. 2.13B). Extensive anterior infarction is denoted by ST elevation in eight or more leads (Fig. 5.7).
- ST elevation in V_3R and V_4R associated with inferior infarction indicates added right ventricular infarction (Fig. 5.8). It is advisable to record V_4R if the patient with an acute inferior infarct has hemodynamic deterioration.
- Tall R waves in V_1 and V_2 associated with ST elevation in II, III, aVF, or V_4R may indicate added posterior infarction. Posterior infarction occurs virtually always in association with inferior or right ventricular infarction. Tall R waves in V_1 and V_2 and T wave upright with no other ECG evidence of MI require cardiac enzyme confirmation.

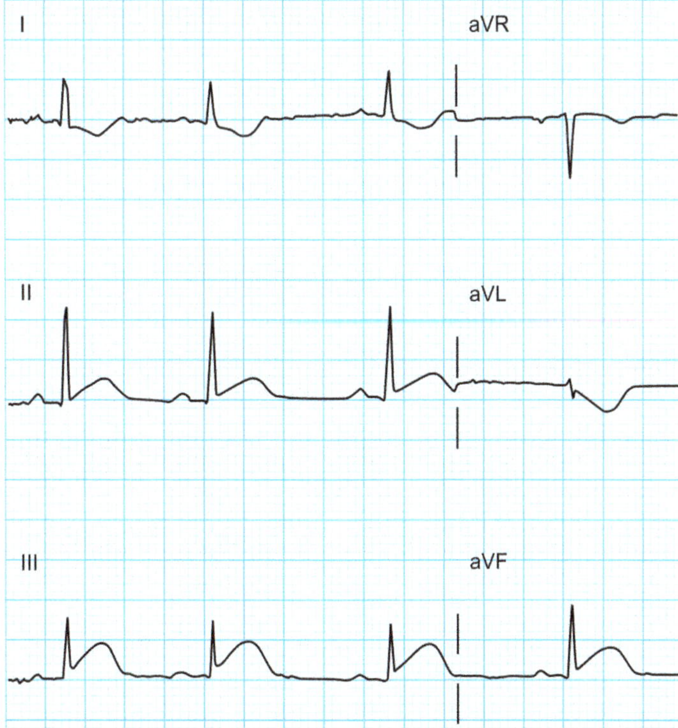

Fig. 5.3: ST segment elevation in leads II, III, and aVF is diagnostic of acute inferior myocardial infarction. Note reciprocal depression in leads I and aVL, which strengthens the diagnosis.

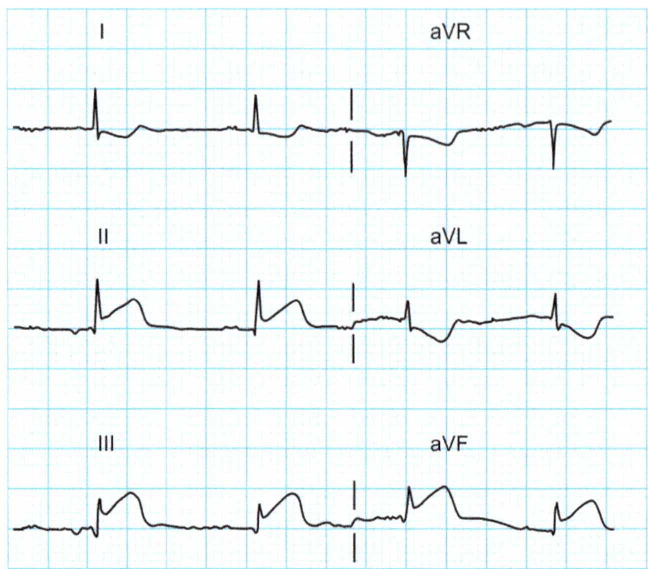

Fig. 5.4: Marked abnormal ST segment elevation in leads II, III, and aVF is diagnostic of acute inferior infarction. Note reciprocal depression in leads I and aVL: this is not diagnostic of STEMI but provides crucial supporting evidence for the presence of STEMI, and excludes mimics such as acute pericarditis, myocarditis and normal variants; this simple sign may prevent expensive testing with CT or MRI.

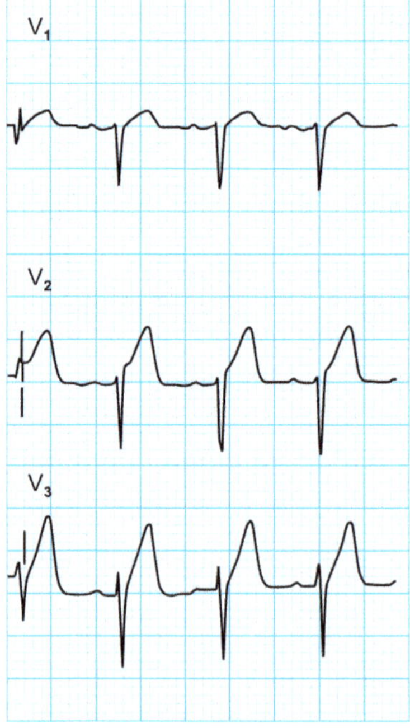

Fig. 5.5: Abnormal ST segment elevation in V_1 through V_3: consider acute anteroseptal or anteroapical myocardial infarction (*see* text for discussion of anteroapical MI). This patient's ECG showed reciprocal depression in leads II, III, and aVF, which strengthens the diagnosis of acute infarction.

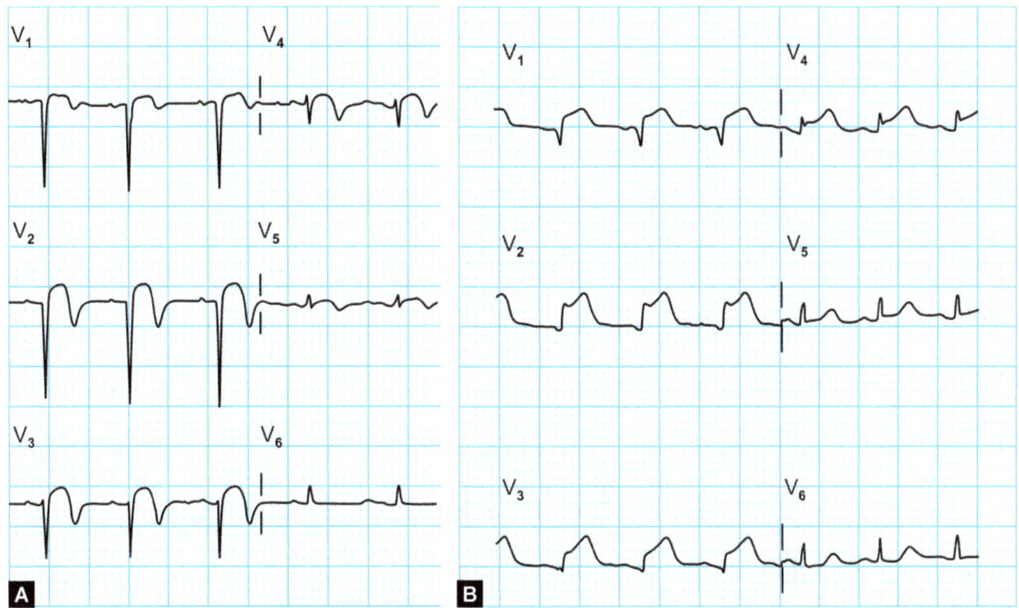

Figs. 5.6A and B: (A) ST segment elevation in V_1 through V_5 and poor R wave progression in V_2 through V_4 typical of recent anterior infarction; (B) Variation in shapes of ST elevation—acute anterior infarct: STEMI.

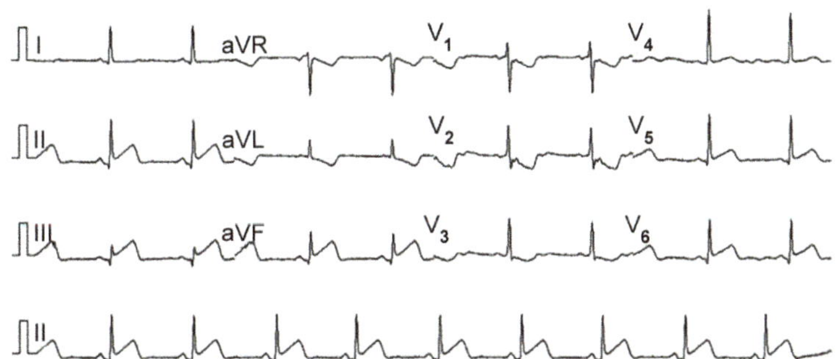

Fig. 5.7: ST elevation in II, III, aVF with reciprocal depression V_1, V_2 diagnostic of acute inferior MI (STEMI); also ST elevation V_5, V_6 = lateral infarction; inferolateral MI.

Other signs that strongly support the diagnosis of acute MI include the following:
- The simultaneous presence of reciprocal depression is not diagnostic for MI but helps confirm the diagnosis (see Fig. 5.7). This is of particular diagnostic importance because ST elevation that may occur as a normal variant is not associated with reciprocal ST depression. With acute pericarditis, ST depression occurs only in lead aVR and sometimes in V_1 (*see* Fig. 2.33, Chapter 10, and further discussion in this chapter).

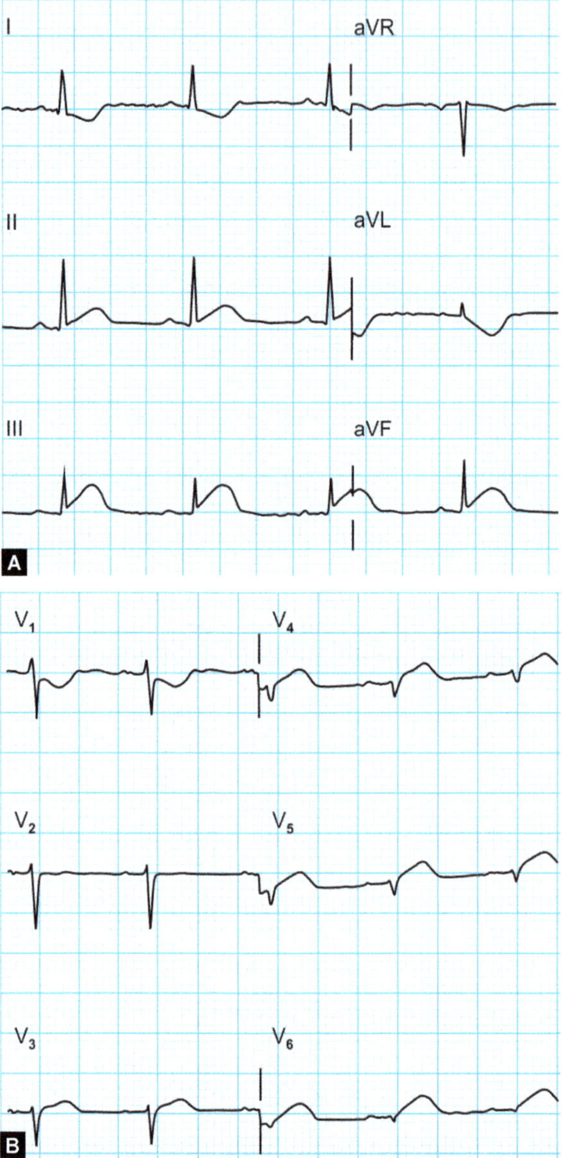

Figs. 5.8A and B: (A) Abnormal ST segment elevation in leads II, III, and aVF indicates recent inferior myocardial infarction. (B) Same patient as in (A). Leads V_4 through V_6 as labeled were appropriately placed on the right side of the chest: leads V_4R and V_5R show abnormal ST segment elevation, which indicates acute inferior and right ventricular infarction. This tracing was read incorrectly by the computer and cardiologist as "widespread ST elevation, consider pericarditis; changes in V_4 through V_6 indicate lateral infarction". (*Note*: V_4 through V_6 were right-sided chest leads and should have been labeled V_4R, $4V_5R$, and V_6R. ST elevation in leads V_3R and V_4R is the main electrocardiographic feature of right ventricular infarction that may occur in association with inferior MI).

- Evolving Q waves. Q waves may become fully developed in 2–24 hours from onset of symptoms (Figs. 5.9 and 5.10). In many patients with acute STEMI, Q waves may not develop, particularly (Figs. 5.11A and B).
- Evolutionary ST-T wave changes that occur during the 10–30 hours after the onset of infarction (*see* Fig. 5.10).
- A decrease in ST segment elevation of 2 mm (0.2 mV) or more may be observed within 30 minutes after the beginning of thrombolytic treatment and may continue for 6 hours.

Infarct Size

An approximation of the size of the infarction can be gauged from the extent of ST elevation:
- *Small MI:* ST elevation in two or three leads
- *Moderate MI:* Four or five leads
- *Large MI:* six or seven leads
- Extensive MI: Eight or nine leads (*see* Fig. 5.7).

Value of Lead aVR in Diagnosis of Acute Myocardial Infarction

- aVR is a lead that is often ignored but recently has gained importance in the diagnosis of left main coronary artery (LMCA) occlusion (*see* Fig. 5.11).

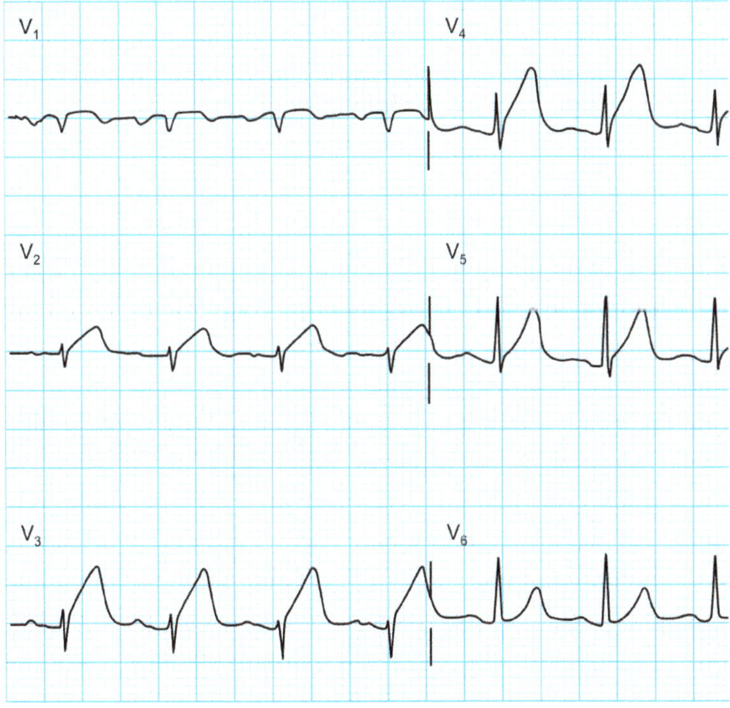

Fig. 5.9: ST segment elevation in V$_1$ through V$_4$ indicates acute anteroseptal infarction, anteroapical MI, or anterior MI.

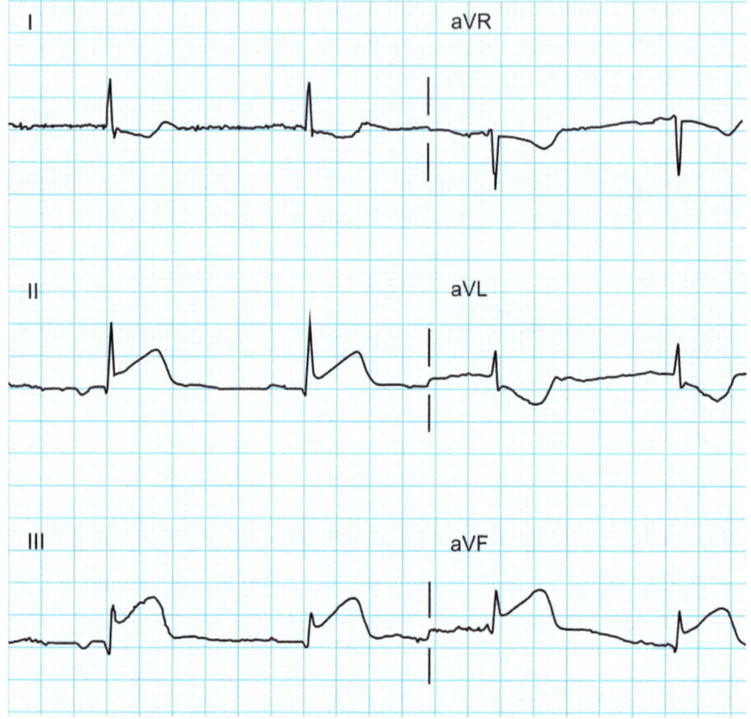

Fig. 5.10: Acute inferior myocardial infarction: ST elevation in inferior leads; note reciprocal depression in leads I and aVL.

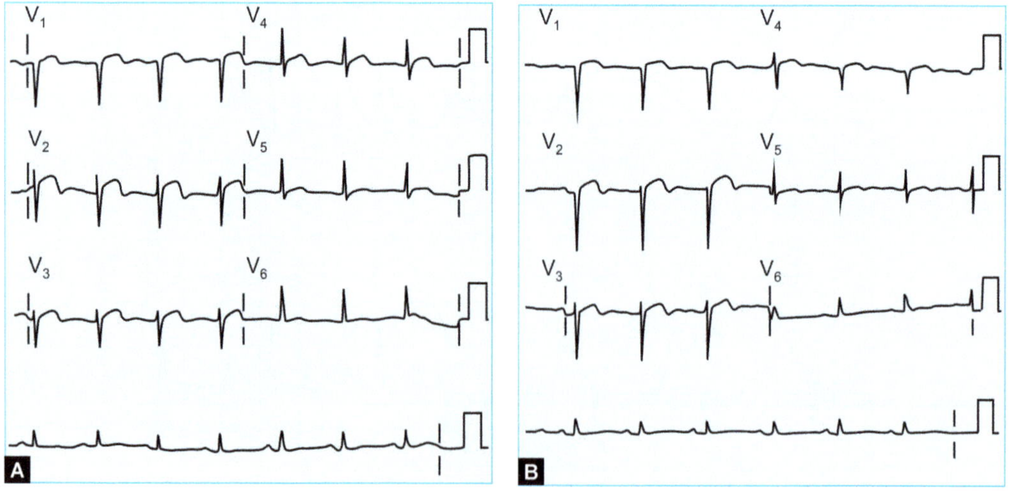

Figs. 5.11A and B: (A) Acute anterior myocardial infarction: ST elevation in leads V_1 to V_4; (B) Acute anterior infarction: same patient as in (A), 8 hours later.

- Figures 5.11 and 5.12 show ST elevation in aVR that is greater than the elevation in V_1, a marker of LMCA obstruction. This criterion is not specific: specificity is 80% and sensitivity is 81%. Circumflex branch occlusion also may cause ST elevation in aVR, but with no elevation in V_1. In addition, right ventricular overload may reveal ST elevation in aVR, but

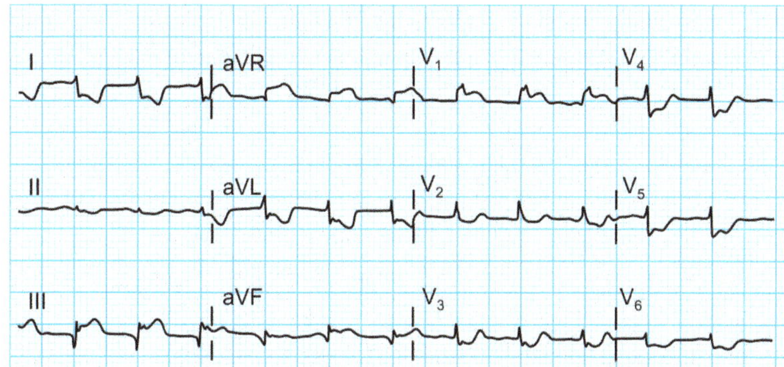

Fig. 5.12: Patient with chest pain for 3 hours. Inferior myocardial infarction and ST elevation in aVR and V_1. Left main occlusion.

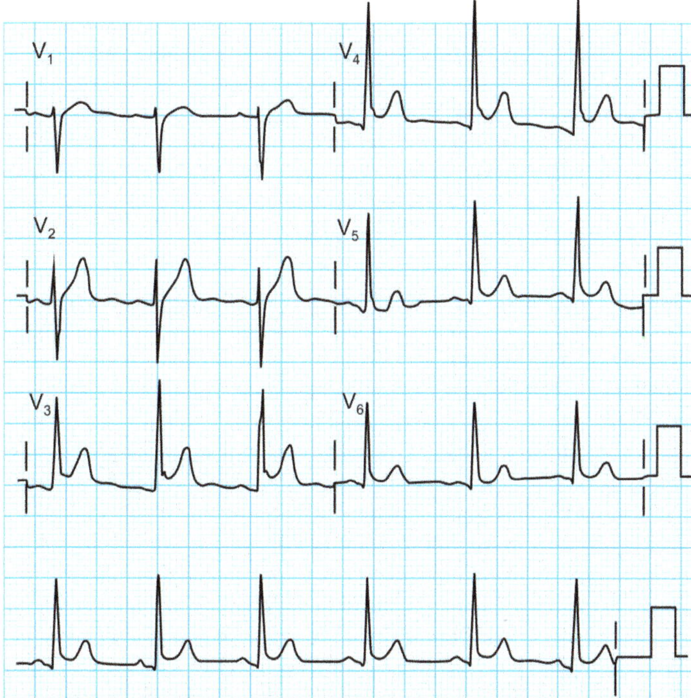

Fig. 5.13: ST segment elevation in a normal 25-year-old: normal variant. Note the notched J-point, fishhook appearance in lead V_3.
Source: Adapted with permission from Khan MG. On Call Cardiology, 3rd edition. Philadelphia: WB Saunders, Elsevier Science; 2006. p. 89.

the clinical scenario is easily differentiated. Subendocardial infarction with marked ST segment depression in V_4 through V_6 that is not caused by left main coronary occlusion may reveal ST segment elevation in aVR, but the elevation may be less than that observed in V_1.

- Because LMCA occlusion is a highly serious condition, any noninvasive diagnostic clue represents a valuable addition to the diagnostic armamentarium.

Reciprocal ST segment depression in aVR with PR segment elevation in aVR with reciprocal PR segment depression in other leads is a feature of acute pericarditis (*see* Chapter 10).

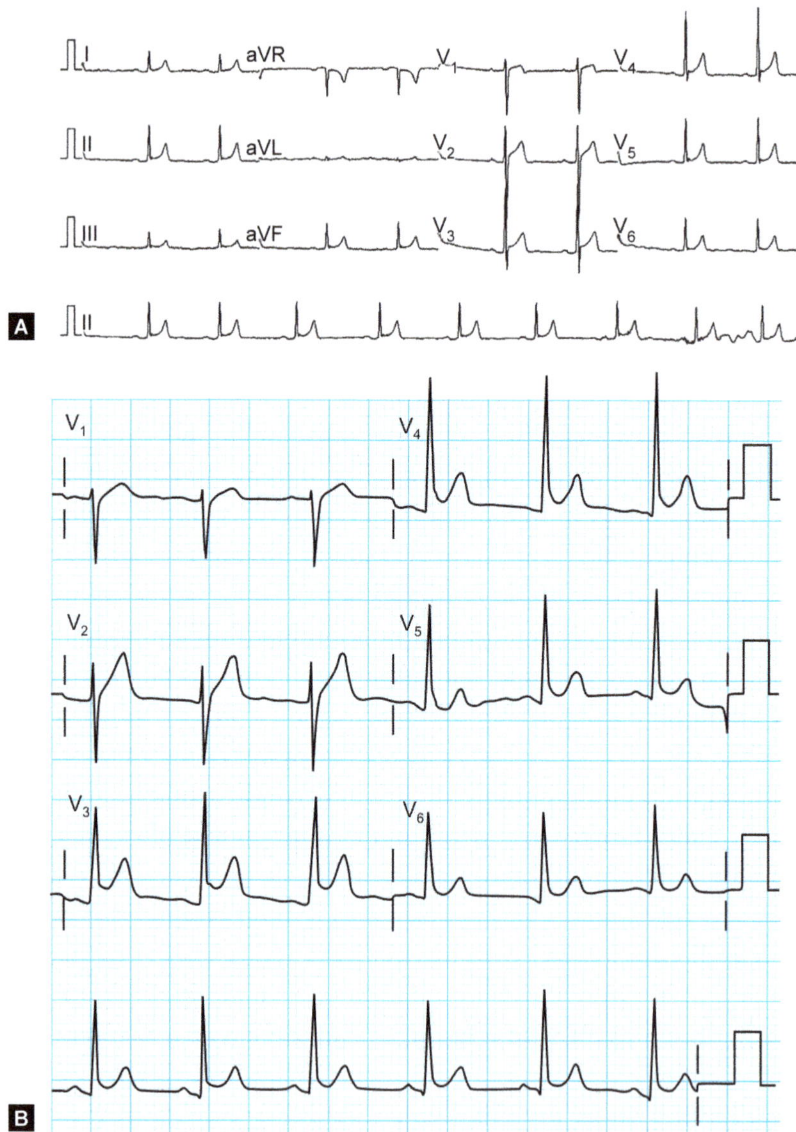

Figs. 5.14A and B: (A) ST elevation V_2 V_4 normal variant, 24-year-old; (B) ST segment elevation in a normal 25-year-old man: normal variant. Note the notched J-point "fishhook" appearance in lead V_3.

Mimics of ST Elevation Infarction

- *Normal variants:* ST segment elevation is often observed as a normal variant in healthy African Americans, Hispanics, and some other ethnic groups. The ST elevation commonly seen in V_2 through V_5 often shows a notched J-point, fishhook appearance (Figs. 5.13 and 5.14). This normal variant is inappropriately termed early repolarization changes. ST elevation may occur in leads II, III, and aVF, but reciprocal depression does not occur. The degree of ST elevation is variable, often 1–4 mm; the normal concave shape remains, but it may end in a prominent, peaked T wave (see Figs. 5.2, 5.13, and Fig. 2.15). Occasionally, ST elevation with T wave inversion is observed in one or two precordial leads in healthy athletes (Figs. 5.14A and B).
- Acute pericarditis causes diffuse ST segment elevation that is not confined to an anatomic coronary blood supply; thus ST elevation is observed in leads I through III, lead aVF, and most precordial leads. The ST segment retains a normal concave shape. Reciprocal depression may be observed in aVR and sometimes in V_1 (*see* Fig. 2.33 and discussion under "Pericarditis" in Chapter 10).
- MI age indeterminate (*see* Fig. 2.18B) in the absence of LV aneurysm may exhibit mild ST elevation, and the differentiation from acute infarction requires clinical correlation and comparison with previous ECGs.
- Coronary artery spasm, Prinzmetal angina, causes ST elevation during the brief period of chest pain (Fig. 5.15).

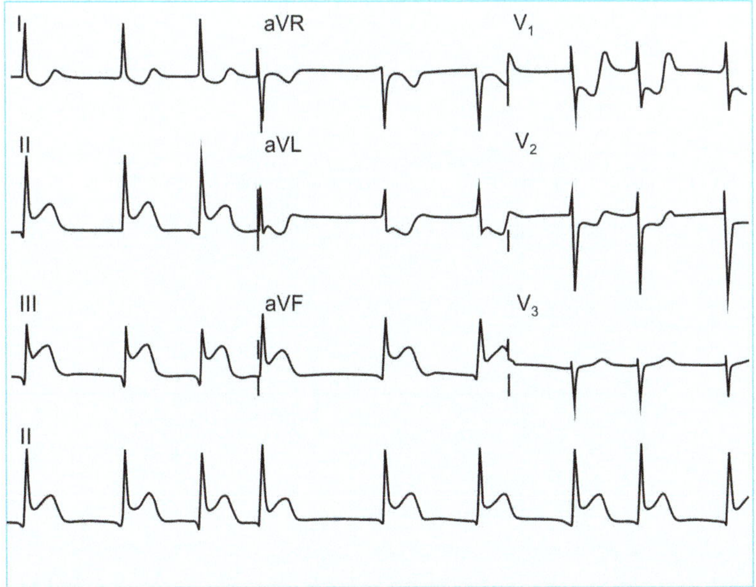

Fig. 5.15: Acute inferior myocardial infarction: ST elevation in leads II, III, and aVF. Note reciprocal depression in leads V_1, V_2, and aVL.

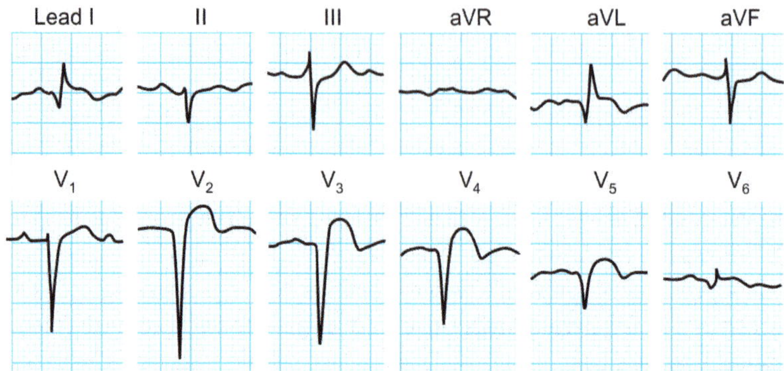

Fig. 5.16: Ventricular aneurysm. The patient is a 52-year-old man who had an acute extensive anterior myocardial infarction 5 months before the recording of this ECG. Note the persistent ST segment elevation in the precordial leads and in leads I and aVL. Left anterior hemiblock also is present.
Source: Adapted with permission from Chou TC. Electrocardiography in Clinical Practice, 4th edition. Philadelphia: WB Saunders, Elsevier Science. 1996.

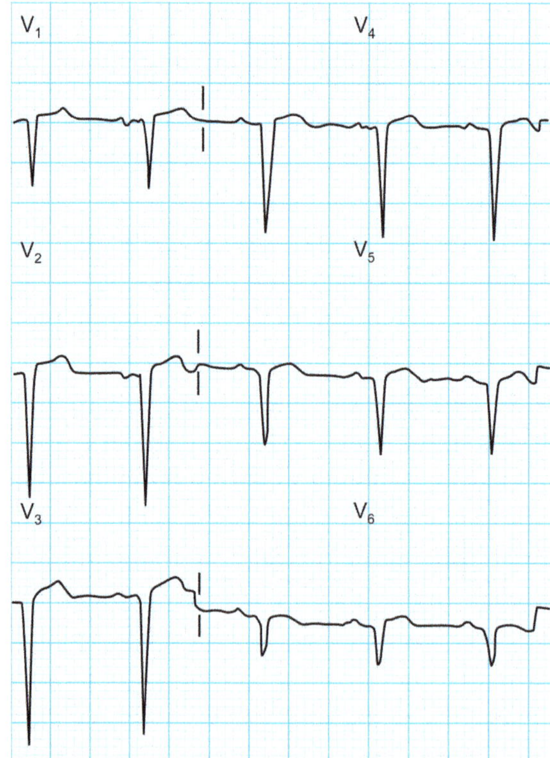

Fig. 5.17: V leads of a patient who sustained an anterior infarction 6 months earlier. Pathologic Q waves are present from V_1 through V_6, and the ST segment is elevated in V_1 through V_5. The tracing is in keeping with an old anterior myocardial infarction with left ventricular aneurysm.

- *LV aneurysm:* ST elevation can persist 3 days to 4 weeks after acute infarction; persistence beyond 4 weeks suggests LV aneurysm (Figs. 5.16 and 5.17).
- Left bundle branch block nearly always causes abnormal ST elevation in leads V_1 through V_4 and can mimic acute or old infarction (*see* Fig. 4.8).
- Left ventricular hypertrophy may cause poor R wave progression in V_1 through V_3, and occasionally ST elevation is observed (*see* Figs. 2.23 and 2.25).
- Hypertrophic cardiomyopathy causes Q waves, but occasionally persistent ST segment elevation is present (*see* Chapter 6).
- Acute myocarditis in persons with acquired immunodeficiency syndrome may cause nonspecific ST-T changes; ST elevation and Q waves may occur (*see* Chapter 6).
- Cocaine abuse may cause ST elevation and, in some individuals, frank infarction (*see* Chapter 6).

NON-ST SEGMENT ELEVATION MYOCARDIAL INFARCTION

- ST segment depression more than or equal to 1 mm in two or more leads in a patient with chest discomfort and an abnormal troponin or creatine kinase-MB (CK-MB) is diagnostic of non-ST segment elevation MI (non-Q wave MI) (*see* Fig. 5.18 and Fig. 2.14A).
- Transient ST segment changes more than 0.05 mm (mV), associated with angina at rest and positive troponin or CK-MB indicate non-ST segment elevation MI. In patients with

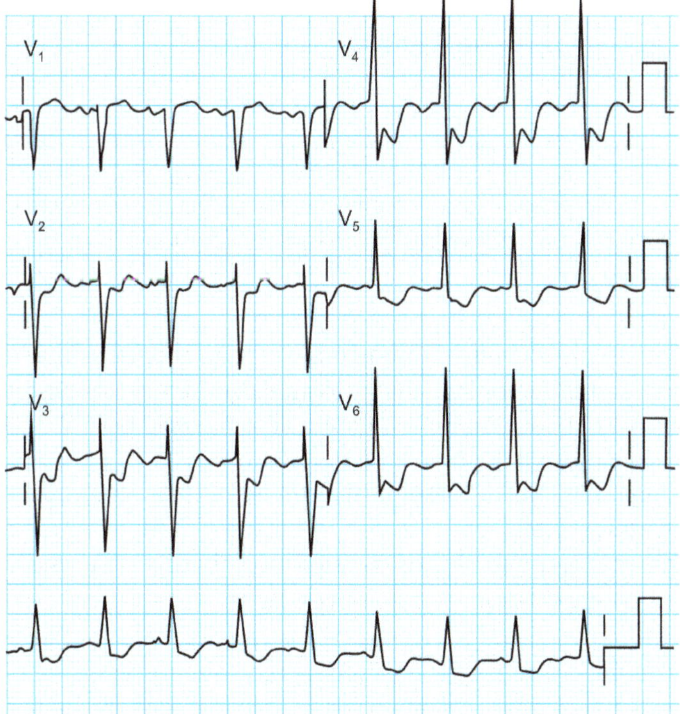

Fig. 5.18A

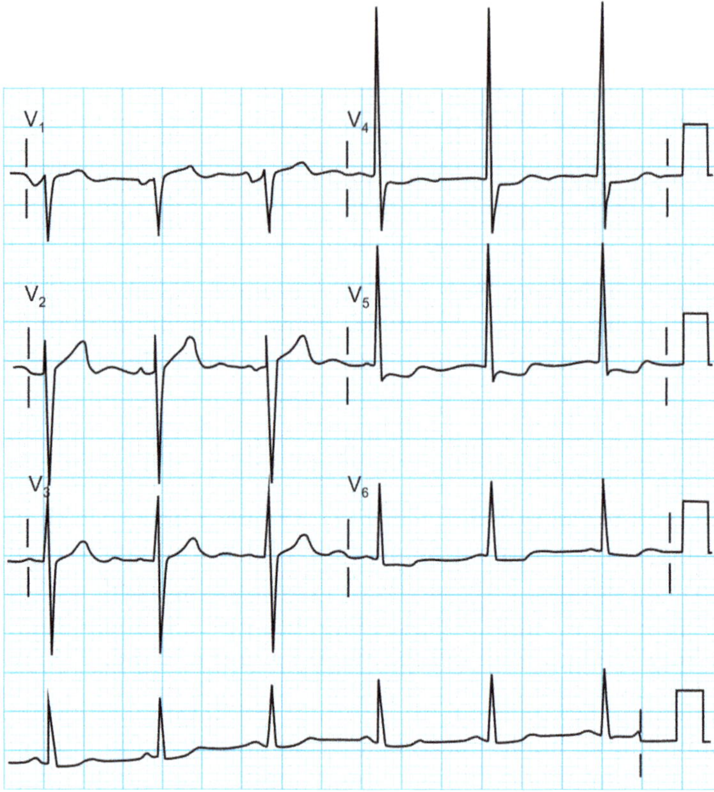

Fig. 5.18B

Figs. 5.18A and B: (A) Non-ST segment elevation myocardial infarction (NSTEMI): non-Q wave infarction (acute subendocardial infarction) in a patient with a clinical picture of infarction and elevated CK-MB. Note widespread ST-T depression in the limb and chest leads but no associated Q waves. (B) The same patient's ECG tracing 18 hours earlier than depicted in (A).
Source: Adapted with permission from Khan MG. On Call Cardiology, 3rd edition. Philadelphia: WB Saunders, Elsevier Science; 2006.

negative cardiac enzymes within 6 hours of onset of pain, another sample should be drawn between 6 hours and 12 hours. Patients with acute coronary syndrome, particularly those with rest pain more than or equal to 20 minutes accompanied by ECG changes are further risk-stratified depending on troponin levels as follows:

1. *High risk:* Troponins (TnT or TnI) more than 0.1 ng/mL (elevated troponin levels indicate myocardial necrosis, MI).
2. *Intermediate risk:* Troponin slightly elevated more than 0.01 but less than 0.1 ng/mL.
3. *Low risk:* Troponin normal.

ISCHEMIA

ST segment depression indicative of definite myocardial ischemia should fulfill the following criteria:

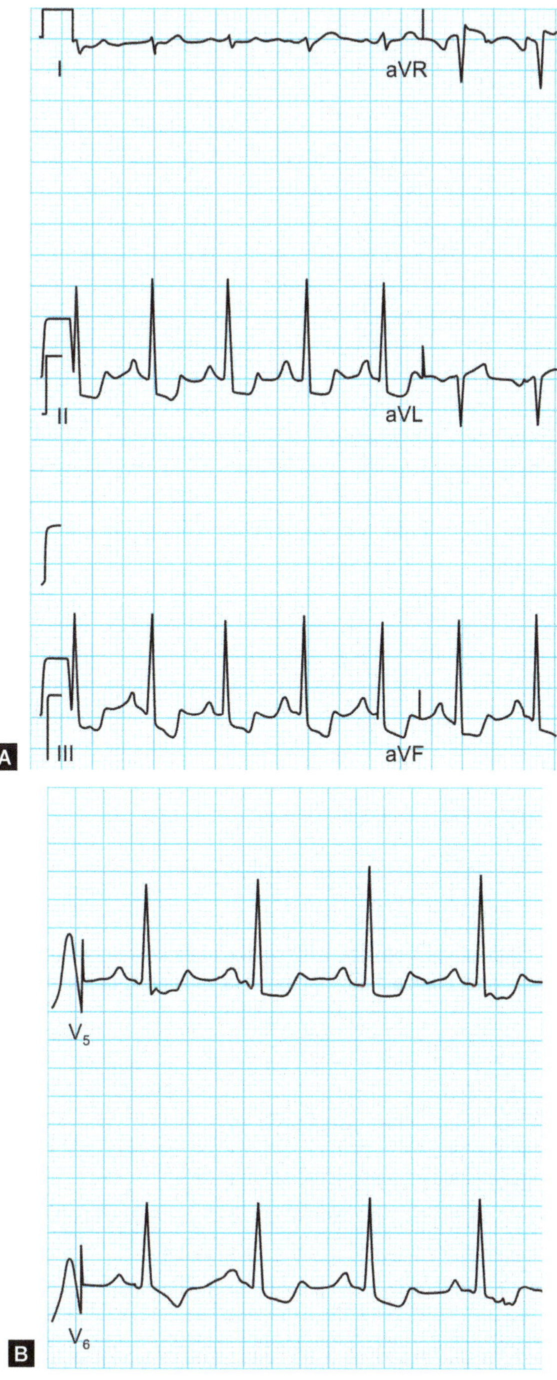

Figs. 5.19A and B: (A) Flat (horizontal) and down-sloping ST segment depression greater than 1 mm in a patient with proven angina and obstructive coronary artery disease. (A) Limb leads; (B) Leads V_5 and V_6.

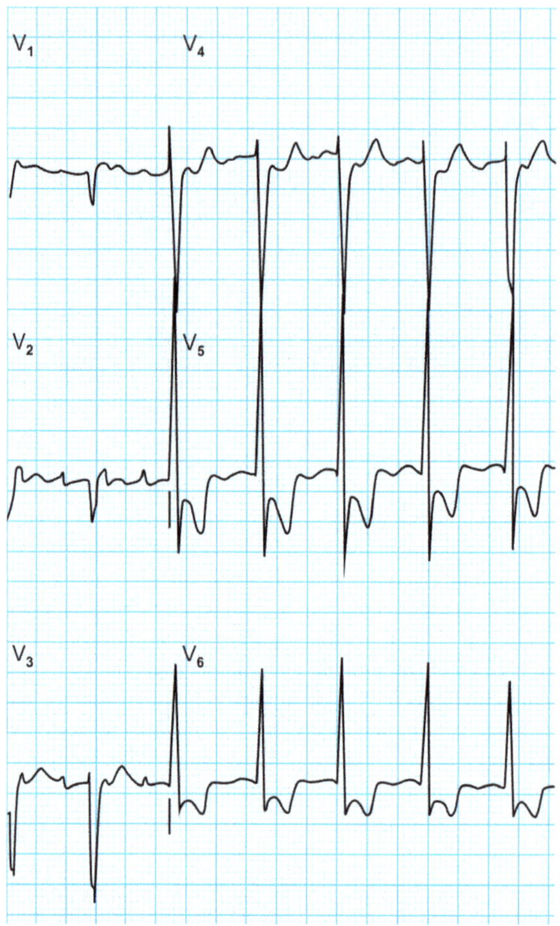

Fig. 5.20: V leads of a patient with severe angina and left ventricular hypertrophy. Note increased voltage and marked ST segment depression in V_4 through V_6.

- Greater than 1 mm depression.
- Present in two or more leads.
- Present in two or more consecutive QRS complexes.
- Flat (horizontal) or down-sloping with or without T wave inversion (these patterns of ischemia are all shown in Figs. 5.19, 5.20, and Fig. 2.14B).
- Abnormal convex coving of the ST segment in V_1 through V_3 or V_2 through V_4 associated with T wave inversion.

The terminal portion of the abnormal ST segment may show a typical hitched-up pattern (Fig. 5.21); this pattern is often caused by a tight obstruction in the proximal left anterior descending artery.

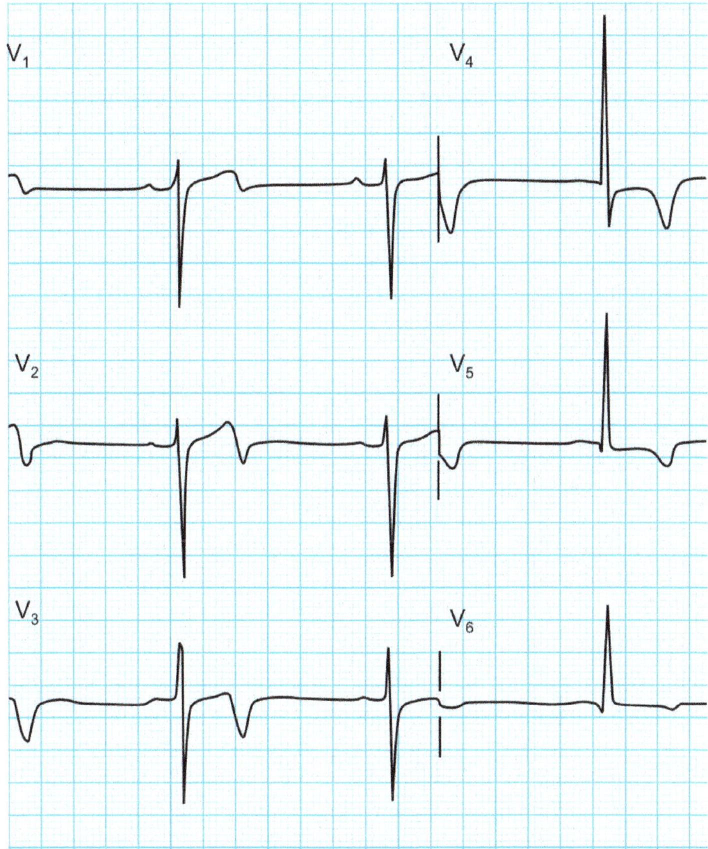

Fig. 5.21: V leads in a patient with unstable angina. ST-T segment abnormalities seen in V_1 through V_4. The tracing was taken when the patient was pain free. Note the "hitched up" ST segment in V_2 and V_3 with deep T inversion: the pattern is typical of significant proximal left anterior descending coronary artery stenosis.

NONSPECIFIC ST CHANGE

Minor ST segment depression less than or equal to 1 mm is not an uncommon finding in normal individuals. Consider ST segment changes to be nonspecific if the following prevails:
- ST depression less than or equal to 1 mm in the absence of typical symptoms of unstable angina, including rest pain more than or equal to 20 minutes (Fig. 5.22)
- Accompanied by baseline drift
- With or without T wave inversion
- Commonly associated with low, flow, or slightly inverted T waves.

T waves normally should be more than or equal to 0.5 mm in height in leads I and II (*see* "T Waves" in Chapter 8). Figure 5.23 depicts nonspecific ST-T changes.

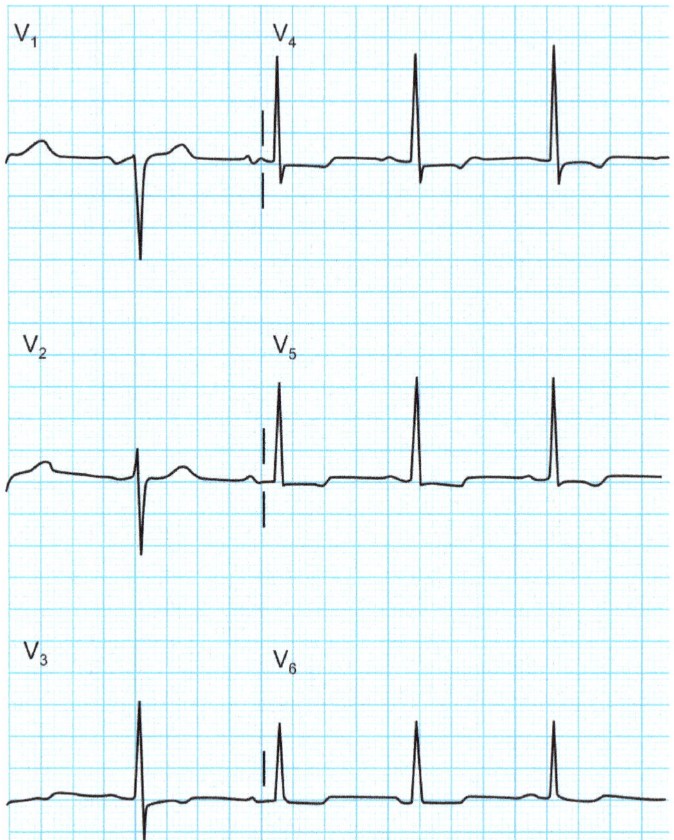

Fig. 5.22: V leads in a patient with no history of heart disease. ST segment is flat in V_4 through V_6 with minimal T wave inversion; similar findings were observed in leads I and aVL: the anterolateral ST-T wave abnormalities are nonspecific; note that ischemia cannot be excluded. Abnormal ECG.

Causes of Nonspecific ST-T Wave Changes

Nonspecific ST-T wave changes can be caused by a number of conditions, such as the following:
- Improper electrode contact
- Ischemia (must be considered; the ECG must be interpreted in regard to the clinical findings)
- Electrolyte abnormalities
- Arrhythmias
- Myocarditis
- Pericarditis, constrictive pericarditis
- Intraventricular conduction defects

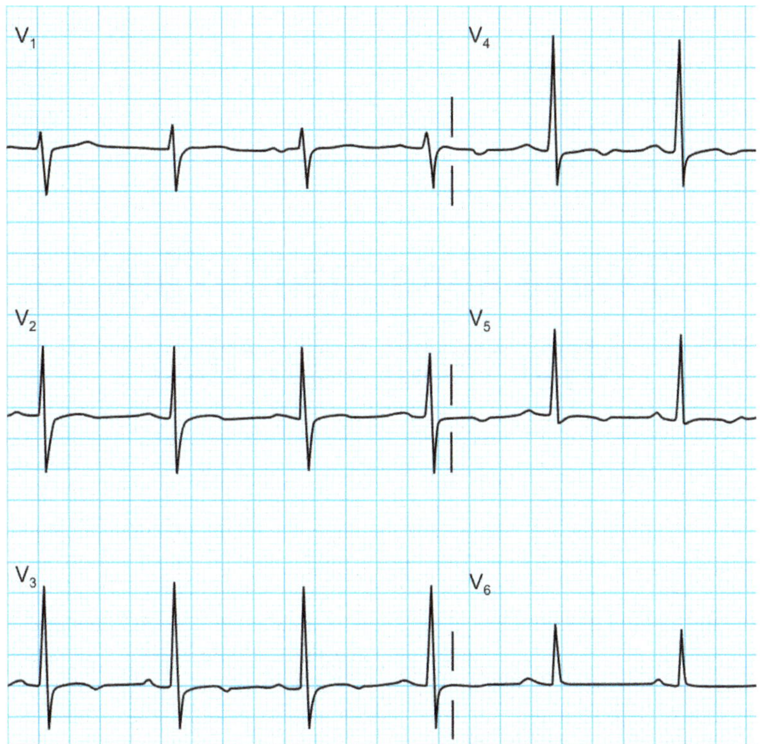

Fig. 5.23: The ST segment is borderline flat but not depressed and is associated with minimal T wave inversion in leads V_3 through V_6; similar findings were present in leads I and aVL: nonspecific ST-T wave changes. Borderline ECG.

- Cardiomyopathy
- Pulmonary embolism
- Drink of cold water
- Hyperventilation
- Drug use, including ethanol abuse
- Digoxin
- Subarachnoid hemorrhage or cerebral hemorrhage.

Q Wave Abnormalities and Myocardial Infarction

CRITERIA FOR NORMAL AND ABNORMAL Q WAVES

The QRS complex should be assessed for the presence of normal and abnormal Q waves and for normal or abnormal R wave progression as outlined in Step 5 of the method for accurate electrocardiogram (ECG) interpretation (Fig. 6.1).

The assessment of pathologic Q or normal q waves should take into account the following:

- Their width
- Their depth
- The leads in which they are observed
- The age of the individual
- Relevant clinical findings.

Normal Parameters

- In general, a Q wave that is wider than 0.03 second is considered abnormal, except in leads III, aVR, and V_1, in which Q waves may be wide and deep in normal individuals (Fig. 6.2A and Table 2.1).
- Lead aVR normally records a negative QRS, QS, or QR complex (*see* Figs. 6.2A to C, and Fig. 2.2).

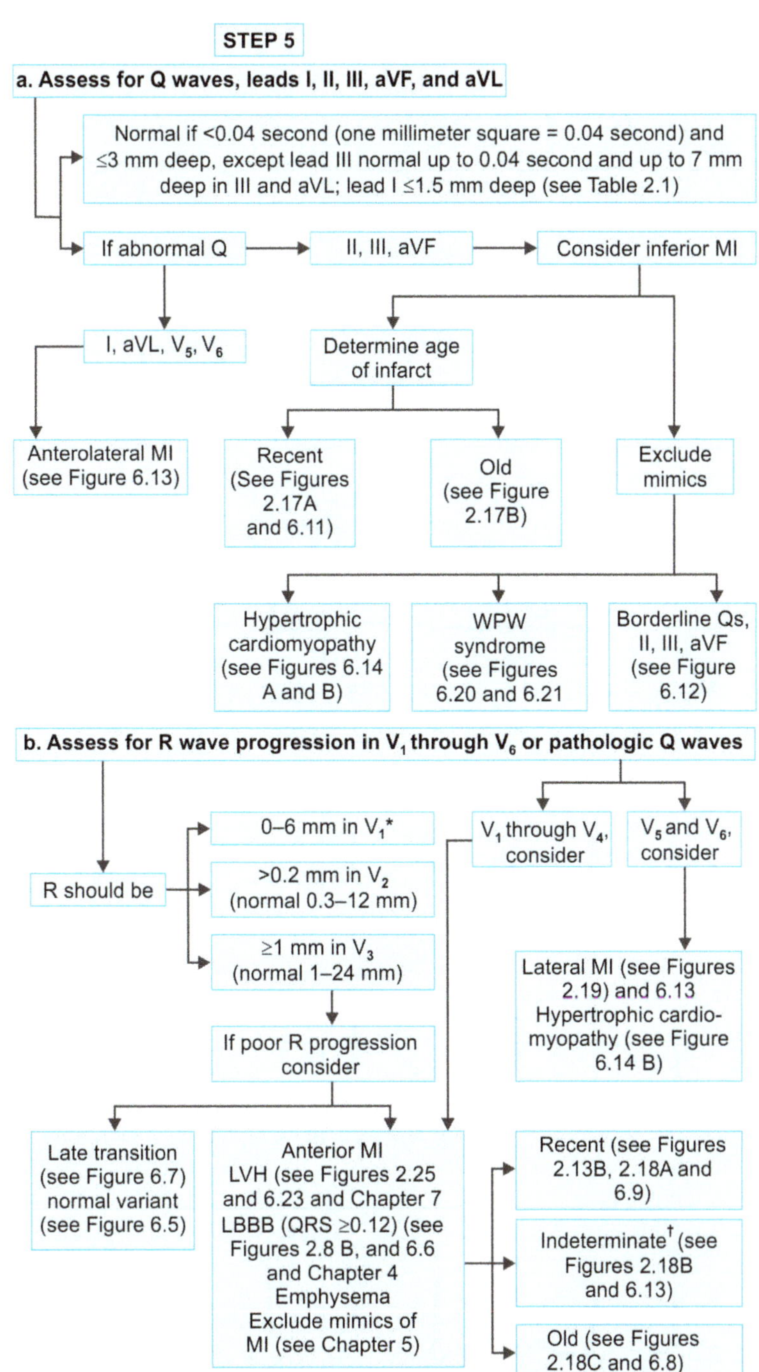

Fig. 6.1: Step-by-step method for accurate ECG interpretation. Step 5: assess for Q waves and R wave progression.
*Age >30; see text and Table 2.1 for exceptions and normal parameters.
†Compare old ECGs.

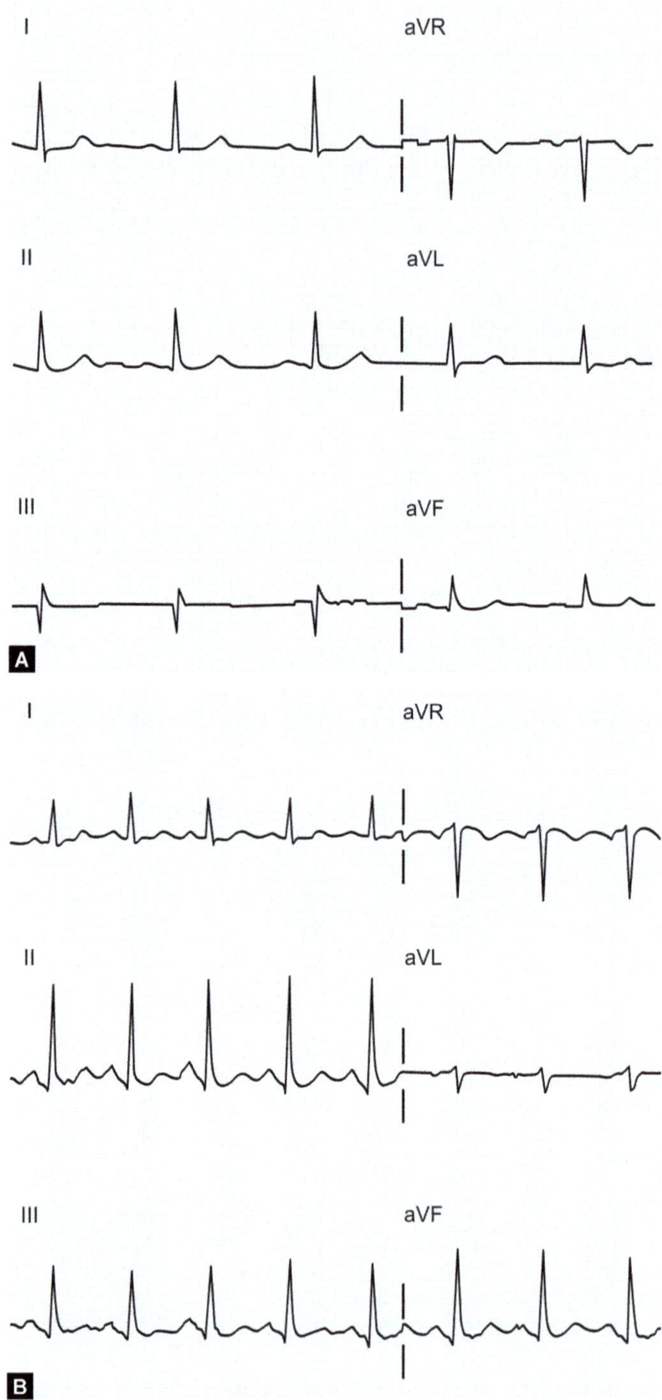

Figs. 6.2A and B

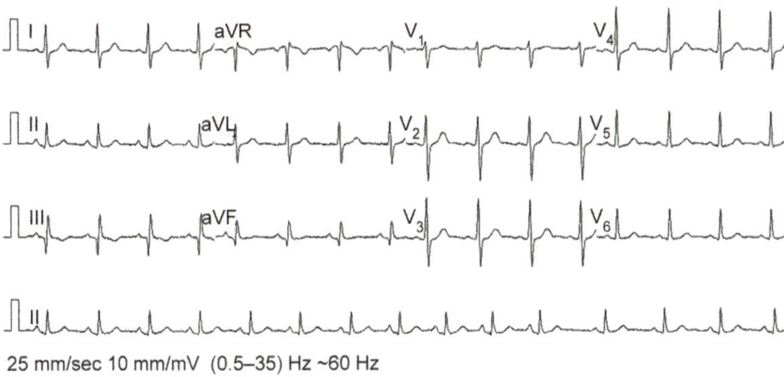

Fig. 6.2C

Figs. 6.2A to C: (A) Isolated, deep, narrow Q wave in lead III is ≤0.04 second as part of a normal ECG. Note the absence of abnormal Q waves in leads II and aVF. (B) Note small, normal q waves <0.04 second and <2 mm deep in duration in leads II and aVF. Normal ECG. (C) A 31-year-old male; computer diagnosis: old inferior MI. Interpretation corrected: nondiagnostic inferior Q-waves noted: 35 < Q < 40 ms in aVF with Q in II III; Q/R > 1/3 in aVF. Clinical correlation required.

- Normal QS complexes occasionally are found in leads III and V_1 and rarely in V_2.
- A narrow Q wave may occur as a normal finding in lead III; this should be less than or equal to 0.04 second in duration (1 square), less than 10 mm deep, and not accompanied by abnormal Q waves in leads II and aVF (*see* Figs. 6.2A to C, and Fig. 2.2D). The depth of the Q wave is not as important as the width.
- Lead aVL may record a Q wave less than 0.04 second and up to 7 mm deep in individuals older than age 30 years and up to 10 mm deep in children. A negative P wave followed by a QS or QR deflection with a negative T wave may be recorded in a normal vertical heart.
- In leads II and aVF, small, narrow Q waves may occur but should be less than or equal to 0.03 second in duration and less than 4 mm deep (*see* Figs. 6.2A and B). Occasionally, the Q waves in leads II, III, and aVF are borderline width and the ECG is interpreted as follows: inferior Qs noted; clinical correlation required; borderline ECG.
- In lead I, the depth of a Q wave should not exceed 1.5 mm in adults older than age 30 years (*see* Fig. 6.2A).
- A small q wave in V_6 less than or equal to 0.03 second is present in more than 75% of normal individuals. In leads V_5 and V_6 and rarely in V_4, normal q waves less than or equal to 0.03 second and less than 3 mm deep may occur (Fig. 6.3). Normal Q waves should be less than 3 mm in adults older than age 40 years; they should not exceed a depth of 4 mm in those younger than age 30 years. Rarely, an amplitude more than 4 mm may be seen in healthy teenagers.
- In contrast, Figure 6.14B shows abnormal Q waves in V_4 through V_6; they are 0.04 second wide and 3 mm deep in a 52-year-old woman with proven hypertrophic cardiomyopathy. Small Q waves may occur in V_2 through V_6 with extreme counterclockwise rotation (Fig. 6.4).

- A Q wave of less than 0.03 second and greater than 2 mm deep in V_2 through V_4 is abnormal if V_1 shows an initial R and there is no significant shift of the transitional zone to the left or right.
- Poor R wave progression may simulate infarction patterns (pseudoinfarction).
- Poor R wave progression in V_2 through V_4 with minute R waves may mimic QS complexes and lead to incorrect diagnoses and uncertainties for cardiologists, the attending physician trainee, or the family physician.

Causes of poor R wave progression include the following:

- In women, and rarely in men younger than age 30 years, minute R waves may be present in leads V_1, V_2, and sometimes, V_3; this poor R wave progression is not uncommon and may lead to an erroneous diagnosis of anteroseptal infarction (Figs. 6.5A and B).
- Improper lead placement of V_2 and V_3, particularly in women, may cause decreased R wave amplitude, often incorrectly assessed as anteroseptal infarction.

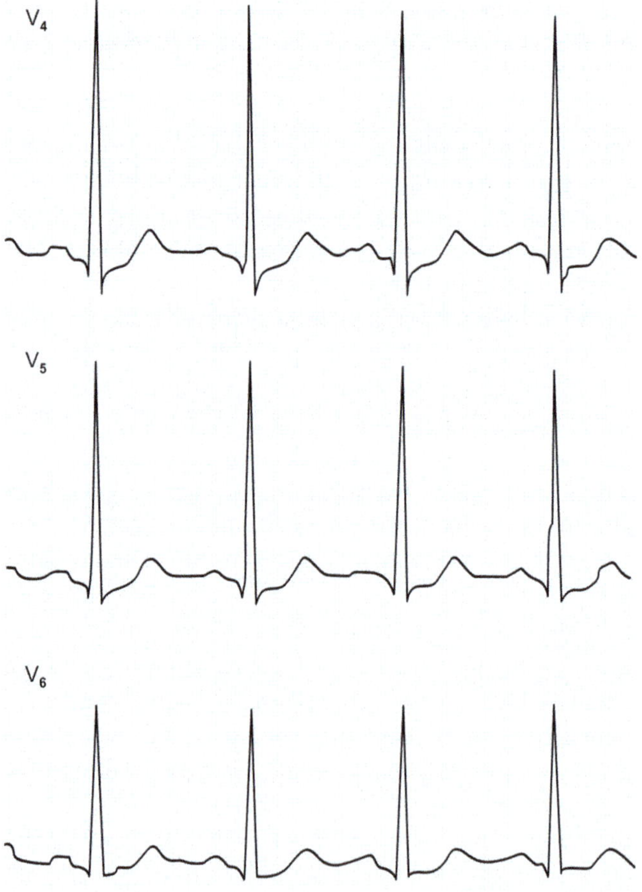

Fig. 6.3: Normal q wave in V_4 through V_6 ≤0.03 second, <4 mm deep.

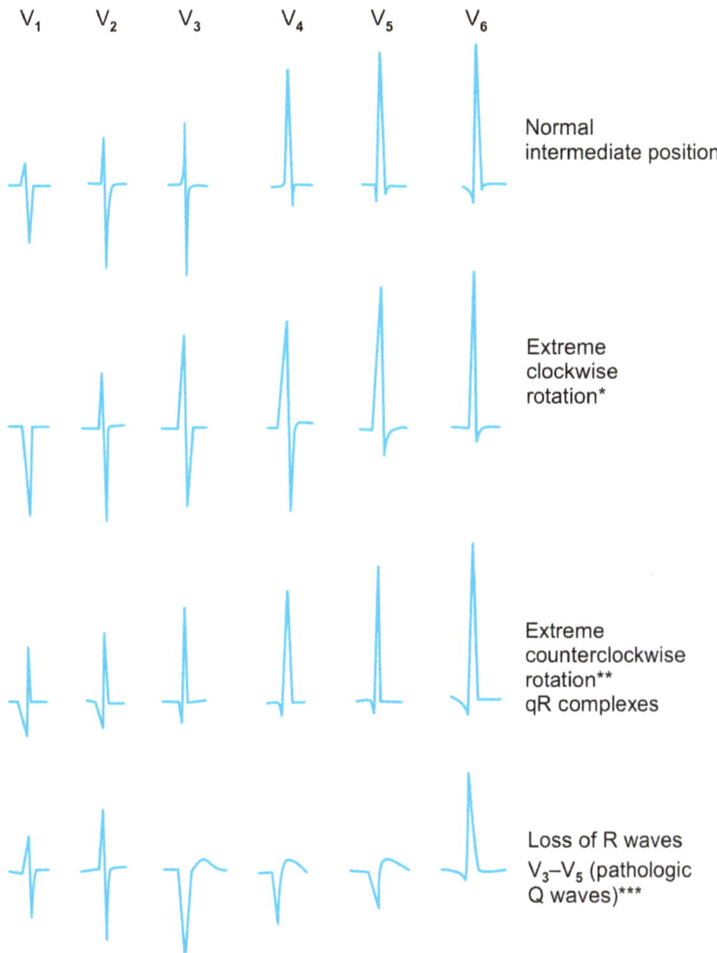

Fig. 6.4: Variations in normal QRS configuration and correlation with abnormals.

*With clockwise rotation, the V_1 electrode, like aVR, faces the cavity of the heart and records a QS complex; no initial q in lead V_6.

**qR complexes; q <0.04 second, <3 mm deep; therefore not pathologic Q waves.

***Loss of R wave in V_3 through V_5 (pathologic Q waves): signifies anterior MI.

Source: Adapted with permission from Khan MG. On Call Cardiology, 3rd edition. Philadelphia: WB Saunders, Elsevier Science; 2006.

- Old anteroseptal and anterior infarction.
- Left bundle branch block (LBBB) (Fig. 6.6).
- Left ventricular hypertrophy (LVH).
- Late transition (Fig. 6.7).
- Severe chronic obstructive pulmonary disease (COPD), particularly emphysema.

Left anterior fascicular block.

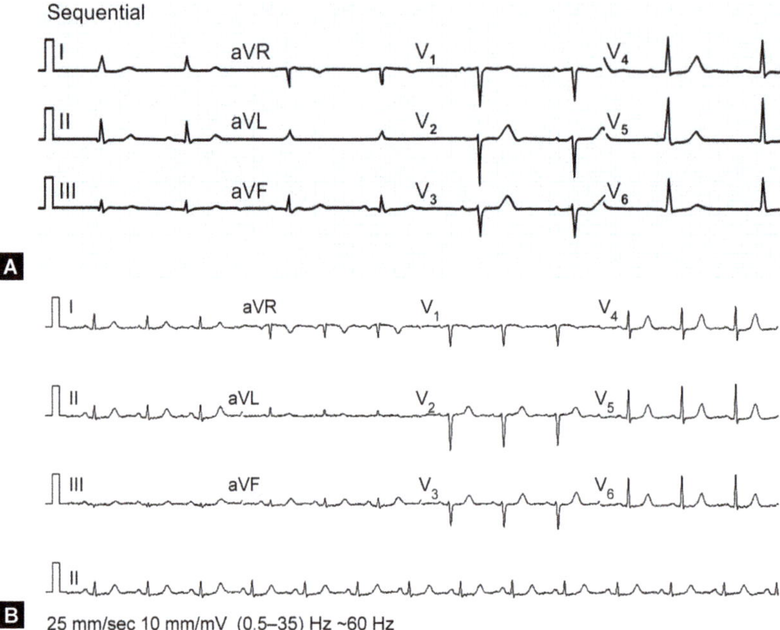

Figs. 6.5A and B: (A) ECG from a healthy 74-year-old female. Poor wave progression V_2–V_3 is a not uncommon finding in females and may mimic old anteroseptal MI. Caution is needed in positioning leads V_1 and V_2 in both females and males. (B) Poor R-wave progression leads V_2–V_3 lead placement in female may cause poor R-wave progression V_2–V_3; computer reported as old anteroseptal MI.

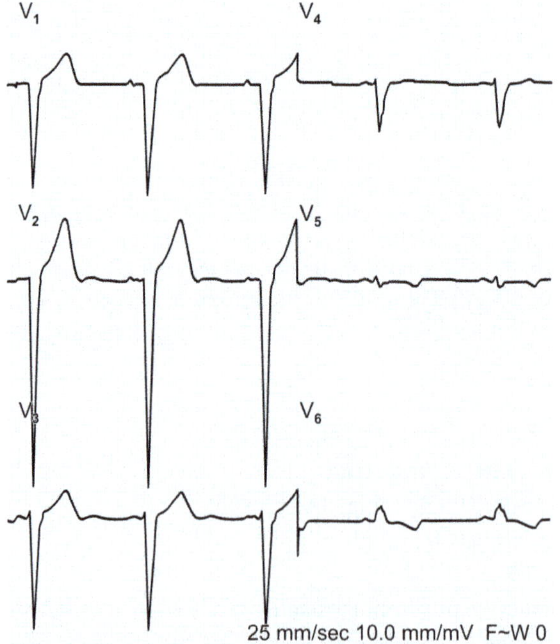

Fig. 6.6: Poor R wave progression in V_1 through V_4 and QRS duration >0.12 second indicate left bundle branch block.

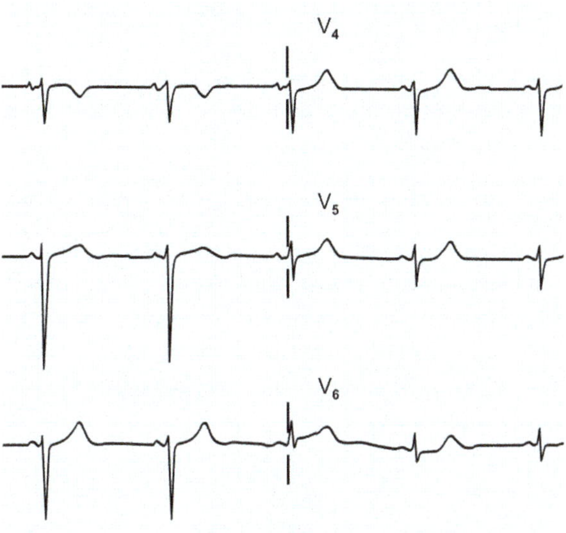

Fig. 6.7: Poor R wave progression in V₂ through V₄ with normal QRS duration. Note that the transition, instead of occurring normally in lead V₃, occurs in V₅ as indicated by a negative QRS in V₅. Tracing from a normal 48-year-old woman—Normal ECG.

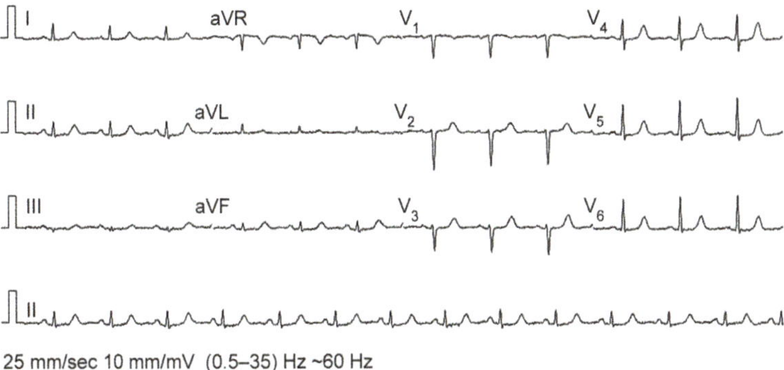

25 mm/sec 10 mm/mV (0.5–35) Hz ~60 Hz

Fig. 6.8: Poor R-wave progression V₁–V₃ that may be incorrectly interpreted by the computer as old anteroseptal MI.

A net negative QRS complex in V_5 or V_6 in the absence of right ventricular hypertrophy (RVH) indicates late transition (Fig. 6.7). Severe COPD is considered if the P wave amplitude is greater than 2.5 mm in any of lead II, III, or aVF. Severe COPD, particularly that caused by emphysema, may reveal poor R wave progression in V_1 through V_4, or Q waves may indicate pseudo-infarction.

- Note that poor R wave progression in V_2 through V_4 in the absence of late transition, LVH, or COPD suggests a diagnosis of anterior infarction (Fig. 6.8), but consideration of lead placement error and clinical correlation is required always.

Q WAVE ABNORMALITIES AND MYOCARDIAL INFARCTION

Abnormal Q waves caused by myocardial necrosis occur as early as 2 hours and as late as 24 hours after the onset of clinical symptoms of acute myocardial infarction (MI). Q waves of acute infarction are always associated with abnormal ST elevation.

Diagnostic Criteria

- The presence of ST segment elevation more than or equal to 1 mm with or without Q waves in two or more contiguous leads in a patient with acute chest discomfort is diagnostic of ST elevation MI (STEMI), probable Q wave MI (Figs. 6.9A and B).
- From 6–12 hours after onset of symptoms, ST segment elevation recedes, but Q waves become more prominent (Figs. 6.10A and B).
- Pathologic Q waves and ST elevation in leads II, III, and aVF indicate inferior infarction (Figs. 6.11A and B).
- The Q waves in leads II, III, and aVF are more than 0.03 second in duration; the Q wave in lead III is more than 0.04 second wide. Figure 6.12 shows acute inferior MI with ST-T wave abnormalities and evolutionary changes.
- An abnormal Q wave in lead III ($\leq$0.04 second in duration) not associated with pathologic Q waves in lead II or aVF should be considered a normal variant.
- Most of the erroneous diagnoses of infarction are made based on findings of nondiagnostic Q waves in leads III and aVF (Figs. 6.10A and B).
- Figures 6.9A to D show features of acute anterior MI.
- Pathologic Q waves of infarction may diminish in amplitude and duration during the years after acute infarction. Pathologic Q waves persist in more than 80% of patients 4–5 years after acute MI. In some patients, abnormal coving of the ST segment and T wave inversion persist for several years and may be difficult to differentiate from a recent infarct. The tracing is often interpreted as infarction age indeterminate (Fig. 6.13). In 10% of patients, Q waves become nondiagnostic but still suspicious; in the remaining 10%, Q waves disappear. In approximately 5% of patients with Q wave infarction, the ECG returns to normal.

Nonatheromatous Cause of Myocardial Infarction

Rarely, infarction may occur in the absence of atherosclerotic coronary artery disease and can be caused by:

- Severe coronary artery spasm.
- Cocaine abuse
- Kawasaki disease may cause coronary artery aneurysm and MI. A Q wave duration more than 0.03 second, depth more than 4 mm in children with symptoms suggestive of an angina can be caused by Kawasaki disease or anomalous left coronary artery arising from the pulmonary artery.

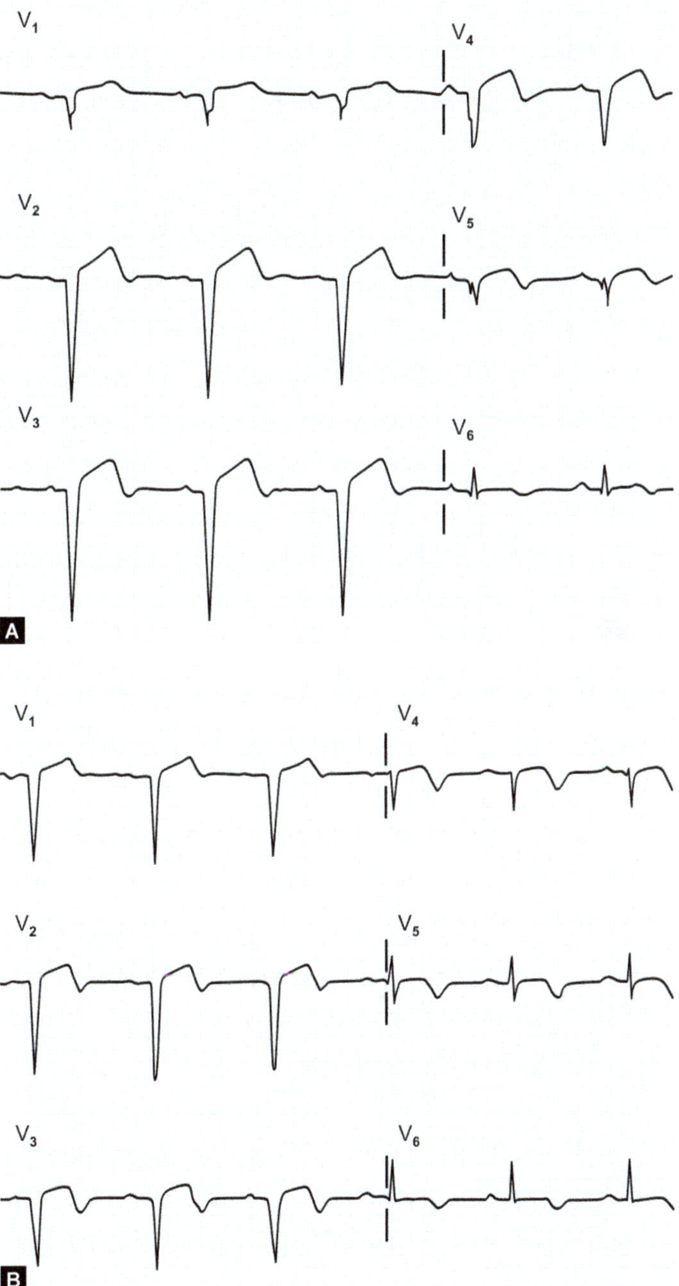

Figs. 6.9A and B

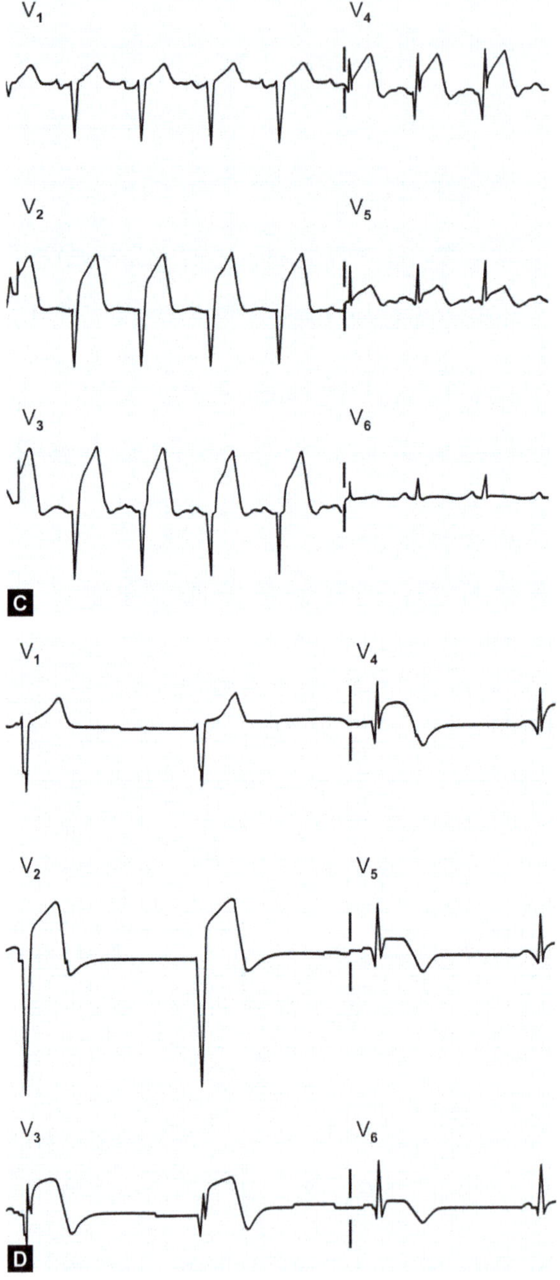

Figs. 6.9C and D

Figs. 6.9A to D: (A) Q waves in leads V_2 with marked abnormal ST segment elevation in V_1 through V_4 indicate acute anterior myocardial infarction; (B) Pathologic Q waves in leads V_1 through V_5 and abnormal ST segment elevation in V_1 through V_5 indicate large acute anterior myocardial infarction; (C) Acute anterior myocardial infarction; (D) Same patient as in (C). Tracing made 1 hour later.

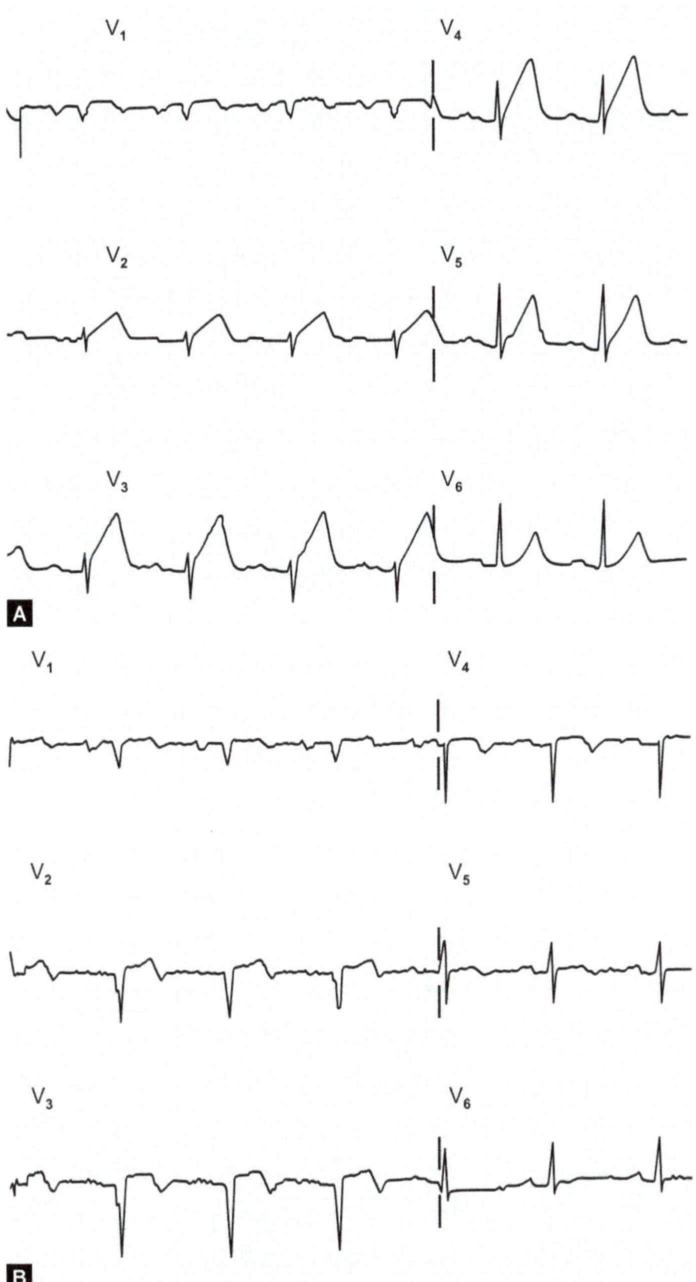

Figs. 6.10A and B: (A) A patient with chest pain and ST elevation in V_1 through V_4, acute anterior myocardial infarction; (B) Same patient as in (A). Tracing taken 10 hours later indicates evolutionary changes: Q waves have developed in V_1 through V_4, and T wave inversion has emerged. Acute anterior infarction confirmed.
Source: Adapted with permission from Khan MG. Heart Disease Diagnosis and Therapy: A Practical Approach, 2nd edition. Totowa, NJ: Humana Press; 2005.

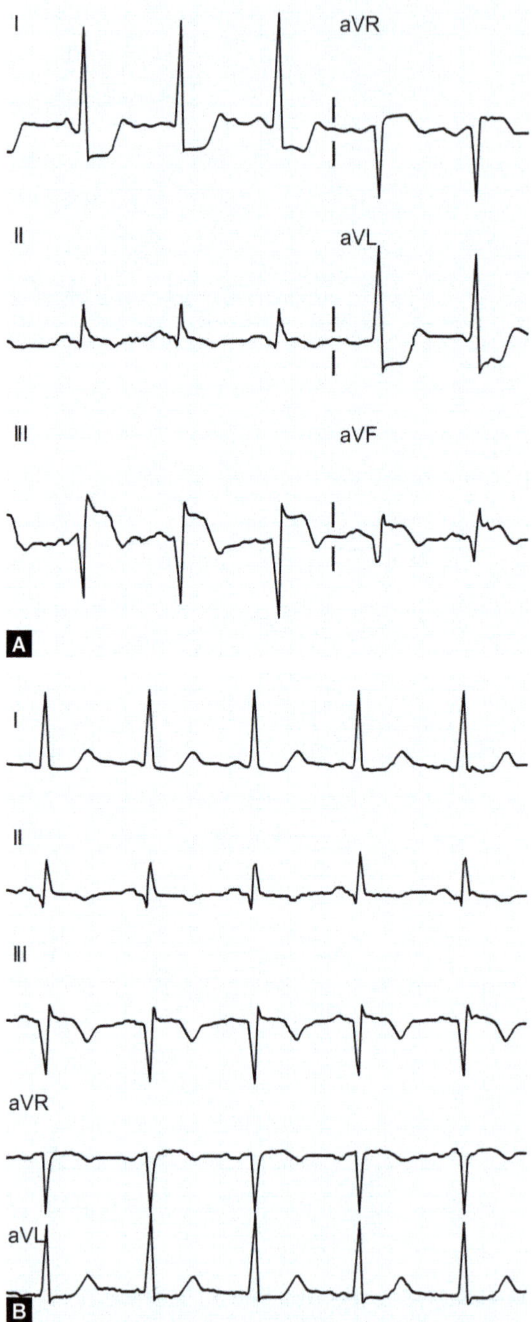

Figs. 6.11A and B: (A) Deep pathologic Q waves in II, III, and aVF with marked ST segment elevation indicate acute inferior myocardial infarction (STEMI). (B) Same patient as in (A). ECG taken 1 hour later shows decrease in ST segment after thrombolytic therapy; ST-T wave abnormality indicative of evolutionary changes.

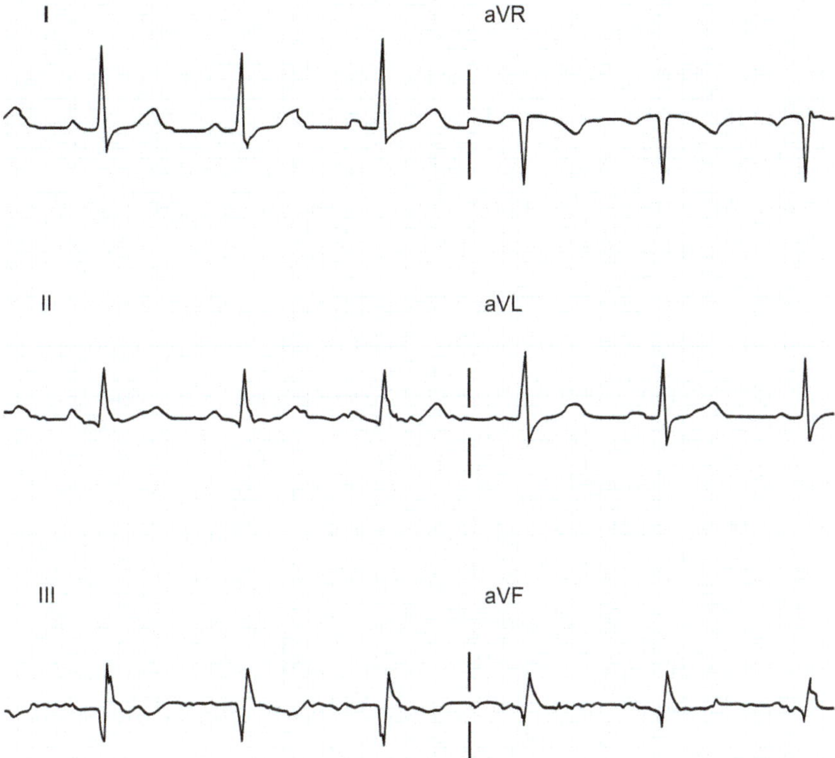

Fig. 6.12: Tracing from a 49-year-old man with no evidence of heart disease; note narrow small Q waves in leads II, III, and aVF <0.04 second. Diagnosis: inferior Q waves noted, nondiagnostic, clinical correlation required: borderline ECG.

Location of Infarction

It is important to emphasize that localization of the infarcted area from the electrocardiographic findings is far from precise, particularly for anterolateral, anteroseptal, and posterior infarctions.

Inferior Infarction

- Pathologic Q waves in leads II, III, and aVF.
- *Acute infarction:* ST segment elevation in II, III, and aVF; diagnostic specificity is enhanced if there is reciprocal depression in leads I, aVL, V_1, and V_2 (*see* Figs. 2.12, 5.3, 5.4, 5.8, and 6.11) during the early hours of infarction. Only ST segment elevation caused by the current of injury may be observed with no Q waves or only small emerging Q waves visible.
- *Old infarction:* Pathologic Q waves may be associated with nonspecific ST-T wave changes in leads II, III, and aVF (*see* Fig. 2.16), but these changes may be minor, being present in only two of the three leads; lead III is the most unreliable lead. The ST segment may be normal;

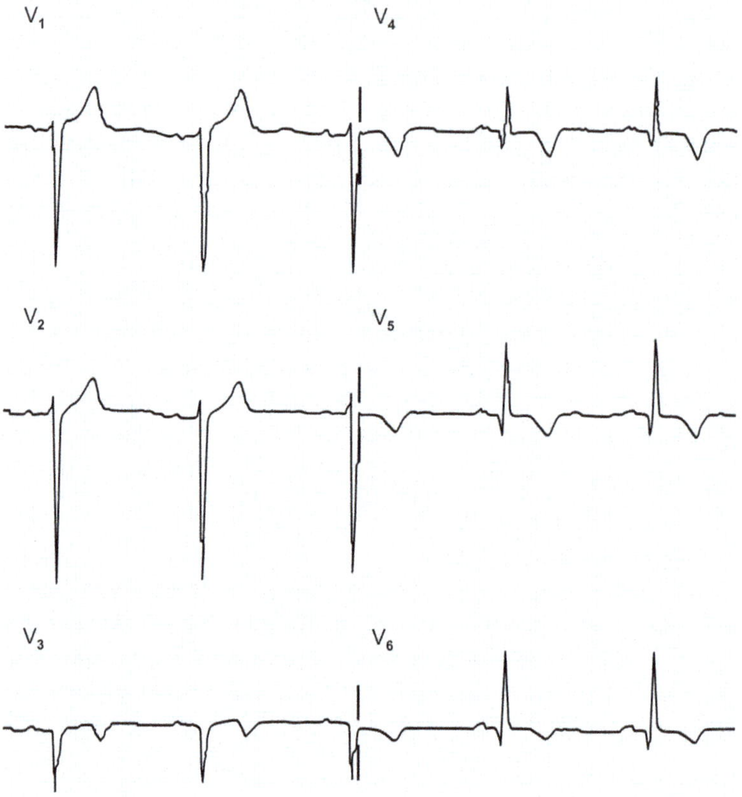

Fig. 6.13: Loss of R wave in V_3 through V_6 indicates anterolateral infarction; note the isoelectric ST segment. However, the ST segment has an abnormal shape with deep T wave inversion, localized to leads I, aVL, and V_3 through V_6, which indicates anterolateral infarction age indeterminate. Comparison with old ECGs and clinical correlation is required to date the time of infarction.

the T wave inversion of acute infarction may persist indefinitely, but the ST segment and T waves may both normalize. The specificity of a Q wave of more than 0.03 second in leads II and aVF is 96% and the sensitivity is approximately 50%.

Anterior Infarction

- Pathologic Q, QS, or QR waves in leads V_2 through V_4 or V_5, or V_1 through V_6, with extensive anterior infarction.
- *Acute infarction*: ST segment elevation in leads V_2 through V_4 or V_5 (*see* Figs. 5.6, 5.9, 6.9, and 6.10). Also, V_1 through V_6 may show ST elevation with extensive anterior infarction. Reciprocal depression may develop in leads II, III, and aVF during the early hours of infarction. Only ST segment elevation caused by the current of injury may be observed with no Q waves or small emerging Q waves visible.

- *Old infarction*: The following: pathologic Q waves, QS complexes in V_2 through V_4 or V_5; the ST segment is usually isoelectric but some deformity of the segment often remains to raise suspicion of an old infarct (*see* Figs. 2.17B and C, 6.8, and 6.13). In most patients, the ST segment is not elevated, but if it persists more than 1 month after infarction and is more than 1 mm in one or more leads, this suggests the presence of a left ventricular aneurysm (*see* Fig. 5.17). T wave inversions may partially normalize but may persist indefinitely (*see* Figs. 2.19, 2.18B and D, and 6.13).

Anteroseptal or Anteroapical Infarction

- Pathologic Q waves, QS deflection in leads V_1 through V_3 in the absence of lead misplacement, and rotational changes that may occur in some conditions, including severe emphysema (*see* Fig. 6.8).
- *Acute infarction:* ST segment elevation in V_1 through V_3 in patients with acute onset of chest pain (*see* Fig. 5.5). This abnormality has long been attributed to anteroseptal infarction. Recent echocardiographic and angiographic findings in patients whose disorders were classified as acute anteroseptal infarction showed that 92% of patients with ST segment elevation in leads V_1 through V_3 had an anteroapical infarct with a normal septum.
- *Old infarction:* QS in V_1 through V_3 with deformity of the ST segment, which may be isoelectric with abnormal or normal T waves (*see* Fig. 6.8).

Anterolateral Infarction

- Pathologic Q waves in leads V_5, V_6, I, and aVL may reflect anterolateral infarction, but the pattern has low specificity. There are many conditions that can produce this electrocardiographic finding. The ECG pattern often reflects an anteroapical infarct; it may be found in patients with septal fibrosis and hypertrophic cardiomyopathy (*see* Figs. 6.14A and B).
- *Acute infarction:* ST segment elevation in leads I, aVL, V_5, and V_6.
- *Old infarction:* Pathologic Q waves associated with an ST segment abnormality. The ST segment may be isoelectric with or without T wave inversion.
- A QS pattern in V_4 increases the specificity (Figs. 2.19 and 6.13).

Right Ventricular Infarction

- Right ventricular infarction is usually associated with inferior infarction. Diagnostic ECG features are ST elevation in V_4R and V_3R in association with ST elevation and emerging Q waves in leads II, III, and aVF. The ST elevation in V_4R recedes within 8 hours of onset of symptoms (Fig. 5.8B).

Posterior Infarction

- True posterior infarction often occurs in association with inferior MI, and this association increases the specificity and makes other possibilities for tall R waves in V_1 and V_2 less likely. The possibilities must always be examined, however (*see* Table 2.3).

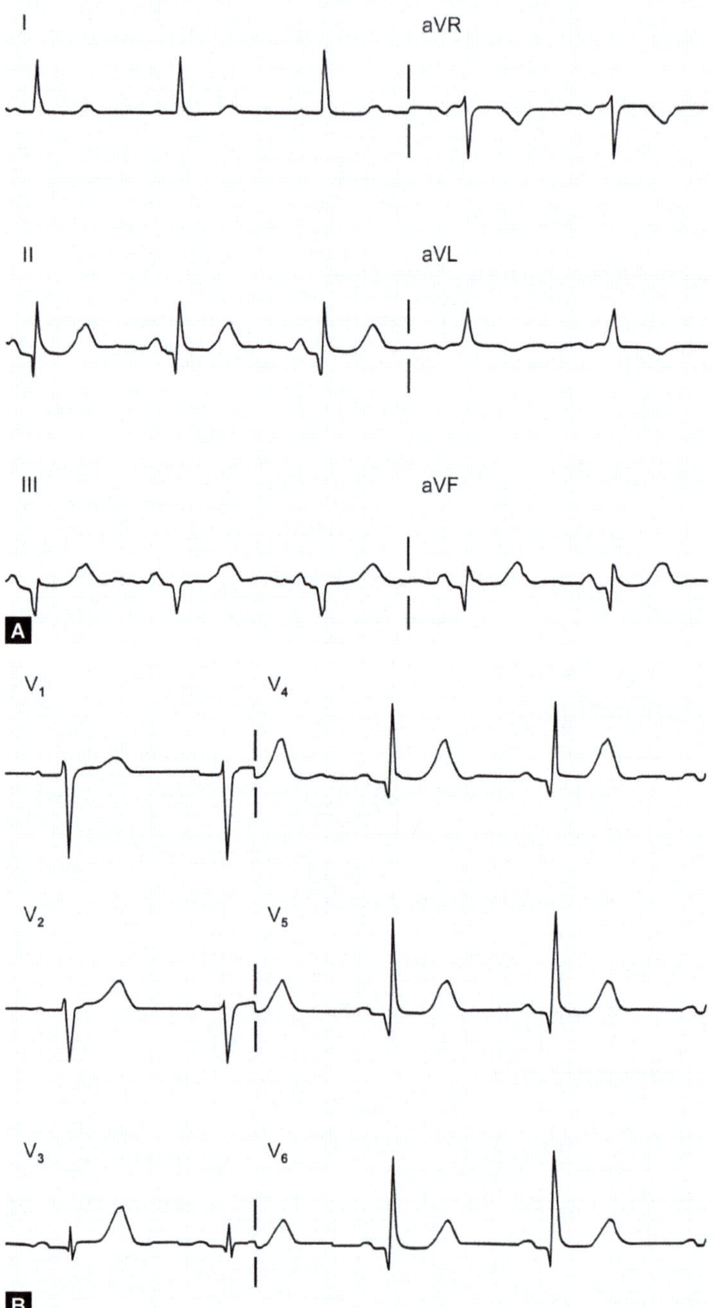

Figs. 6.14A and B: (A) Deep, wide pathologic Q waves in leads II, III, and aVF in a 52-year-old woman with known hypertrophic cardiomyopathy. (B) Same patient as in (A). Wide, deep pathologic Q waves in leads V_4 through V_6.

Old Myocardial Infarction

Figures 6.15 to 6.19 show examples of old myocardial infarction.

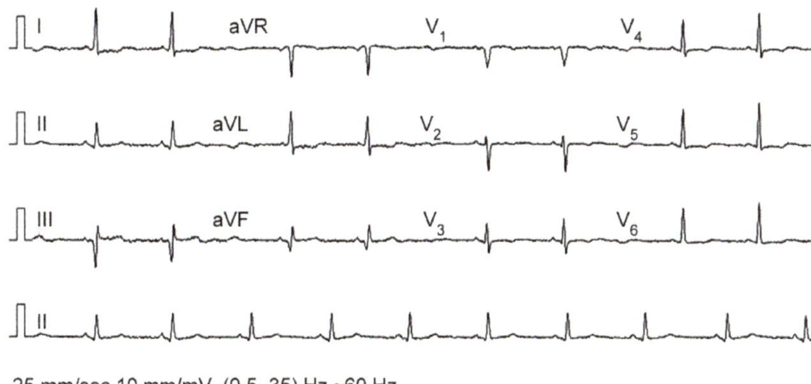

25 mm/sec 10 mm/mV (0.5–35) Hz ~60 Hz

Fig. 6.15: Sinus bradycardia; Q > 40 ms in aVF with Q in II III; Q/R > 1/3 in aVF; old inferior infarct.

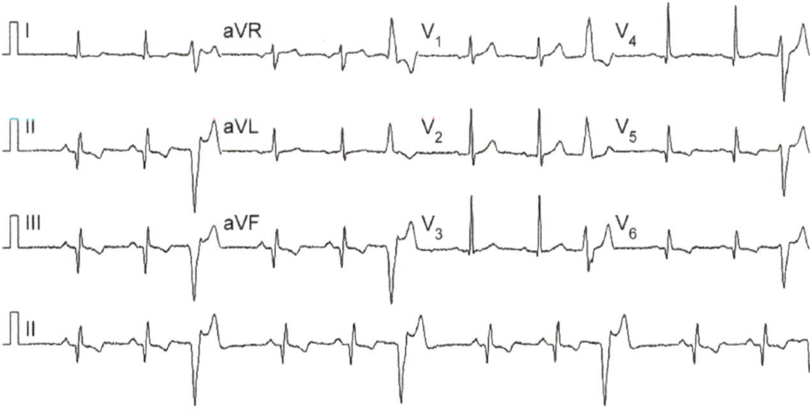

25 mm/sec 10 mm/mV (0.5–35) Hz ~60 Hz

Fig. 6.16: Sinus rhythm; premature ventricular complexes, Q > 40 ms in aVF; with Q in II III; Q/R > 1/3 in aVF; 35 < Q < 40 ms in V_5–V_6; Q/R > 1/3 in V_5–V_6; R/S > 1 in V_1–V_2 with Q in V_5–V_6; old inferoposterolateral infarct.

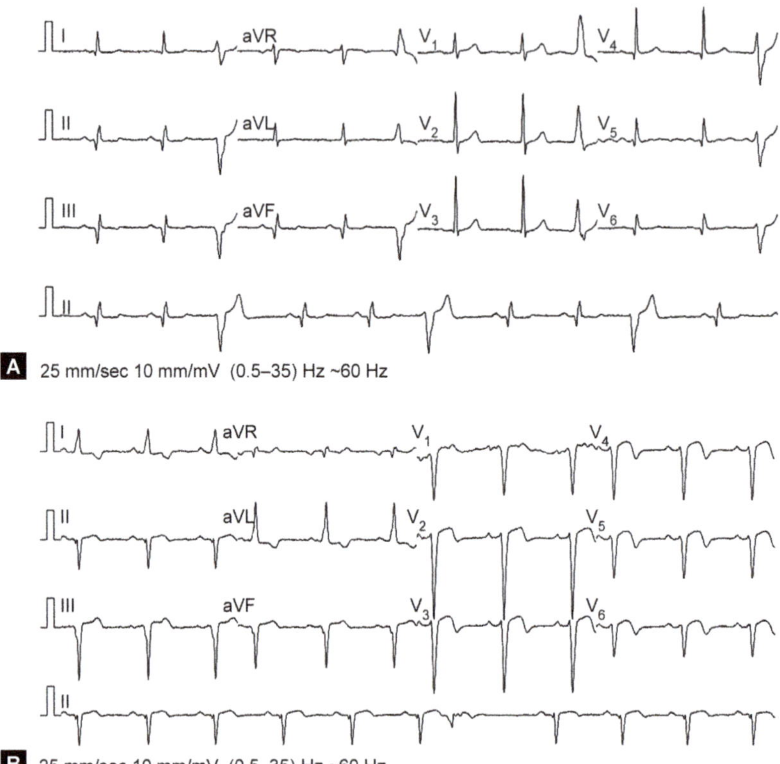

Figs. 6.17A and B: (A) Sinus rhythm; old inferior—posterolateral myocardial infarction. Tall R waves V_1 due to posterior involvement; (B) Sinus rhythm; premature ventricular complexes. Large negative T in aVL V_4–V_5, with negative T in I V_3–V_6 abnormal Q waves V_1–V_6. Old anterior infarct, QS in II III aVF, old inferior infarct.

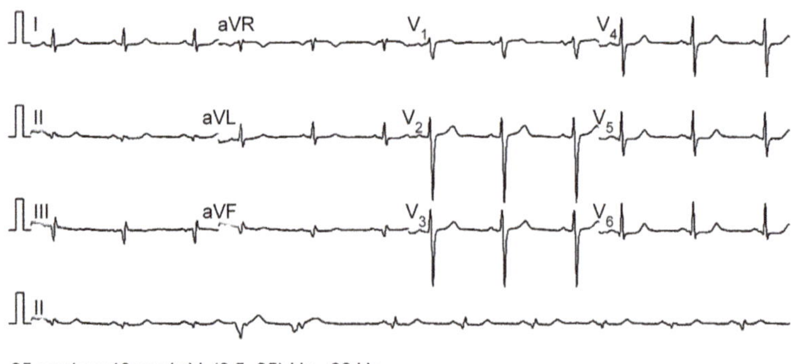

Fig. 6.18: Sinus rhythm; premature ventricular complexes, doublets of multiform premature ventricular complexes. Although the Q waves in inferior leads are not deep they are wider than normal; Q > 40 ms in aVF; with Q in II III, Q/R > 1/3 in aVF; A proven old inferior infarct.

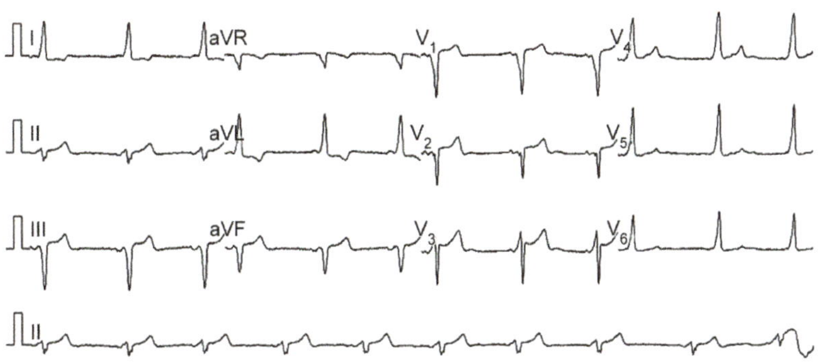

A   25 mm/sec 10 mm/mV (0.5–35) Hz ~60 Hz

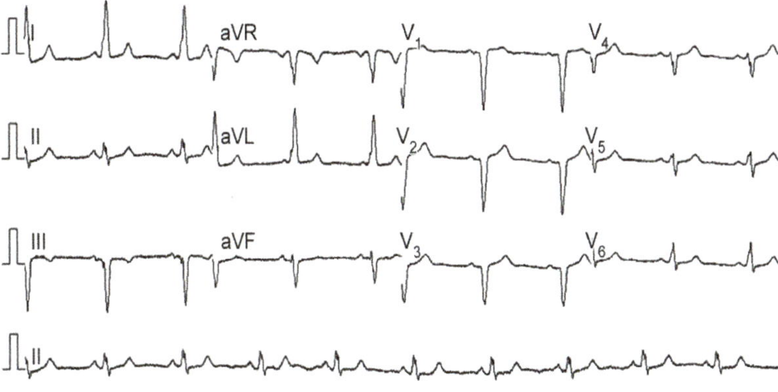

B   25 mm/sec 10 mm/mV (0.5–35) Hz ~60 Hz

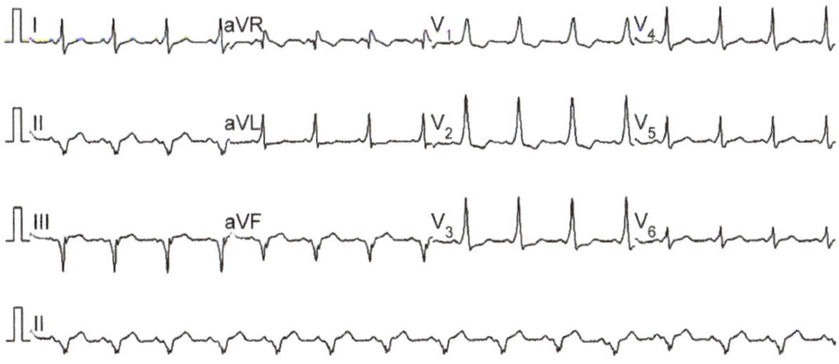

C   25 mm/sec 10 mm/mV (0.5–35) Hz ~60 Hz

Figs. 6.19A to C: Anterior myocardial infarction. (A) WPW mimic old inferior and anteroseptal MI. (B) WPW; delta wave leads 1, 11 aVL, V_6; note no R wave V_1–V_3; small R V_4 mimic anteroseptal, MI; (C) WPW mimic old inferior MI and note tall R waves in V_1–V_3.

MIMICS OF Q WAVE MYOCARDIAL INFARCTION

- Myocarditis, including Chagas disease and acquired immunodeficiency syndrome, may cause pathologic Q waves.
- Pathologic Q waves may occur in patients with hypertrophic cardiomyopathy (Figs. 6.14A and B).
- Pseudo-Q waves in leads II, III, and aVF in Wolff-Parkinson-White syndrome may mimic inferior MI (Figs. 6.20 to 6.22).
- In LVH, QS may occur in lead V_1, V_2, or V_3 and simulate MI (Fig. 6.23).
- Typically in LBBB, R waves are absent or minute in V_1 through V_3. LBBB can simulate anteroseptal infarction (*see* Figs. 2.8B and 6.6). In addition, Q waves may occur in leads II, III, and aVF in the absence of infarction.
- In some patients with emphysema, a QS pattern may be recorded in leads V_1 through V_4 and mimic anterior MI. The precordial leads should be placed one intercostal space lower than usual.

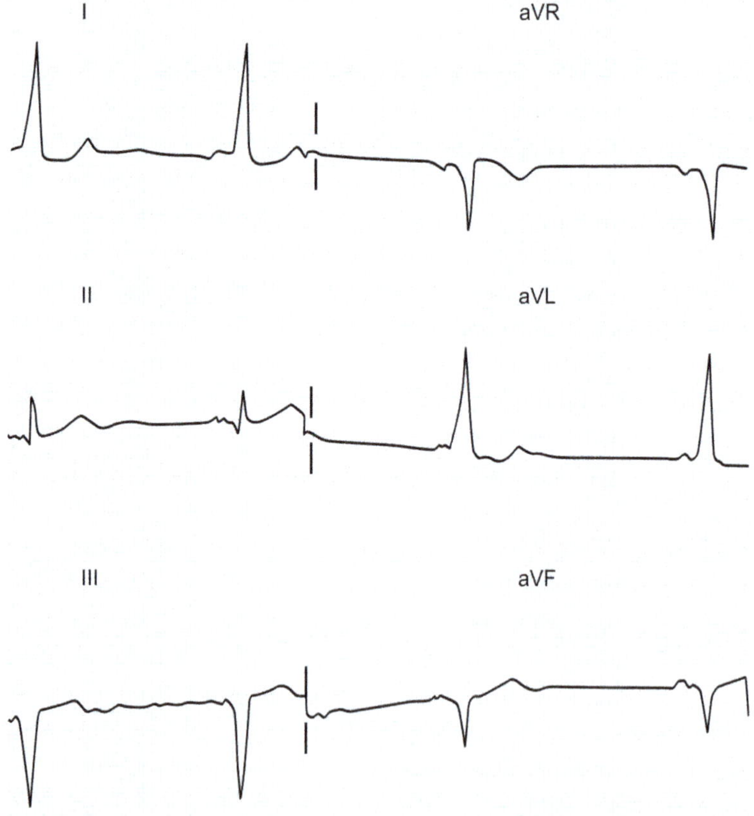

Fig. 6.20: Tracing from a 42-year-old woman with Wolff-Parkinson-White syndrome; note pseudo-Q waves in leads II, III, and aVF, which can mimic inferior myocardial infarction.

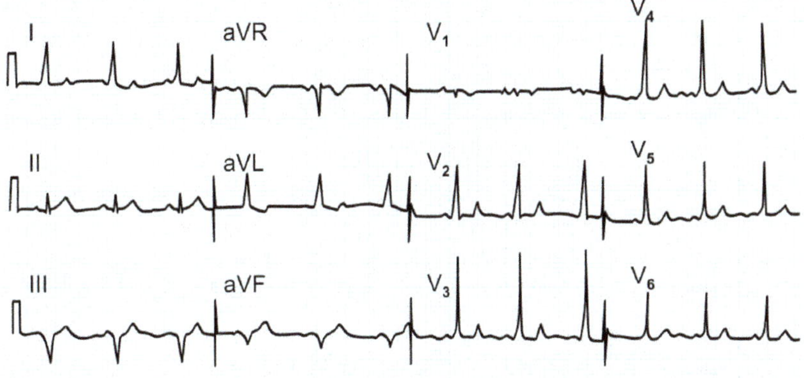

Fig. 6.21: Wolff-Parkinson-White syndrome mimics inferior myocardial infarction

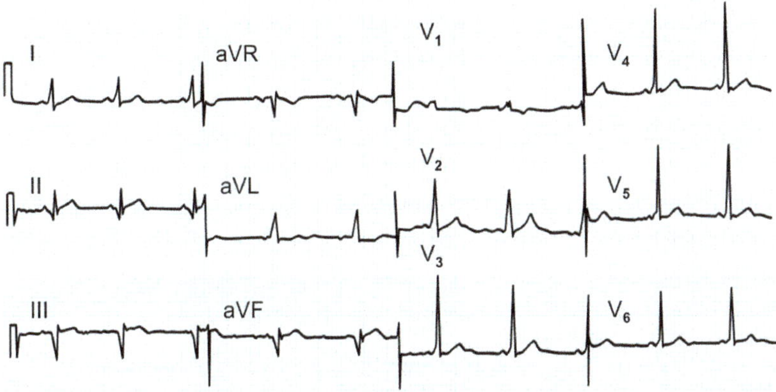

Fig. 6.22: Wolff-Parkinson-White syndrome (WPW); deep Q waves in leads II, III, and aVF. Mimics inferior MI. See Step 3 of the step-by-step method for accurate ECG interpretation. See also discussion in Chapter 2 regarding the necessity to include WPW syndrome early in the interpretive sequence, at the same time as assessment for blocks.

- A left-sided pneumothorax may cause a QS pattern in leads V_1 through V_4.
- Massive pulmonary embolism may cause a QS pattern in leads V_1 through V_4 (*see* Chapter 10).
- Nonpenetrating chest trauma may cause Q waves simulating MI. Conditions that may cause pseudoinfarction patterns are given in Table 6.1.

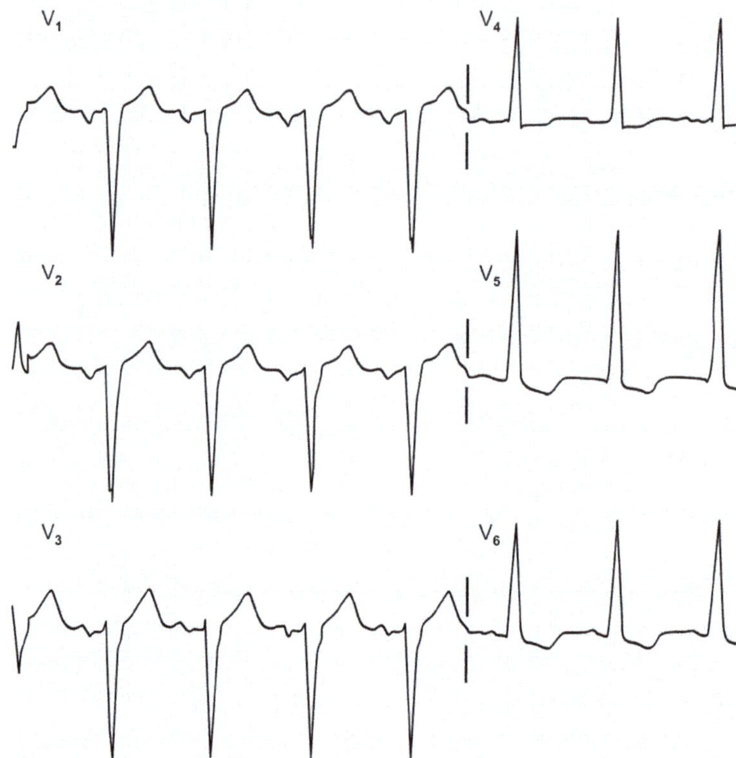

Fig. 6.23: Left ventricular hypertrophy: QS complexes in V_1 and V_2 and a minute R wave in V_3. The tracing can mimic old anteroseptal myocardial infarction, a common error of interpretation.

TABLE 6.1: Noncardiac conditions causing pseudoinfarction.

- Cardiac tumors, primary and secondary
- Cardiomyopathy, particularly hypertrophic (*see* Figs. 6.14A and B) and dilated
- Chagas disease
- Chest deformity
- Chronic obstructive pulmonary disease, particularly emphysema
- HIV infection
- Hyperkalemia
- Left anterior fascicular block
- Left bundle branch block (*see* Figs. 2.9 and 6.6)
- Left ventricular hypertrophy (*see* Fig. 6.23)
- Myocarditis and pericarditis
- Normal variant (*see* Figs. 5.13 and 6.5)
- Pneumothorax
- Poor R wave progression, rotational changes (*see* Fig. 6.7), and lead placement errors
- Pulmonary embolism
- Trauma to the chest (nonpenetrating)
- Wolff-Parkinson-White syndrome (*see* Figs. 6.21 and 6.22)
- Other causes, although rare, include acute pancreatitis, amyloidosis, sarcoidosis, scleroderma

LEFT BUNDLE BRANCH BLOCK AND INFARCTION

The diagnosis of MI in the presence of LBBB is difficult but often can be made. The usual finding in LBBB is a QS pattern in V_1 and V_3 or very small R waves in V_1 through V_3 simulating infarction or LVH.

ECG Features Suggestive of Left Bundle Branch Block with Infarction

- Q waves in leads I, aVL, V_5, and V_6 indicate an anterior (anterolateral or anteroseptal) infarction, but a false-positive diagnosis is common. These findings often occur in the absence of infarction and may occur in patients with severe LVH or nonspecific fibrosis.
- A reversal of R wave progression in the right and midprecordial leads (R waves in V_1 and V_2 that decrease in amplitude in V_3 and V_4) may indicate anterior infarction, but false-positive diagnoses are common.

New Diagnostic Information

Abnormal ST segment deviations occur during infarction and ischemia in patients with LBBB, and these deviations having been documented during percutaneous interventions in patients with LBBB.

- Discordant ST segment deviations are an exaggeration of normal ST segment elevation in leads V_1 to V_4 that possess a dominant S wave. Extensive ST segment elevation in leads V_2, V_3, and V_4 indicating acute injury pattern manifested by discordant ST segment elevation, which is equal to or exceeds the QRS amplitude in leads V_2 through V_4.
- In patients with LBBB and acute onset of chest pain, electrocardiographic features of inferior infarction are reflected by ST segment elevation observed in inferior leads with concordant reciprocal ST segment depression in leads V_1 through V_4. The concordant reciprocal ST segment depression is in the opposite direction to the usual secondary ST segment elevation observed in V_1 through V_4 in patients with LBBB. These discordant and concordant patterns appear to have a specificity of 92–96%; the sensitivity is, however, low.

RIGHT BUNDLE BRANCH BLOCK AND INFARCTION

- Right bundle branch block (RBBB) occurs in approximately 15% of patients with acute MI.
- RBBB may be associated with deep Q waves in leads III and aVF without infarction. MI is likely only if there is an added Q wave in lead II.
- RBBB with infarction is often accompanied by left anterior fascicular block (*see* Fig. 9.8).
- RBBB can be associated with Q waves in leads V_1 and V_2 without infarction. Added Q waves in V_3 and beyond suggest infarction.

LOW-VOLTAGE QRS

ECGs should be recorded with the graph paper moving at 25 mm/s. At this speed, a 1 mm square on the horizontal plane equals 0.04 second. The voltage of the P wave, QRS complex, and T wave are measured vertically with reference to the calibration or standardization, which should be set at 1 mV = 10 mm. With this universal standardization, a 1 mm square in a vertical direction measures 0.1 mV.

Criteria for Low-Voltage QRS

- In all limb leads, the amplitude of the entire QRS complex (R + S) is less than 5 mm.
- In each of the precordial leads, the amplitude of the entire QRS complex (R + S) is less than 10 mm.

Causes of Low-Voltage QRS

- Obesity
- Pericardial effusion
- Constrictive pericarditis
- Myxedema
- Amyloidosis and other restrictive cardiomyopathy and diffuse myocardial diseases
- Pleural effusion
- Chronic obstructive pulmonary disease.

Hypertrophy: Atrial and Ventricular

ATRIAL HYPERTROPHY

Left Atrial Hypertrophy

Diagnostic Criteria

- The P wave duration is more than or equal to 0.12 second (3 small squares) in leads II, III, or aVF. The P wave may be widely notched. These features are most apparent in lead II.
- The terminal deflection of the P waves in V_1 is downward and its duration is prolonged more than or equal to 0.04 second (Figs. 7.1A and B).
- The depth of the terminal negative deflection in V_1 is more than or equal to 1 mm.
- The product of the depth of the terminal negative deflection in V_1 (in millimeters) and the duration in seconds (the P terminal force) is more than or equal to -0.04 mm.s
- The P terminal force (PTF-V_1) is determined rapidly by observation of the P wave in V_1. The P wave terminal negative duration equal to 1 small square (0.04 second) and a depth of 1 small square (1 mm) yield a P terminal force of -0.04 mm.s (Figs. 7.1A and 7.2).

Reliability of Criteria

The diagnostic changes are observed in patients with left atrial enlargement or hypertrophy without significant enlargement and in patients with an increase in left atrial pressure and volume.

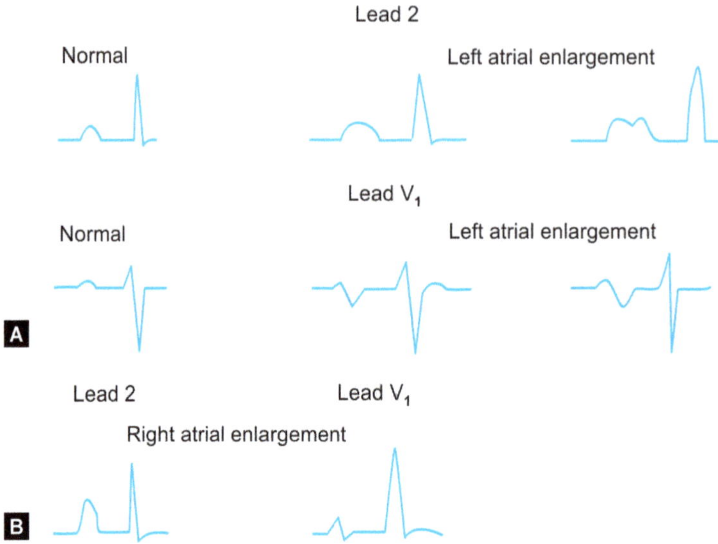

Figs. 7.1A and B: (A) Left atrial enlargement: P wave duration ≥3 mm (0.12 second) in lead 2. In lead V_1, the negative component of the P wave occupies 50% of one small box = 1 mm × 0.04 = P terminal force more than −0.04 mm.s (*see* Figs. 7.2A and B). (B) Right atrial enlargement: lead 2 shows P amplitude ≥3 mm. In V_1, the first half of the P wave is positive and >1 mm wide.
Source: Adapted with permission from Khan MG. On Call Cardiology, 3rd edition. Philadelphia: WB Saunders, Elsevier Science; 2006.

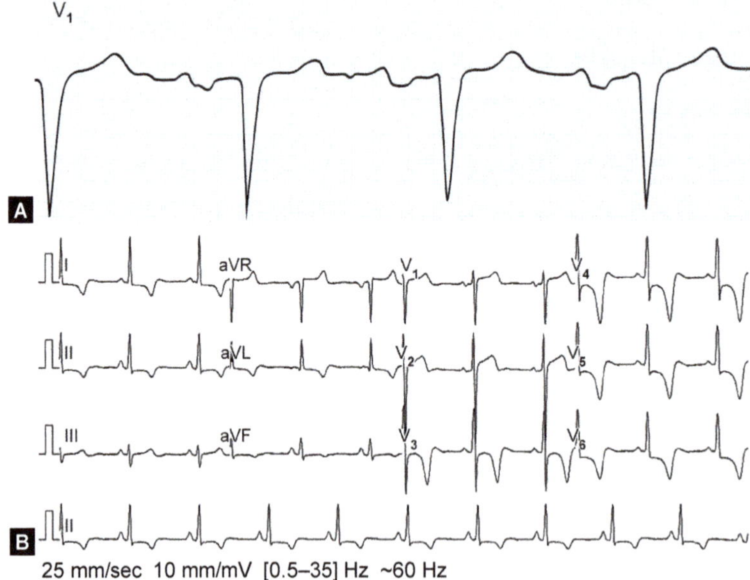

Figs. 7.2A and B: (A) Lead V_1 shows typical P wave pattern of left atrial enlargement. (B) Left ventricular hypertrophy; often there is also evidence for left atrial abnormality usually seen I V_1. See Chapter 3 for detailed discussion of P wave abnormalities and how important it is to study lead V_1 early in the interpretative sequence.

- The combined sensitivity of PTF-V_1 more than or equal to –0.04 mm.s and P wave duration in II, III, or aVF more than 0.10 second (100 ms) has been shown to be 82%.
- A PTF-V_1 of more than –0.06 has been shown to correctly predict left atrial enlargement in 80% of cases.
- P wave duration more than 0.10 second appears to have a specificity of approximately 85% but with a low sensitivity of less than 33%.

Importantly, these relationships relate to echocardiographic left atrial enlargement more than 4 cm; left atrial hypertrophy may occasionally occur without significant echocardiographic enlargement, and the electrocardiographic findings may be the only sign of left ventricular disease caused by hypertension and other cardiac diseases. Thus, the term left atrial abnormality is preferred to cover enlargement, hypertrophy, or increase in atrial volume or pressure.

Causes

It is most important to assess for the electrocardiographic features of left atrial hypertrophy, because this may be the only abnormality in the electrocardiogram (ECG) in patients with various forms of heart disease. It may be the only clue to the diagnosis of underlying left ventricular hypertrophy (LVH), valvular heart disease, congenital heart disease, ischemic heart disease that has caused heart failure, left ventricular dysfunction, the various cardiomyopathies, or constrictive pericarditis. Left atrial hypertrophy is a common ECG finding. Causes of left atrial abnormality include the following:

- Mitral stenosis.
- Mitral regurgitation.
- Left ventricular failure, particularly acute pulmonary edema in which the abnormality may decrease or disappear after approximately 1 week of successful therapy.
- Left ventricular hypertrophy (the atrium hypertrophies in response to altered left ventricular compliance).
- Aortic valve disease.

Right Atrial Hypertrophy

Diagnostic Criteria

- The P wave is tall and peaked with a height more than or equal to 2.5 mm in lead II, III, or aVF and is of normal duration (Figs. 7.3A and B).
- The positive component of the P wave in lead V_1, V_2, or V_3 is tall and peaked with a height more than or equal to 1.5 mm.

Helpful Guides

- An abnormally tall P wave in leads V_1, V_2, and sometimes V_3 more than or equal to 1.5 mm is a more specific electrocardiographic sign for right atrial hypertrophy than the usual diagnostic criteria based on peaked P waves in leads II, III, or aVF (P pulmonale).
- An initial positive component of the P wave in V_1 or V_2 more than or equal to 0.04 second is an indication of right atrial hypertrophy. The findings in the right chest leads are not common with cor pulmonale; however, it is more commonly seen in children with significant congenital heart disease and in individuals with right ventricular hypertrophy (RVH).

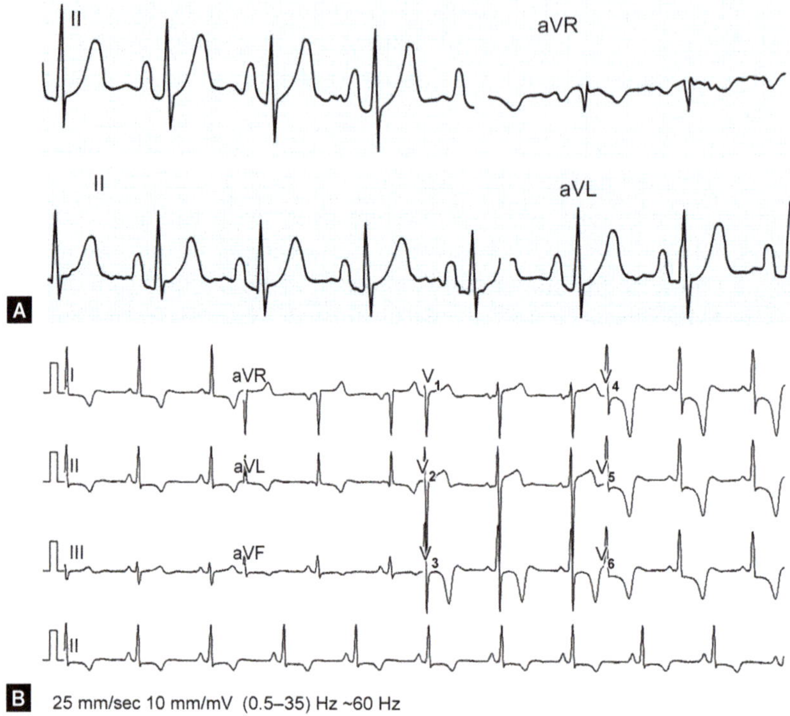

Fig. 7.3A and B: (A) Leads II, III, and aVF show tall, peaked P waves >2.5 mm right atrial hypertrophy. (B) P waves are tall and d peaked particularly in lead II. See Figure right ventricular hypertrophy with atrial hypertrophy.

- The typical pattern of P pulmonale seen in leads II, II, and aVF is less specific for right atrial hypertrophy than the findings in the right chest leads, but because cor pulmonale and some conditions may show no abnormalities in leads V_1 to V_3, it is absolutely necessary to pay attention to findings in leads II, III, and aVF.
- Right atrial hypertrophy is not a common disorder, but it is important to search diligently for electrocardiographic signs of right atrial hypertrophy because the finding may lead to the discovery of significant underlying congenital heart disease and is an important clue to the presence of RVH.

Causes

The causes of right atrial hypertrophy include the following:
- Congenital heart disease (some forms)
- Cor pulmonale
- Pulmonary stenosis
- Pulmonary hypertension
- Tricuspid stenosis
- Tricuspid regurgitation
- Right ventricular hypertrophy.

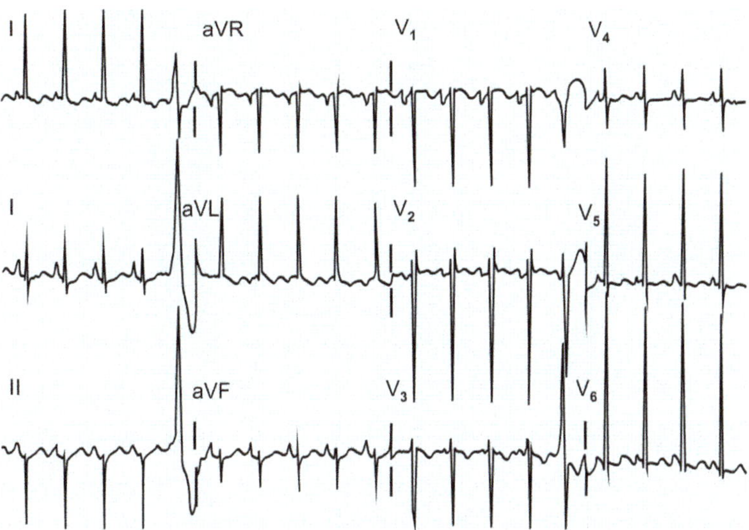

Fig. 7.4: Sinus tachycardia 120 beats/minute, ventricular premature beats, RSR′, V_1, and V_2. Lead V_1 shows characteristics of right and left atrial hypertrophy. Voltage increased V leads that satisfies the criteria for LVH; ST-T changes V_4 and V_5, which can be caused by LVH or ischemia.

Bilateral Atrial Hypertrophy

Bilateral enlargement is indicated by the following:

- A large biphasic P wave in lead V_1, with the positive component more than 1.5 mm and the initial terminal negative deflection reaching 1 mm in depth and with a duration of 0.04 second (Figs. 7.1, 7.2 and 7.4).
- Peaked P waves more than or equal to 1.5 mm in V_1, V_2, and V_3.
- Notched P waves in V_4 to V_6.
- P wave amplitude more than or equal to 2.5 mm and duration more than or equal to 0.12 second in the limb leads.

VENTRICULAR HYPERTROPHY

Left Ventricular Hypertrophy

The genesis of the normal QRS complex is described in Chapter 1, and the genesis of the QRS complex in LVH is shown in Figure 7.5. In LVH, the left atrium becomes hypertrophied to compensate for decreased compliance of the compromised left ventricle. Left atrial hypertrophy is an early ECG manifestation of LVH.

Diagnostic Criteria for Patients Older than 35 Years of Age

The electrocardiographic voltage criteria for the diagnosis of LVH are imprecise and unreliable and have a low sensitivity of approximately 50%; the specificity approaches 94%.

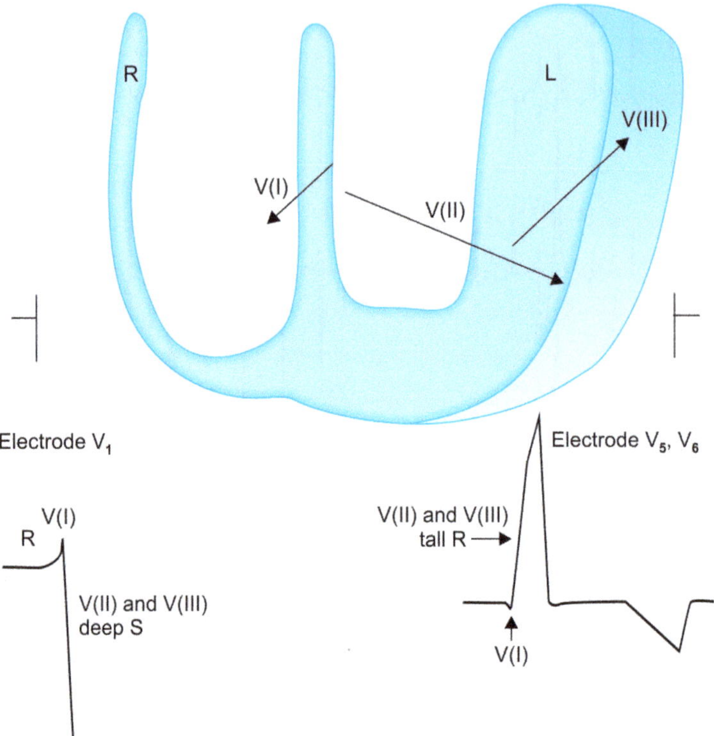

Fig. 7.5: The contribution of vector II to the ECG features of left ventricular hypertrophy. The thicker the left ventricular muscle, the greater the magnitude of vector II; thus, the deep S wave in lead V_1 and tall R wave in leads V_5 and V_6. Note that the T wave has a gradual descending and a steep ascending limb "strain pattern".
Source: Adapted with permission from Khan MG. On Call Cardiology, 2nd edition. Philadelphia: WB Saunders, Elsevier Science; 2001.

Supporting Evidence

Asymmetric ST segment depression and T wave inversion in V_5 and V_6: left ventricular strain pattern; the proximal descending limb of the inverted T wave has a slow descent, and the ascending limb rises steeply. These changes should be maximal in V_5 and V_6 and minimal in V_4 (Fig. 7.6). Note that ST-T changes that are prominent in V_3 and V_4 may reflect ischemia. Changes in V_5 and V_6 with no changes in V_3 and V_4 may be caused by LVH, ischemia, or both (*see* Figs. 8.12A and B).

The QRS duration must be less than 0.12 second.

1. *Sokolow-Lyon voltage criteria:*
    - R wave in lead I + S wave in lead III more than 25 mm (2.5 mV)
    - R wave in aVL more than 11 mm (1.1 mV)
    - R wave in V_6 more than 26 mm (2.6 mV)
    - R wave in V_6 + S wave in V_1 more than 35 mm (3.5 mV) (Figs. 7.6 and 2.25).

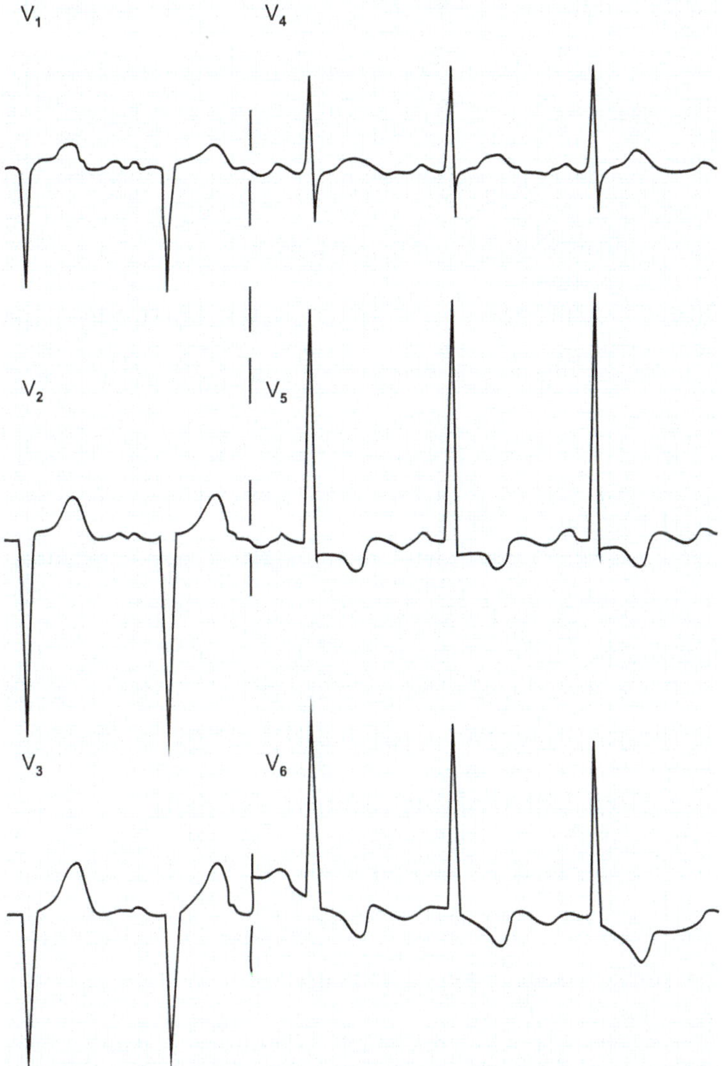

Fig. 7.6: Significant increase in voltage of R wave in V_5 or V_6 and S wave in V_1 or V_2 >35 mm. There is asymmetric ST segment depression and T wave inversion in V_5 and V_6, features typical of left ventricular hypertrophy; note the lack of ST-T changes in V_4.

The criteria reportedly have a sensitivity of 49% and a specificity of approximately 90%:
- Left axis is supportive of LVH but is not necessary for the diagnosis.
- Onset of intrinsicoid deflection in V_5 or V_6 more than 0.05 second.

2. *Cornell voltage criteria:*
   - S wave in V_3 + R wave in aVL more than 28 mm (2.8 mV) in men or more than 20 mm (2.0 mV) in women; the sensitivity is approximately 49% and the specificity is approximately 90%.

3. *Author's criteria for patients older than 35 years of age: 3 points = probable LVH; 4 points = significant LVH:*
   - S wave in V_1 + R wave in V_6 more than or equal to 35 mm = 2 points
   - R wave in aVL + S wave in V_3 more than 28 mm in men or more than 20 mm in women = 3 points
   - Left atrial enlargement with P terminal force more than or equal to –0.04 mm.s or P wave duration more than or equal to 0.12 in leads II, III, or aVF = 2 points
   - Asymmetric ST depression in V_5 and V_6 = 2 points.
4. *Romhilt-Estes scoring system:*
   - R wave in the limb leads more than or equal to 20 mm, S wave in lead V_1 or V_2 more than or equal to 30 mm, or R wave in lead V_5 or V_6 more than or equal to 30 mm = 3 points
   - Negativity of P wave in V_1 more than 1 mm in depth with duration more than 0.03 second = 3 points
   - ST-T wave changes (if patient is not taking digoxin) = 3 points (if patient is taking digoxin = 1 point)
   - Presence of left axis = 2 points
   - A score of 4 points indicates probable LVH, and a score of 5 or more points indicates LVH. The sensitivity is approximately 30% and the specificity is approximately 90%.

Pitfalls in Diagnosis of Left Ventricular Hypertrophy

The preceding criteria do not apply in subjects younger than age 35 years, because QRS voltage can be notably increased in healthy young individuals (Fig. 7.7A; *see* Table 2.1).
- QRS voltage appears to be increased by left anterior fascicular block.
- QRS voltage is higher in African-Americans than in Caucasians.
- Conditions that decrease QRS voltage and that may mask the ECG signs of LVH include severe chronic obstructive pulmonary disease; pericardial effusion; large, old anterior infarctions; myxedema; and heart muscle diseases such as dilated cardiomyopathy, amyloidosis, and scleroderma.

Other examples of LVH are shown in Figures 7.7B and C, and Figure 7.7D shows apical left ventricular hypertrophy.

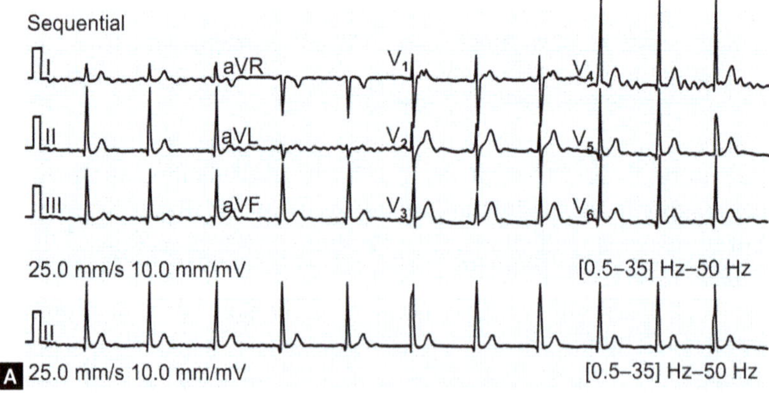

Fig. 7.7A

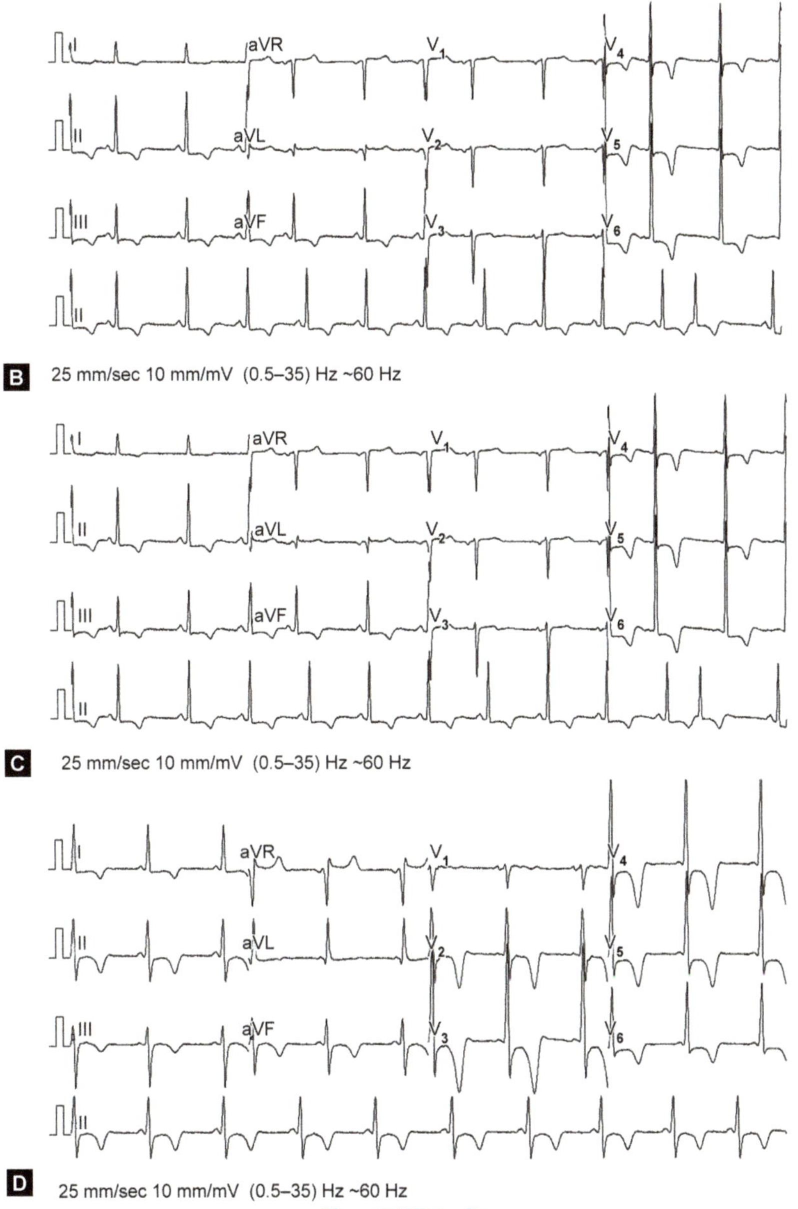

Figs. 7.7B to D

Figs. 7.7A to D: (A) High QRS voltage: S in V_1 + R in V_5 or V_6 = 54 mm (5.4 mV) in a normal 24-year-old male. Caution with voltage criteria in individuals younger than age 30 and think of LVH only if additional features are present (left atrial hypertrophy, and/or ST-T changes, the strain pattern). (B) Left ventricular hypertrophy (LVH); (C) LVH sinus arrhythmia. LVH; age-corrected Sokolow index (SV1 + RV_5 or V_6) = 6.2 mV, very large negative T in V_4, V_5, V_6. Abnormal S-T, T wave changes/also consider ischemia. (D) LVH; age-corrected Sokolow index (SV$_1$ + RV_5 or V_6) = 4.2 mV, age-corrected R in left precordial leads = 3.3 mV, age-corrected vectorial R in extremity leads = 2.5 mV, consider apical hypertrophic cardiomyopathy.

Right Ventricular Hypertrophy

The QRS duration must be less than 0.12 second because the diagnosis of RVH cannot be made accurately in the presence of right bundle branch block (RBBB) or Wolff-Parkinson-White (WPW) syndrome, posterior myocardial infarction (MI), dextroposition.

Diagnostic Criteria for Patients Older than 30 Years of Age

Two or more of the following criteria are required for the diagnosis of RVH:
- Right-axis deviation greater than +110° (Fig. 7.8)
- Tall R wave in V_1 more than or equal to 7 mm (can be a normal variant), S wave in V_1 less than or equal to 2 mm, R/S ratio in V_1 more than 1, R/S ratio in V_5 or V_6 less than or equal to 1 (Fig. 7.8), patient older than age 30 years (*see* Table 2.1)
- S wave in V_5 or V_6 more than 2 mm
- qR pattern in V_1 (not commonly observed but increases specificity).
- Most important is scrutiny for right atrial hypertrophy: peaked P waves with an amplitude in V_1, V_2, or V_3 more than or equal to 1.5 mm or more than or equal to 2.5 mm in II, III, or aVF (this increases specificity).

Supporting Evidence

- Onset of intrinsicoid deflection in V_1 = 0.035–0.055 second.
- ST-T strain pattern in V_1 through V_3 (Fig. 7.8).
- Right atrial enlargement.

Pitfalls in Diagnosis of Right Ventricular Hypertrophy

Right ventricular hypertrophy and right atrial enlargement are uncommon ECG diagnoses; cardiologists should refrain from making an ECG diagnosis of RVH in the presence of the following conditions:

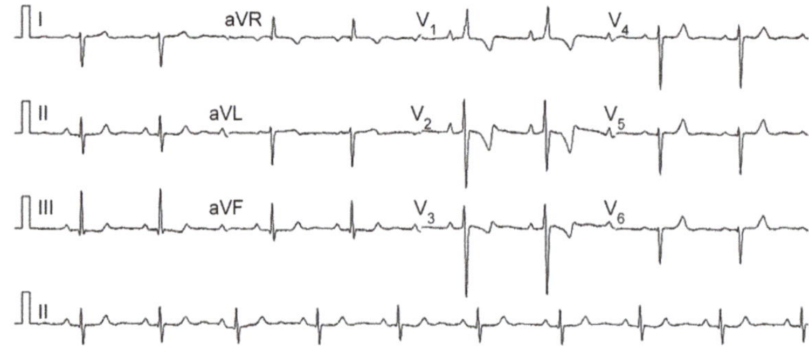

Fig. 7.8: A high P voltage: right atrial hypertrophy; right axis deviation 160°; RVH (right ventricular hypertrophy): R > 1 mV in V_1; R/S > 1 in V_1; R/S < 1 in V_2–V_6, very marked right-precordial repolarization disturbance secondary to RVH; very large negative T in V_2 with negative T in V3R; ST-T right ventricular strain pattern in V_1 through V_3. From a patient with Eisenmenger syndrome.

- Right bundle branch block
- WPW syndrome
- True posterior MI
- In children, the preceding ECG findings can be a normal variant
- Early transition (the R wave is increased in V_1 and V_2, but the R/S ratio in V_5 or V_6 is >1)
- Dextroposition (*see* Table 2.3)
- Hypertrophic cardiomyopathy (a tall R wave in V_1 with an R/S ratio >1 may be observed).

T Wave Abnormalities

INTRODUCTION

The T wave represents repolarization, the recovery period of the ventricles. As emphasized in Chapter 5, the skillful interpreter focuses on the ST segment and does not try to make diagnoses based on T wave changes. T wave changes often are nonspecific and always should be interpreted in light of associated abnormalities of the ST segment and clinical findings. An algorithmic approach for the interpretation of T wave changes is depicted in Figures 8.1A and B.

NORMAL DIRECTION OF T WAVE

- The T wave is always upright (positive) in leads I(1), II(2), and V_4 through V_6 (Figs. 8.2 and 8.3).
- The T wave is normally upright in lead aVF if the QRS complex is less than 5 mm tall, but the T wave can be flat or inverted.
- The T wave is variable in leads III and aVL.
- The T wave is always inverted in aVR (*see* Fig. 8.2).
- The T wave in V_1 is inverted in approximately 50% of women and in less than 33% of men (*see* Fig. 8.2).
- In women with a persistent juvenile pattern, the T wave is inverted in V_1 and V_2 and sometimes in V_3 (Fig. 8.4). This finding is common in African-American women.
- Diagnoses based solely on the appearance of abnormal-looking T waves are fraught with danger. Figures 8.4 to 8.6 indicate errors that can be made in the interpretation of T or ST-T wave changes.

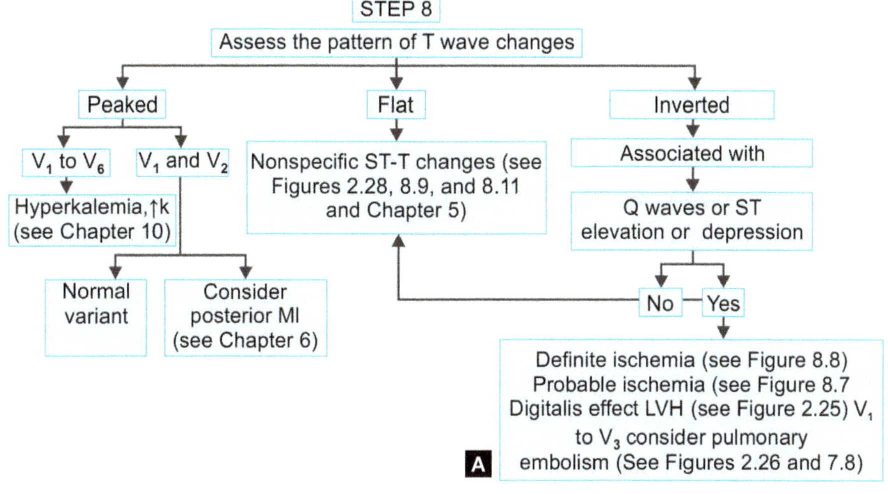

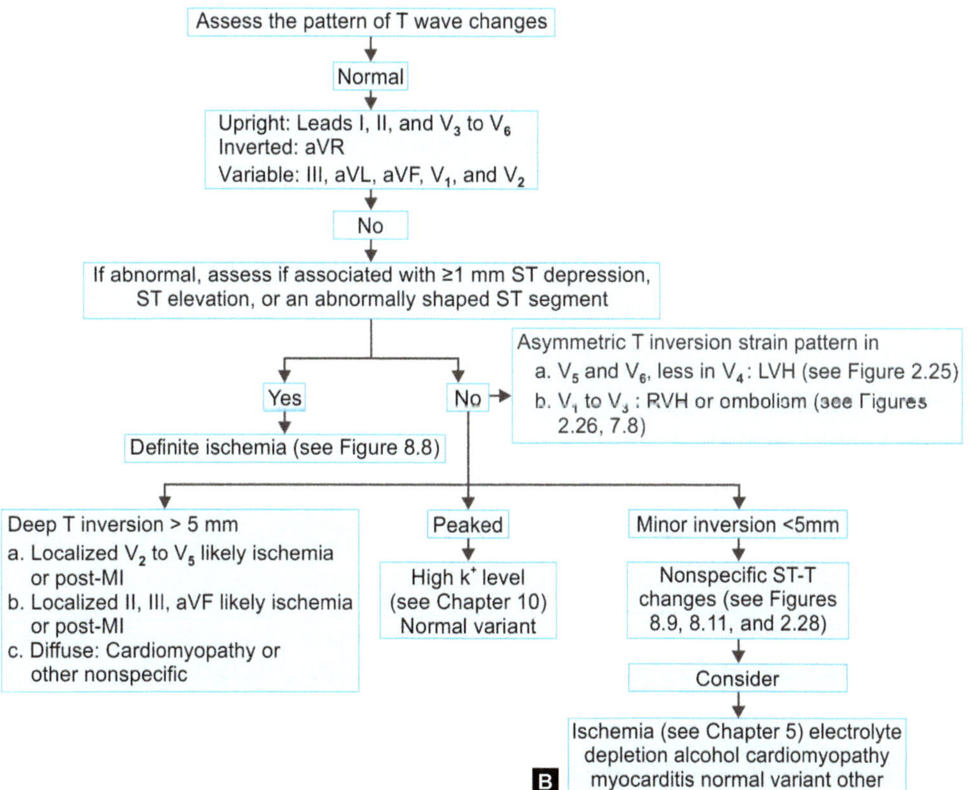

Figs. 8.1A and B: Step-by-step method for accurate ECG interpretation. (A) Step 8: assessment of T wave changes; (B) Step 8: alternative methods for the assessment of T wave changes. (LVH, left ventricular hypertrophy; MI, myocardial infarction; RVH, right ventricular hypertrophy)

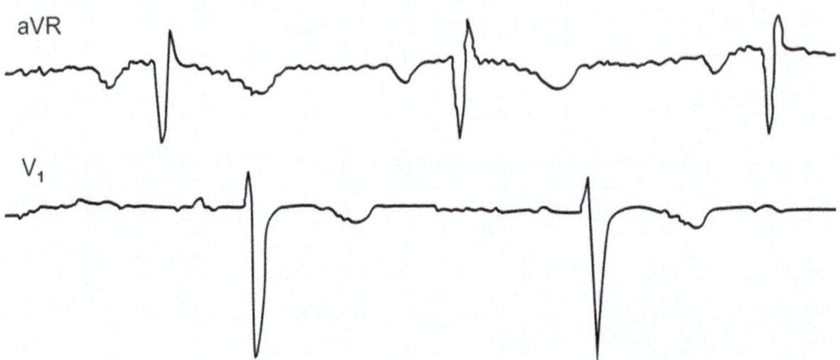

Fig. 8.2: Normally occurring negative T waves in a VR and V_1.

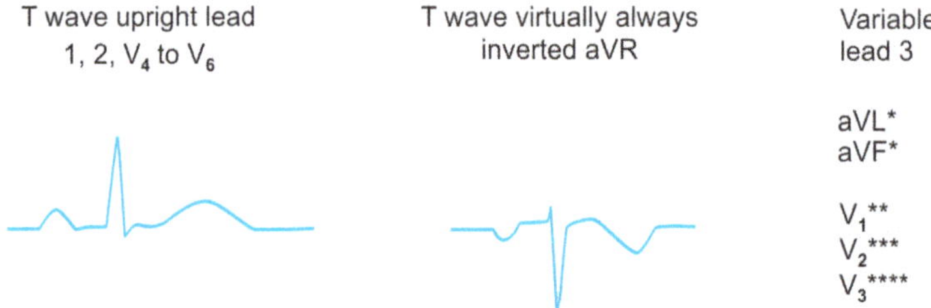

T wave upright lead 1, 2, V_4 to V_6	T wave virtually always inverted aVR	Variable lead 3
		aVL* aVF*
		V_1** V_2*** V_3****

Fig. 8.3: T wave, normal variability.
*Usually upright; can be inverted if R wave <5 mm.
**Inverted in >50% of women and <20% of men who are >30 years of age.
***Usually upright; can be inverted with juvenile pattern.
****Usually upright; rarely flat or biphasic in women or with juvenile pattern.

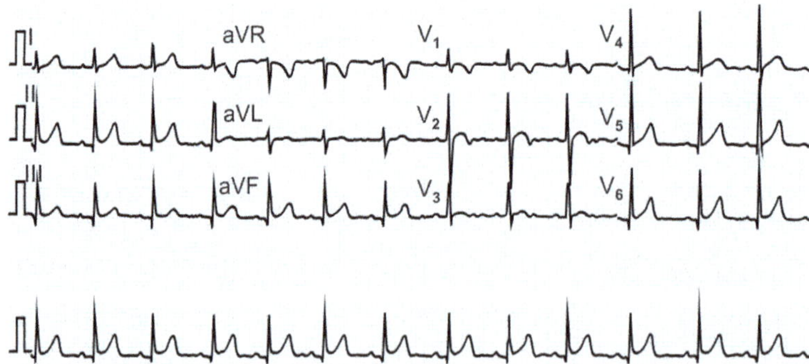

Fig. 8.4: Sinus rhythm 80/minute; ST segment coving with juvenile T wave inversion in leads V_1-V_3: normal variant in this 10-year-old male. Also, normal variant ST elevation in II, III aVF, V_5, and V_6 (so-called early repolarization changes). The diffuse ST segment elevation and PR elevation in aVR might suggest pericarditis. But, in pericarditis the, J-point level almost equals the height of the T wave in V_6. Clinical correlation required.

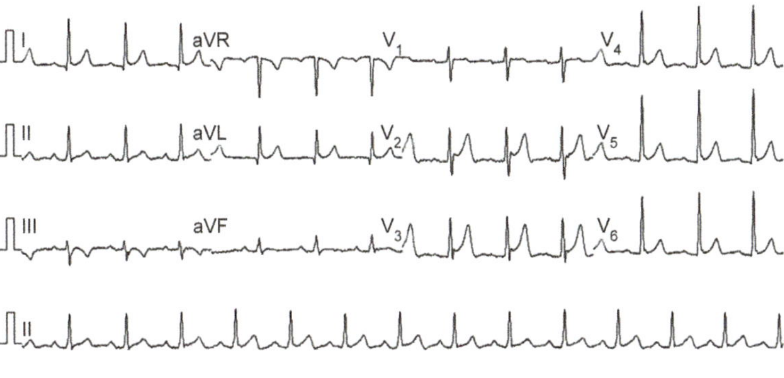

25 mm/sec 10 mm/mV (0.5–35) Hz ~60 Hz

Fig. 8.5: Prominent, tall T waves V_2, V_3 with minor ST elevation V_2, V_3 and a tiny fish-hook like abnormality on the commencement of the ST segment V_2; normal variant in a healthy young adult.

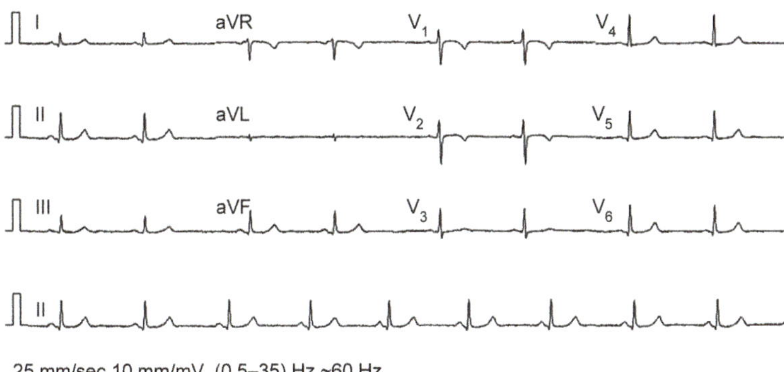

25 mm/sec 10 mm/mV (0.5–35) Hz ~60 Hz

Fig. 8.6: T wave inversion V_1, V_2, in a healthy 39-year-old female. This finding may occur in ~1–2% of females, and may involve V_3; termed by some as female variant.

ABNORMALITIES OF T WAVE

Inverted T Wave

- T wave inversion in leads I, II, and V_3 through V_6 is abnormal.
- If T wave inversion is accompanied by abnormal coving of the ST segment (horizontal or down-sloping ST segment depression greater than 1 mm (Figs. 8.7 and 8.8), a diagnosis of ischemia can be made with confidence. T wave inversion with ST segment elevation and abnormal coving is a feature of evolving recent infarction.
- If T wave inversion is associated with less than 1-mm ST depression or an up-sloping depression, the finding is nonspecific (Fig. 8.9) and can be caused by a host of cardiac and noncardiac conditions.

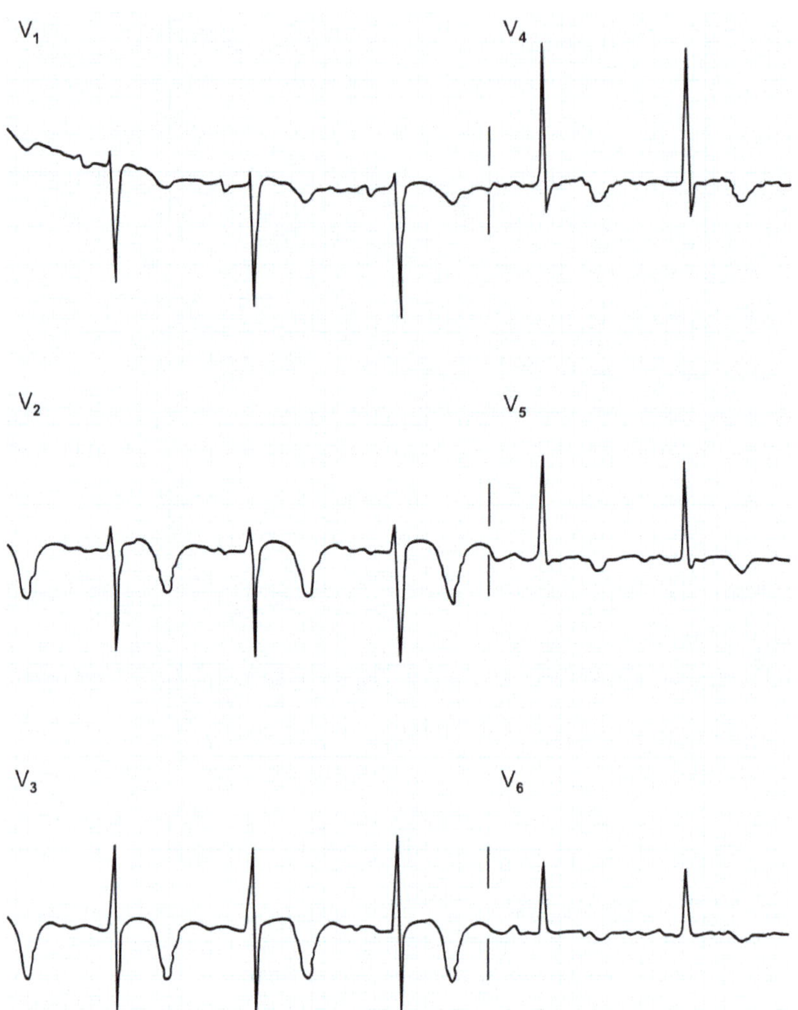

Fig. 8.7: T wave inversion in V_2 through V_5 associated with abnormal curvature of the ST segment; likely caused by ischemia.

- Isolated T wave inversion is nonspecific (Figs. 8.10 and 8.11), but ischemia cannot be excluded.
- The 5-year mortality rate in patients with moderate T wave inversion associated with the presence of heart disease reportedly is 21% versus 3% when heart disease is absent.

  Diffuse, deep T wave inversion in the absence of ST segment elevation or significant depression is not diagnostic (*see* Fig. 8.10), and can be associated with the following:
- Ischemia
- Post-MI evolutionary changes—Takotsubo stress cardiomyopathy

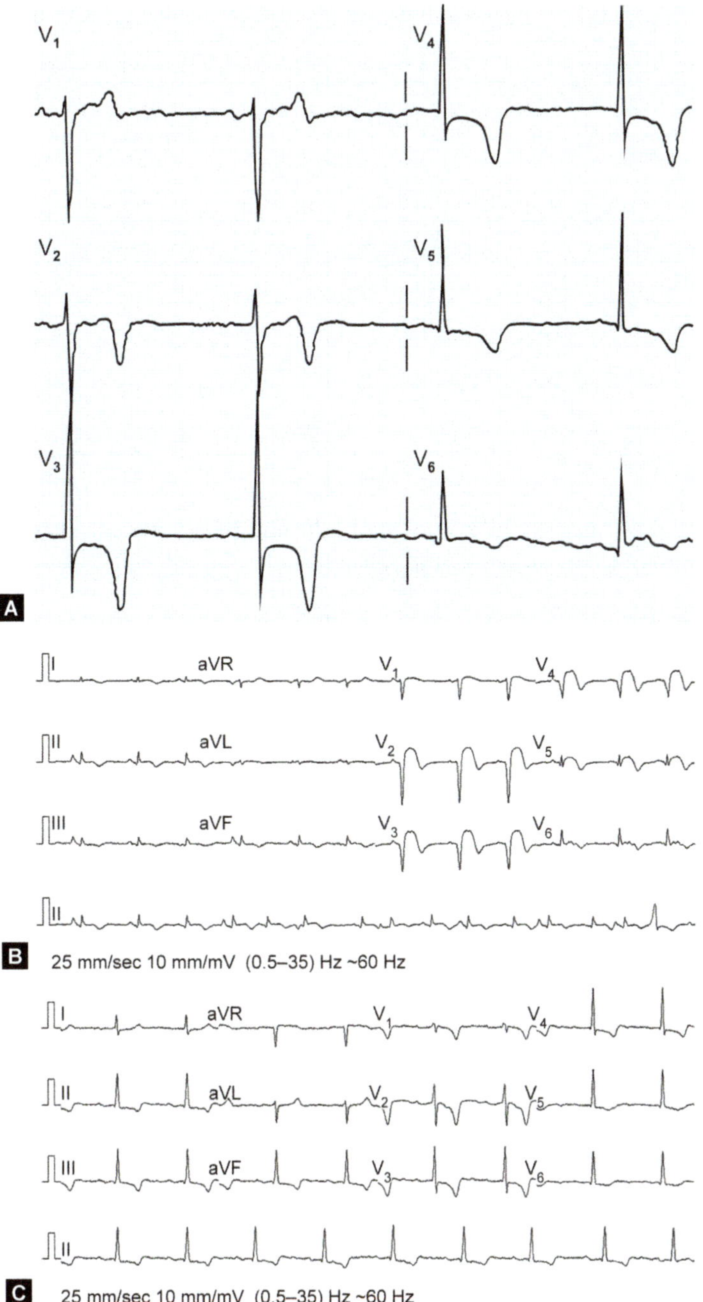

Figs. 8.8A to C: (A) Tracing from a 53-year-old woman with a 1-week history of unstable angina. Tracing taken in the absence of pain. Deep T wave inversion in V_2 through V_4. Note the abnormal coving of the ST segment and "hitched-up" ST segment in V_1 and V_2. (B) T wave inversion accompanying evolving anterior MI with ST elevation and deep abnormal Q waves V_2-V_5; (C) Diffuse T wave inversion, with abnormally coved ST segment without elevation but down-sloping: suggests ischemia.

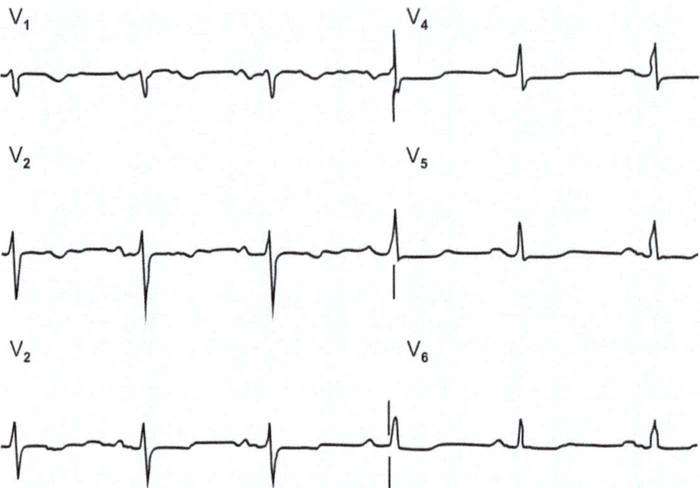

Fig. 8.9: Minimal T wave inversion in V_2 through V_4 with less than 1 mm ST depression: nonspecific ST-T changes; cannot exclude ischemia, especially since the ST segment depression is horizontal.

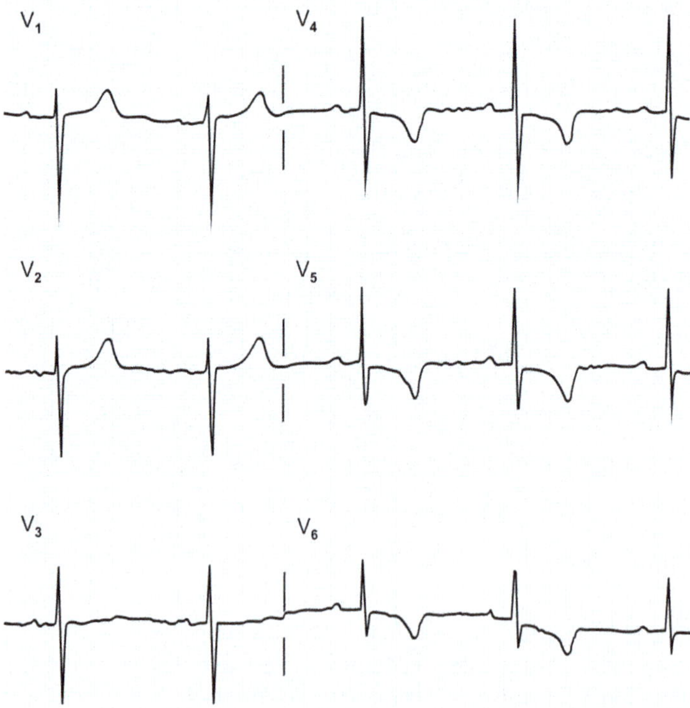

Fig. 8.10: T wave inversion in V_4 through V_6; similar changes were observed in leads aVL, II, III, and aVF: nonspecific ST-T changes; cannot exclude ischemia.

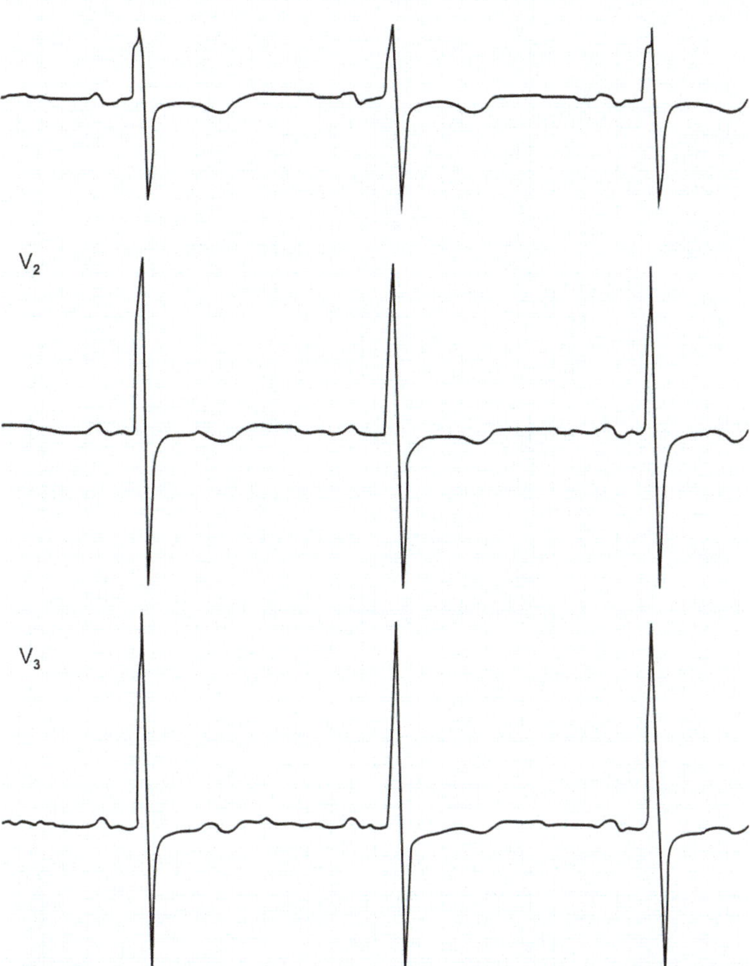

Fig. 8.11: Tracing from a 50-year-old man with no history of heart disease; nonspecific ST-T wave changes as seen from V₁ through V₃; the limb leads show no abnormality. Abnormal ECG: clinical correlation needed.

- Left ventricular hypertrophy with or without ischemia (Figs 8.12A to C)
- Post-Stokes-Adams attack
- Post-supraventricular tachycardia or ventricular tachycardia
- Myocarditis
- Pericarditis
- Apical cardiomyopathy (causes giant T wave inversion) (Figs. 8.13A and B)
- Pulmonary embolism

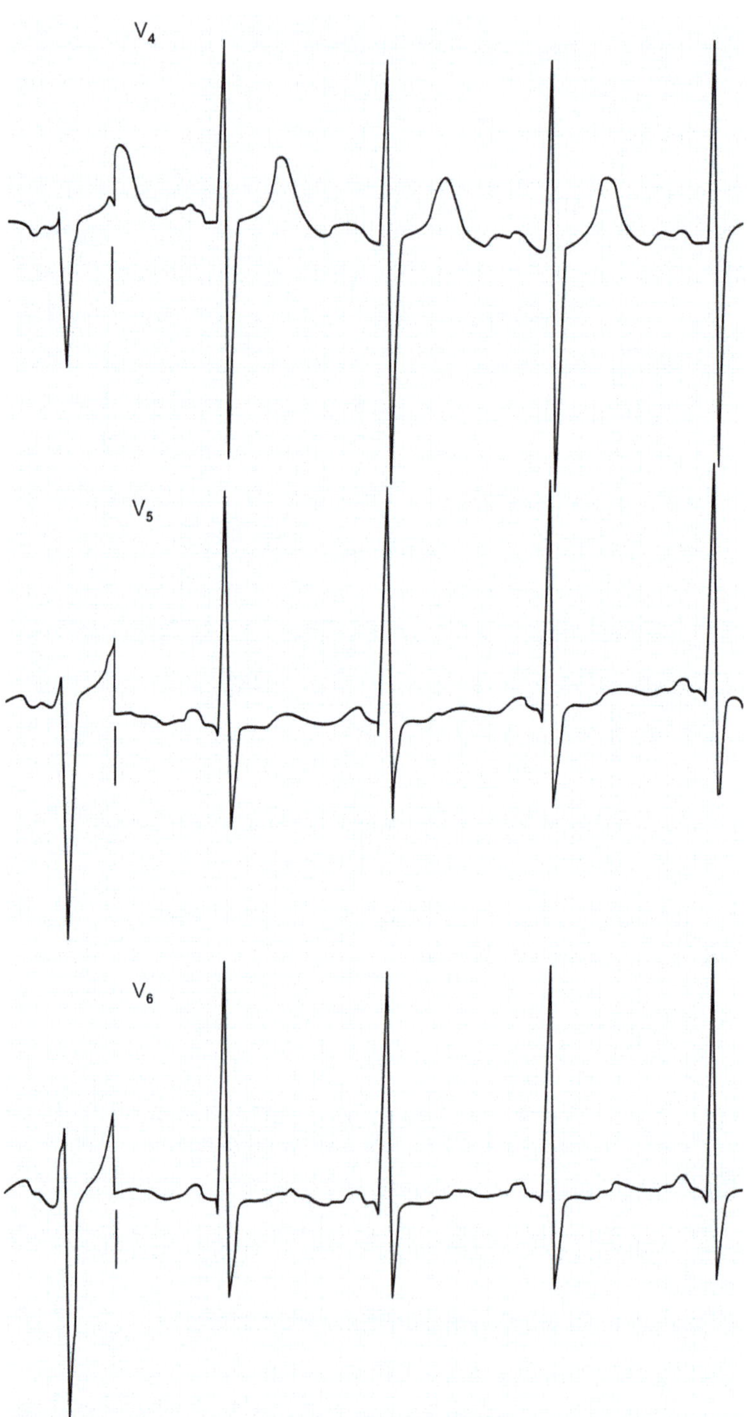

Fig. 8.12A

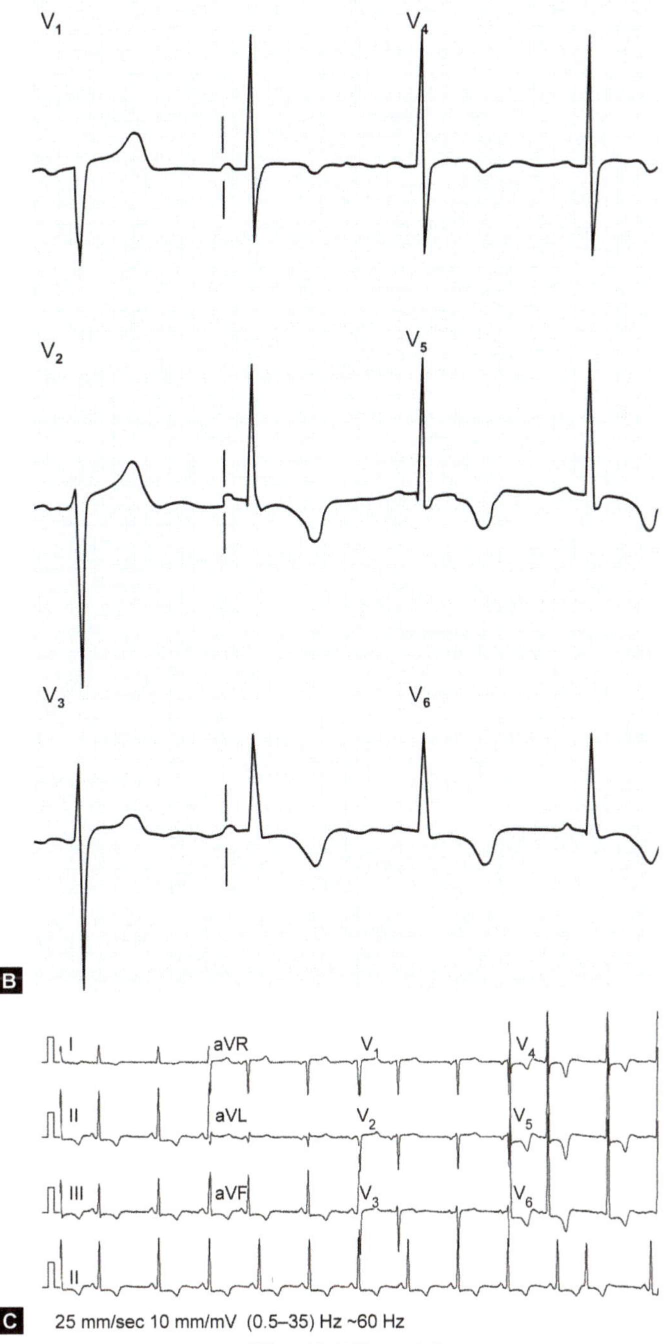

Figs. 8.12B and C

Figs. 8.12A to C: (A and B) Voltage increase: probable left ventricular hypertrophy; (C) Definite voltage increase change. Note diffuse deep T wave inversion, in keeping with hypertrophy but cannot exclude ischemia.

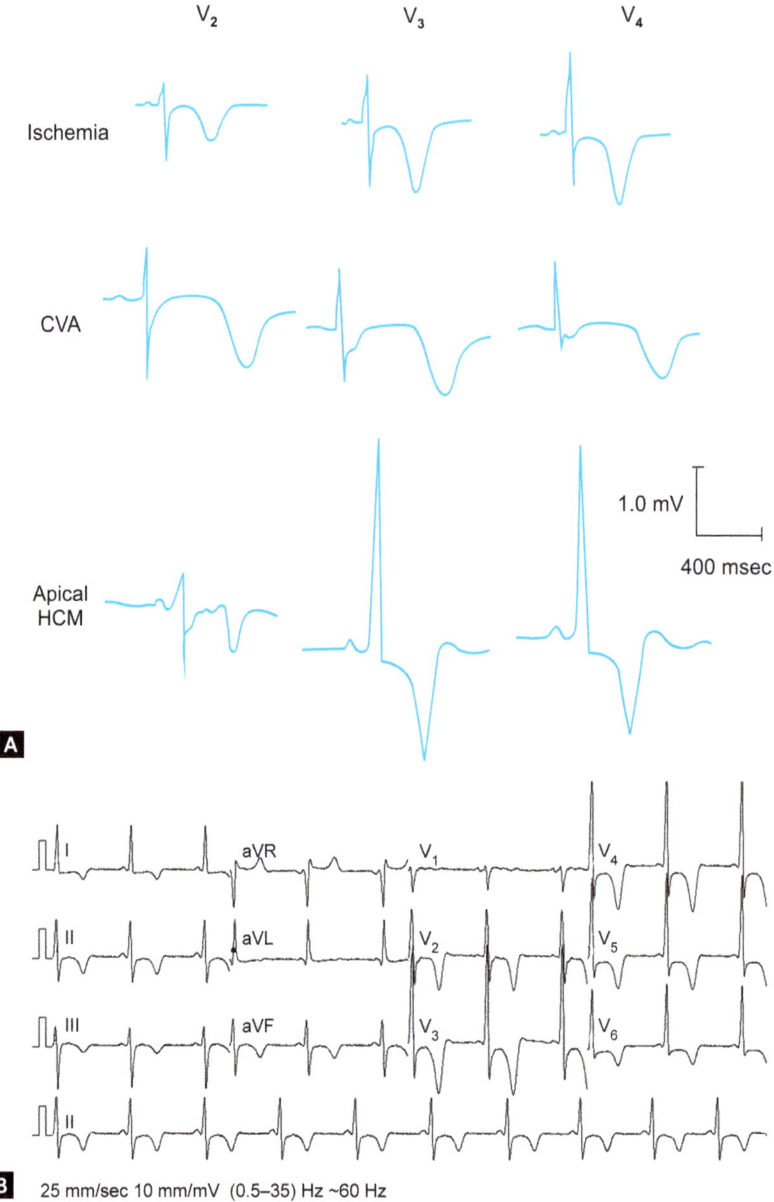

Figs. 8.13A and B: (A) Deep T wave inversion can result from a variety of causes. Note the significant QR prolongation in conjunction with the cerebrovascular accident (CVA) T wave pattern caused here by subarachnoid hemorrhage. Apical hypertrophic cardiomyopathy (HCM) is another cause of deep T wave inversion that can be mistaken for coronary disease. (B) Deep T waves in a patient with apical hypertrophic cardiomyopathy.

Source: Adapted with permission from Goldberger AL. Deep T wave inversions: ischemia, cerebrovascular accident, or something else. ACC Curr J Rev. 1996

- Cardiomyopathies
- Primary or secondary cardiac tumors
- Cocaine abuse
- Alcohol abuse
- Electrolyte imbalance
- Subarachnoid hemorrhage
- Acute pancreatitis and gallbladder disease
- Pheochromocytoma
- Other causes.

Symmetric T wave inversion is four times more common in women than it is in men. Interpreting symmetric, deep T wave inversion as a sign of ischemia without considering other diagnoses is a common error.

Minor T wave inversion not associated with significant ST segment changes can be caused by all of the aforementioned conditions, as well as by the following:

- Hyperventilation
- Postprandial (after the patient has a meal or a cold drink, the tracing normalizes in the fasting state)
- Mitral valve prolapse
- Intraventricular conduction defects
- Pneumothorax
- Ventricular hypertrophy (*see* Chapter 7).

Minor T wave inversion not associated with significant ST segment changes also can be a normal variant. T wave inversion occurs in V_1 through V_3 in some young adults as a persistent juvenile pattern; this is more common in women (*see* Fig. 8.4). Benign T wave inversion in V_4 through V_6 may be observed in healthy young adults and may be associated with ST elevation as a normal variant (*see* Chapter 5).

Tall T Waves

The height of the normal T wave is usually less than 5 mm in the limb leads and less than 10 mm in any precordial lead. T waves that are greater than 6 mm in the limb leads or greater than 10 mm in the precordial leads may occur as follows:

- In V_2 through V_5 in some normal individuals. Note the base of normal peaked T waves is not narrow, as it is with hyperkalemia (*see* Fig. 8.5). Peaked T waves occasionally may be associated with ST elevation occurring as a normal variant; the ST elevation is commonly and inappropriately interpreted as repolarization changes (*see* Chapter 5).
- In patients with severe myocardial ischemia or acute MI (hyperacute T waves may occur).
- In patients with hyperkalemia.
- In patients with left ventricular overload, as in severe mitral regurgitation.
- Occasionally, in patients with cerebrovascular accidents.

U WAVES

Normal U Waves

- The U wave is a very small wave that follows the T wave and is observed only in some individuals. In the normal subject, the U wave is virtually always upright if the T wave is upright.
- The U wave is best visible in leads V_3 and V_2 (looks like the hump on a camel's back). It is barely visible in other leads, and its electrophysiologic source remains uncertain.
- The U wave may merge with the T wave, and the QU interval may be measured, causing a falsely lengthened QT interval.
- The U wave coincides with the phase of supernormal excitability during ventricular recovery, and most ventricular premature beats occur around the time of the U wave.

Causes

U waves are considered large when the amplitude is greater than or equal to 1.5 mm. The causes of prominent U waves include the following:
- Hypokalemia
- Digitalis use
- Quinidine use
- Hypercalcemia
- Intracranial hemorrhage
- Thyrotoxicosis.

Abnormal U Waves

A negative U wave is rarely recorded in normal individuals.
- The most common cause of U wave inversion is severe hypertension, systolic or diastolic overload.
- Rarely, U wave inversion may be the earliest ECG sign of acute coronary syndrome.
- U wave inversion may be the only ECG finding in acute ischemia.
- Exercise-induced transient U wave inversion has been correlated with left anterior descending artery stenosis.

Electrical Axis and Fascicular Block

ELECTRICAL AXIS

The electrical axis is discussed early and extensively in most books on electrocardiogram (ECG) interpretation. Although the electrical axis is an important parameter that should be documented, it provides little or no assistance in the diagnosis of most cardiac conditions, particularly those that require specific therapy.

Determination of the electrical axis is useful mainly in the supporting diagnosis of 4 of the 100 or more diagnoses made from ECG tracings:

1. Left anterior fascicular block (LAFB) (hemiblock).
2. Right ventricular hypertrophy (RVH). Right-axis deviation (RAD) is usually a feature. The electrical axis is of minor assistance in the diagnosis of left ventricular hypertrophy (LVH); left axis is not necessary for the diagnosis of LVH.
3. Ventricular tachycardia (VT). Some forms of VT are associated with left-axis deviation (LAD) or an axis in "no man's land", but RAD may occur in some.
4. Left posterior fascicular block (LPFB). Criteria for the diagnosis of LPFB are imprecise and unreliable.

Figure 9.1 shows the vectorial genesis of the QRS complex and axis. The addition of all the vectors of ventricular depolarization produces one large mean QRS vector. The QRS axis represents the direction of the mean QRS vector in the frontal plane. The electrical axis is determined by using the hexaxial reference system, which was derived from Einthoven's equilateral triangle (Figs. 9.2A to C).

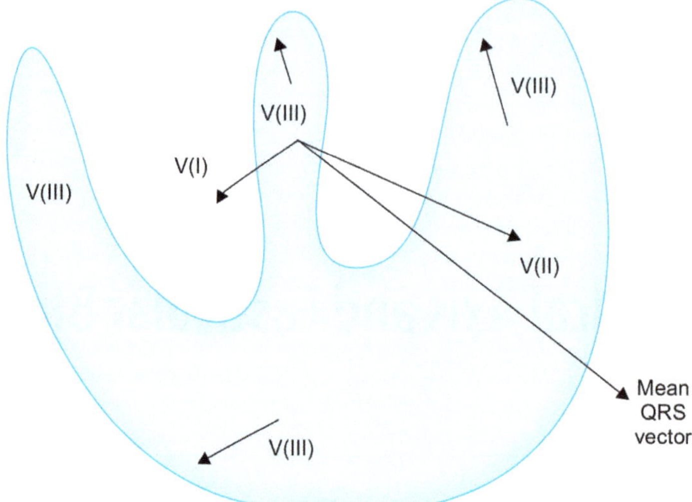

Fig. 9.1: The mean QRS vector.

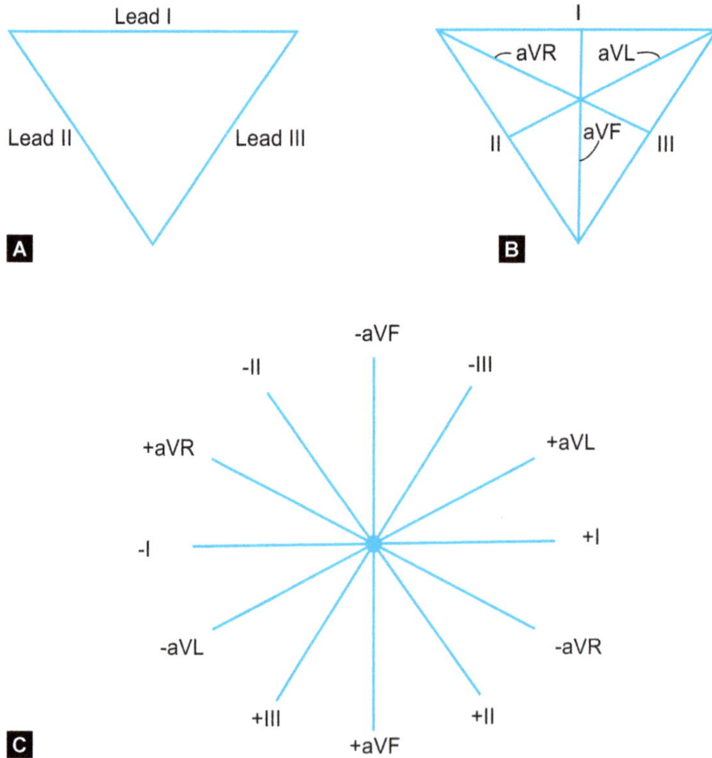

Figs. 9.2A to C: (A) Einthoven's equilateral triangle formed by leads I, II, and III; (B) The unipolar limb leads are added to the equilateral triangle; (C) The hexaxial reference system derived from (B).

Because of the minor contribution of the electrical axis to clinical cardiologic diagnosis, this topic is discussed late in this text and is relegated to Step 9 in the 11-step method for accurate ECG diagnosis. *See* Figures 9.3A and B, Table 9.1, and instructions given in Chapter 2 for the determination of the electrical axis.

- The range of the electrical axis in the majority of normal adults older than the age of 40 years is −30° to +90° (*see* Figs. 9.3A and B); for those younger than age 40, the range is 0° to +105°. Normal children may have an axis of up to +110°. Most normal individuals have values between +30° and +75°.

Left-axis Deviation

An axis of −15° to ~−30°, which is relatively normal for individuals older than the age of 40 years, is sometimes termed leftward axis to distinguish it from LAD. An axis of −30° to −45° is termed LAD (Fig. 9.4).

Causes

- Normal variation

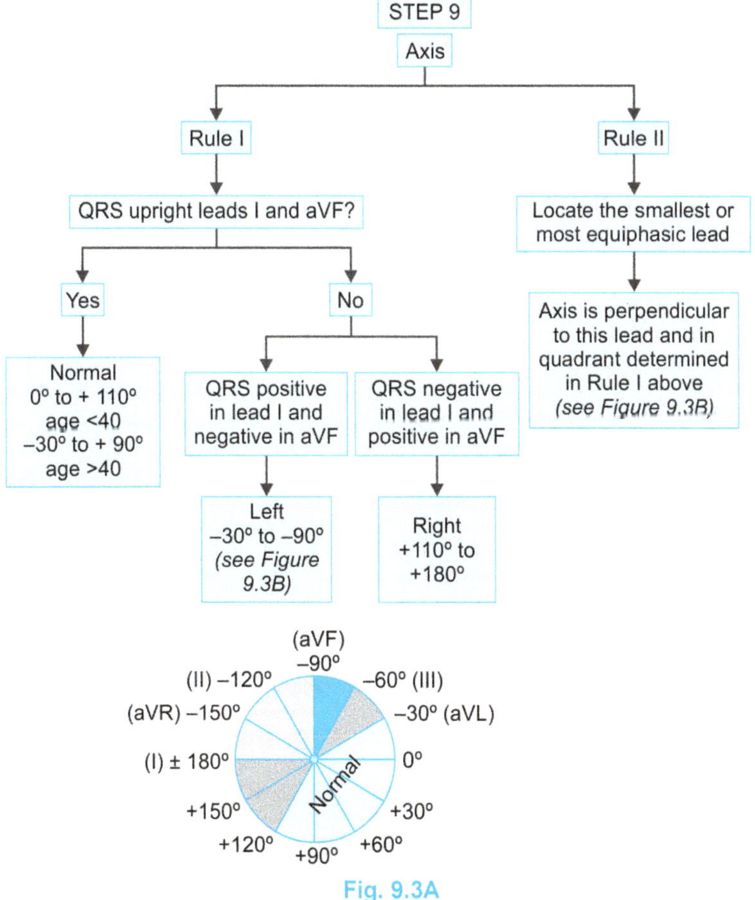

Fig. 9.3A

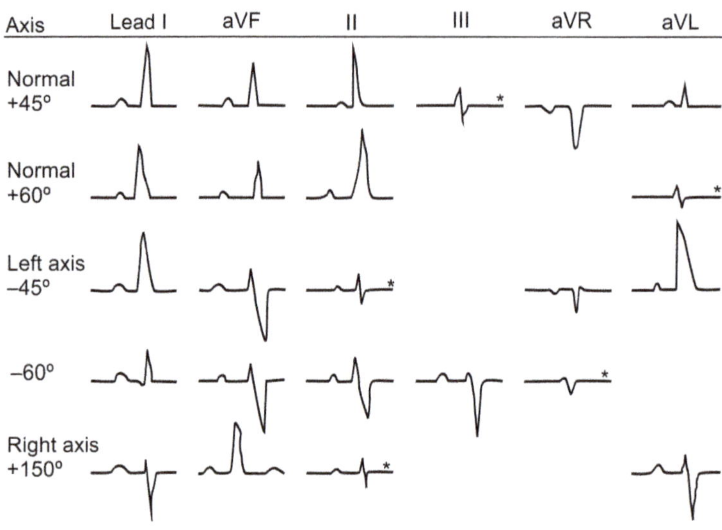

Fig. 9.3B

Figs. 9.3A and B: Step-by-step method for accurate ECG interpretation. (A) Step 9: detection of the electrical axis. Leads are indicated in parentheses. *See* Table 9.1; (B) *See* Table 9.1, and figures. 9.4 and 9.5. *Most equiphasic lead

TABLE 9.1: Electrical axis.		
Most equiphasic lead	*Lead perpendicular**	*Axis*
		Leads I and aVF positive = normal axis
III	aVR	Normal = +30°
aVL	II	Normal = +60°
		Lead I positive and aVF negative = left axis
II	aVL (QRS positive)	Left = −30°
aVR	III (QRS negative)	Left = −60°
I	aVF (QRS negative)	Left = −90°
		Lead I negative and aVF positive = right axis
aVR	III (QRS positive)	Right = +120°
II	aVL (QRS negative)	Right = +150°

*Lead perpendicular (at right angle) to the most equiphasic (isoelectric) lead usually has the tallest R or deepest S wave.

- Left anterior fascicular block (hemiblock)
- Left bundle branch block
- Left ventricular hypertrophy

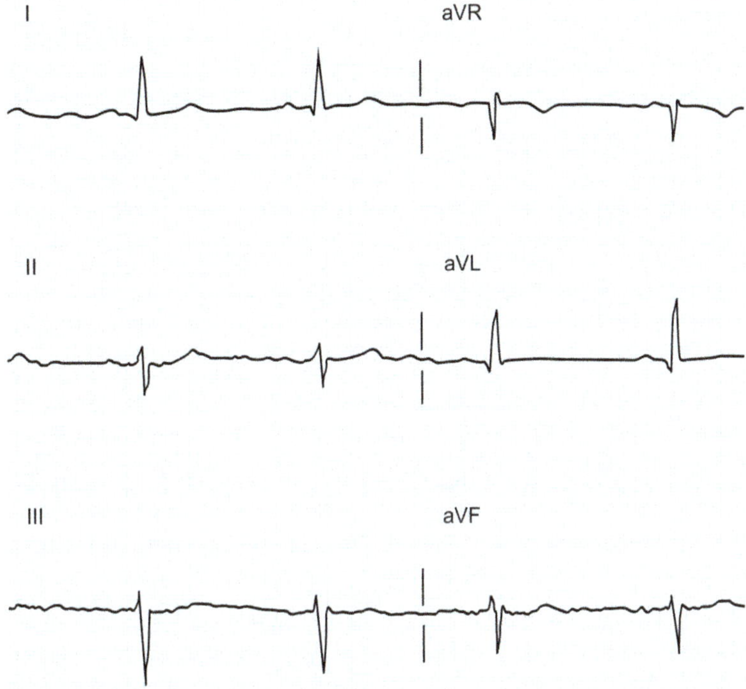

Fig. 9.4: Left-axis deviation −45°; lead II is the most equiphasic QRS; aVL is perpendicular and lies at −30°; aVR is the next most equiphasic; lead III is perpendicular at −60°; therefore, the axis that lies between = −45° (*see* Fig. 9.3B).

- Mechanical shifts causing a horizontal heart; high diaphragm; pregnancy, ascites
- Some forms of VT
- Endocardial cushion defects and other congenital heart disease.

Right-axis Deviation

Criteria for RAD in adults include an axis of +100° to +180° (Figs. 9.5A and B).

Causes

- Normal variation
- Right ventricular hypertrophy
- Left posterior fascicular block
- Lateral myocardial infarction (MI)
- Pulmonary embolism
- Dextrocardia
- *Normal variants*: Mechanical shifts or emphysema causing a vertical heart.

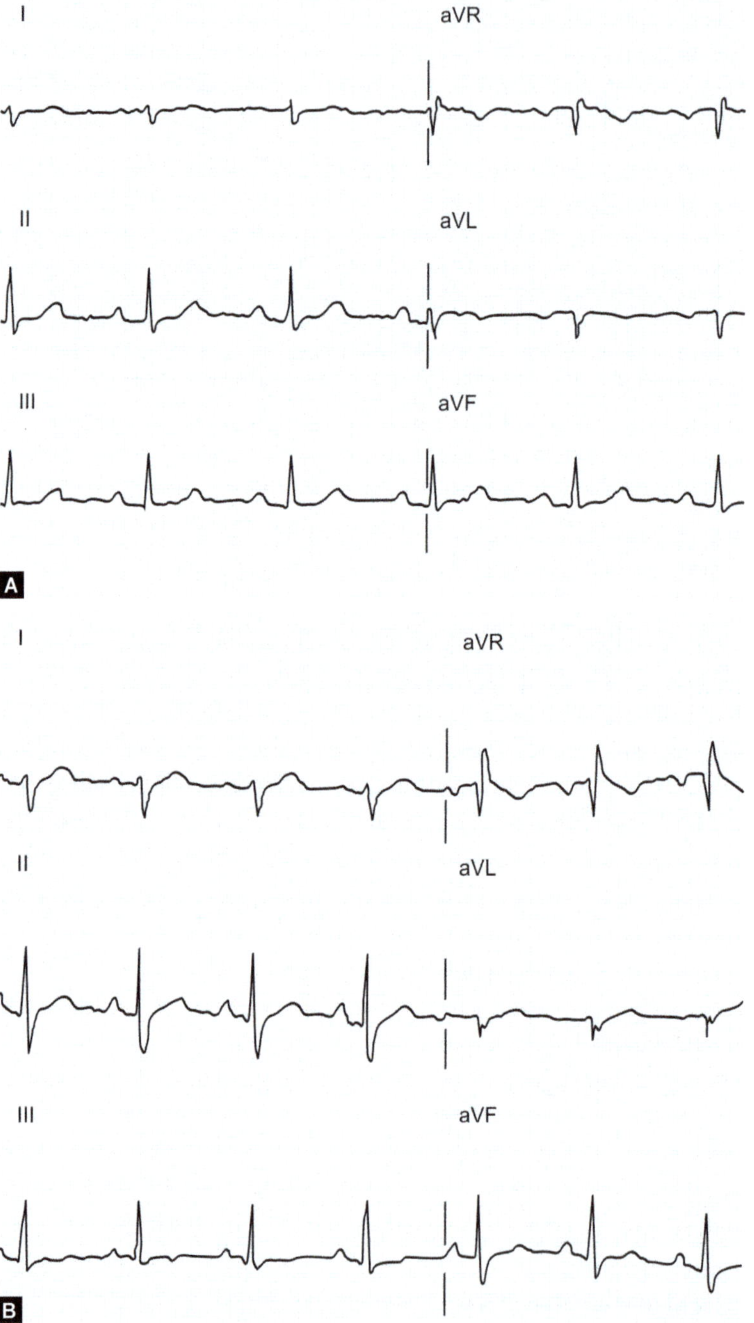

Figs. 9.5A and B: (A) Right-axis deviation; QRS axis +110°; lead I is the most equiphasic; aVF is perpendicular at +90°; aVR is the next most equiphasic, with lead III being perpendicular at +120°. The exact axis lies somewhere between +90° and +120° (i.e. at +110°). Patient is older than 40 years of age; (B) Right-axis deviation. ECG from a 26-year-old healthy man.

FASCICULAR BLOCK

Left Anterior Fascicular Block (Left Anterior Hemiblock)

Division of the left bundle branch into: (1) the anterior and (2) posterior fascicles (Fig. 9.6). The anterior fascicle traverses an anterosuperior course and ends at the base of the anterior papillary muscle. The anterior fascicle is thin and long, has a single blood supply, and is commonly damaged by ischemic-disease fibrosis and other pathologic processes, resulting in LAFB. Rosenbaum initially called the block, left anterior hemiblock (LAH), and many cardiologists use it rather than LAFB.

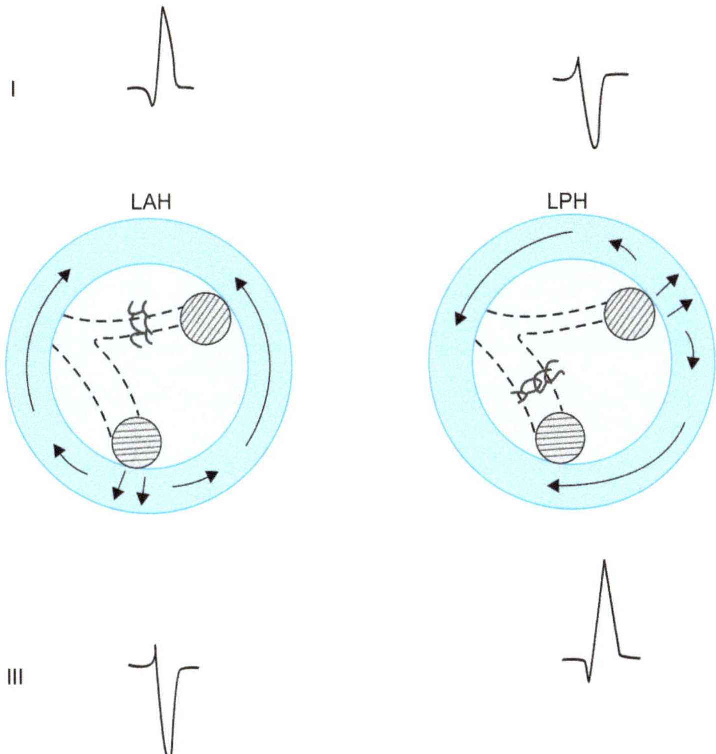

Fig. 9.6: Hemiblock patterns in the limb leads: left anterior hemiblock (LAH) and left posterior hemiblock (LPH). The "anterior" papillary muscle is above and lateral to the "posterior" papillary muscle, and the two divisions of the left bundle branch course toward their respective papillary muscles. Thus, if the anterior division is blocked, initial electromotive forces are directed downward and to the right, inscribing a small Q wave in leads I and aVL and an S wave in leads II, III, and aVF. The subsequent forces are directed mainly upward and to the left, writing an R wave in I and aVL and an S in II, III, and aVF, to produce a left-axis deviation. In LPH, the initial forces spread upward and to the left to write an R in I and aVL and a small Q in II, III, and aVF while subsequent forces are directed downward and to the right to produce right-axis deviation.
Source: Adapted with permission from Marriott JL. Practical Electrocardiography, 8th edition. Baltimore: Williams & Wilkins; 1988.

Diagnostic Criteria

- Left-axis deviation, −45° to −90° (preferably −60° to −90°).
- A small q wave, 0.5 to less than 2 mm deep in lead I, qR in I (Fig. 9.7).
- A small r wave, 1–4 mm tall in lead III, rS in III.
- A normal QRS duration, provided right bundle branch block (RBBB) or other conduction defects are absent (other fascicles conduct normally; thus, depolarization of the ventricles is not delayed).

Figure 9.6 shows how the ECG configuration of LAFB is derived. With block of the anterior fascicle, depolarization starts at the posterior papillary muscle and inferior wall and proceeds upward, superiorly and to the left to activate the left ventricular muscle mass that lies above the papillary muscle. Thus, the electrical axis is directed strongly to the left at −60° to −90°. Because the electrical impulse originating from the posterior papillary muscle travels initially downward from endocardium to epicardium, it registers a small r wave of less than 4 mm in lead III.

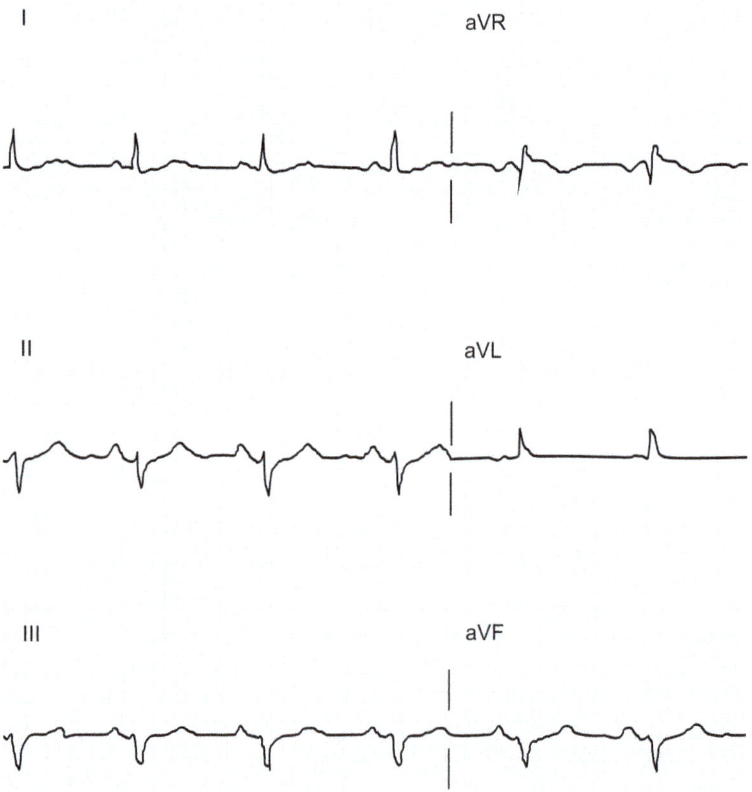

Fig. 9.7: Left-axis deviation −60°. There is a small q wave in lead I and a small r wave in lead III. These are the criteria for the diagnosis of left anterior fascicular block: borderline ECG.

The small impulse is directed away from lead I and thus causes a small q wave in lead I. The current then travels upward to the left and causes an r wave in lead I and an s wave in lead III, because electrical impulse travels away from the inferior leads (*see* Figs. 9.4 and 9.6).

Causes

- Acute or chronic ischemic heart disease
- Cardiomyopathy and specific heart muscle disease
- Chagas disease
- Myocarditis.
  Left anterior fascicular block is a normal finding in approximately 1% of men older than age 40 years.

Pitfalls in Diagnosis of Left Anterior Fascicular Block

- *Acute or old MI:* When LAFB occurs during acute inferior MI, the initial small r wave caused by LAFB in leads II, III, and aVF masks the Q wave of infarction.
- *Hypertensive heart disease:* LAFB lowers the QRS voltage in the precordial leads and may mask LVH; conversely, LAFB increases QRS voltage in the limb leads and may mimic LVH.

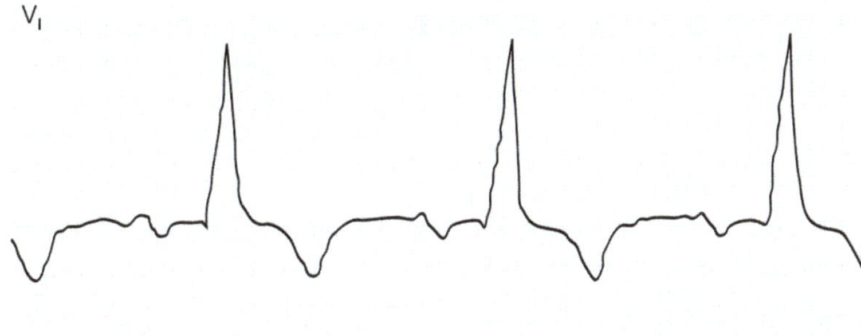

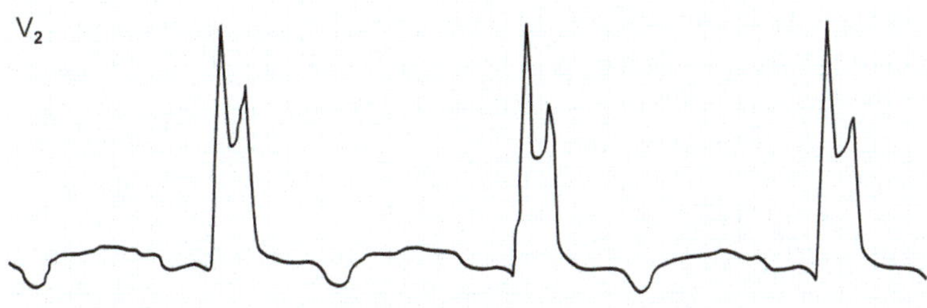

Fig. 9.8A

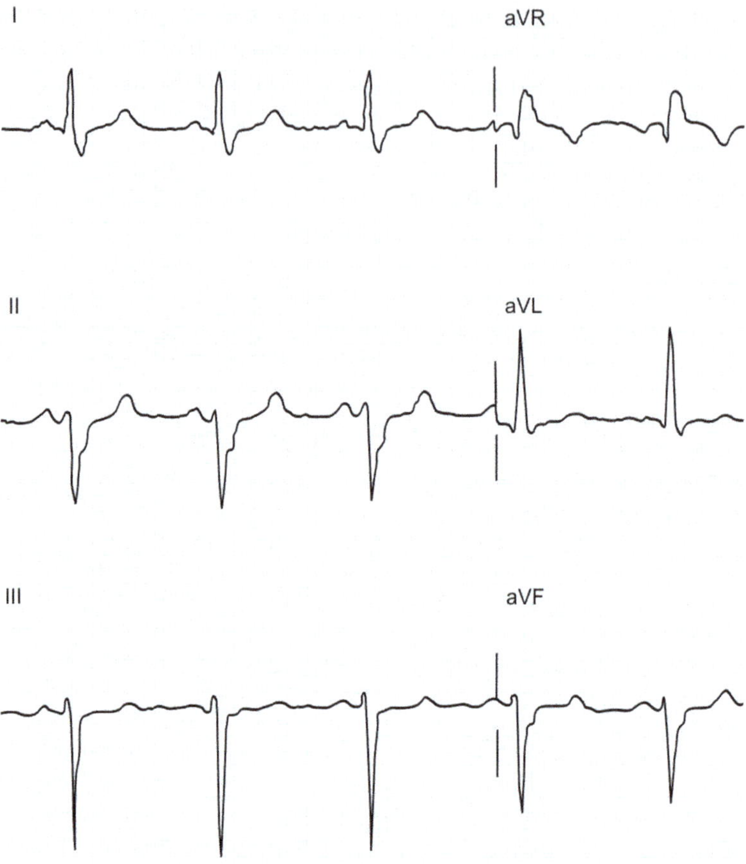

Fig. 9.8B

Figs. 9.8A and B: (A) V leads from a patient with right bundle branch block (RBBB); (B) Features of left anterior fascicular block (LAFB). The QRS axis is −75° with a small Q wave in lead I and a small R wave in lead III, which is in keeping with LAFB. Diagnosis: bifascicular block: RBBB and LAFB.

Left Posterior Fascicular Block

Left posterior fascicular block or left posterior hemiblock occurs rarely, because the posterior bundle is thick and short and has a double blood supply. The fascicle runs to the base of the posterior papillary muscle (*see* Fig. 9.6). The diagnosis can be made only after excluding RVH and chronic obstructive pulmonary disease (COPD). The following are criteria for the diagnosis of LPFB:

- Right-axis deviation, +120° to +180° (*See* Fig. 9.9B).
- A small r wave less than 4 mm in leads I and aVL and an S wave (mainly negative) in lead I (*See* Fig. 9.9B)
- A small q wave in lead II or III
- A normal QRS duration
- Absence of RVH or cor pulmonale, COPD, a vertical heart, and other causes of RAD (thus, a confident diagnosis of LPFB is not often made).

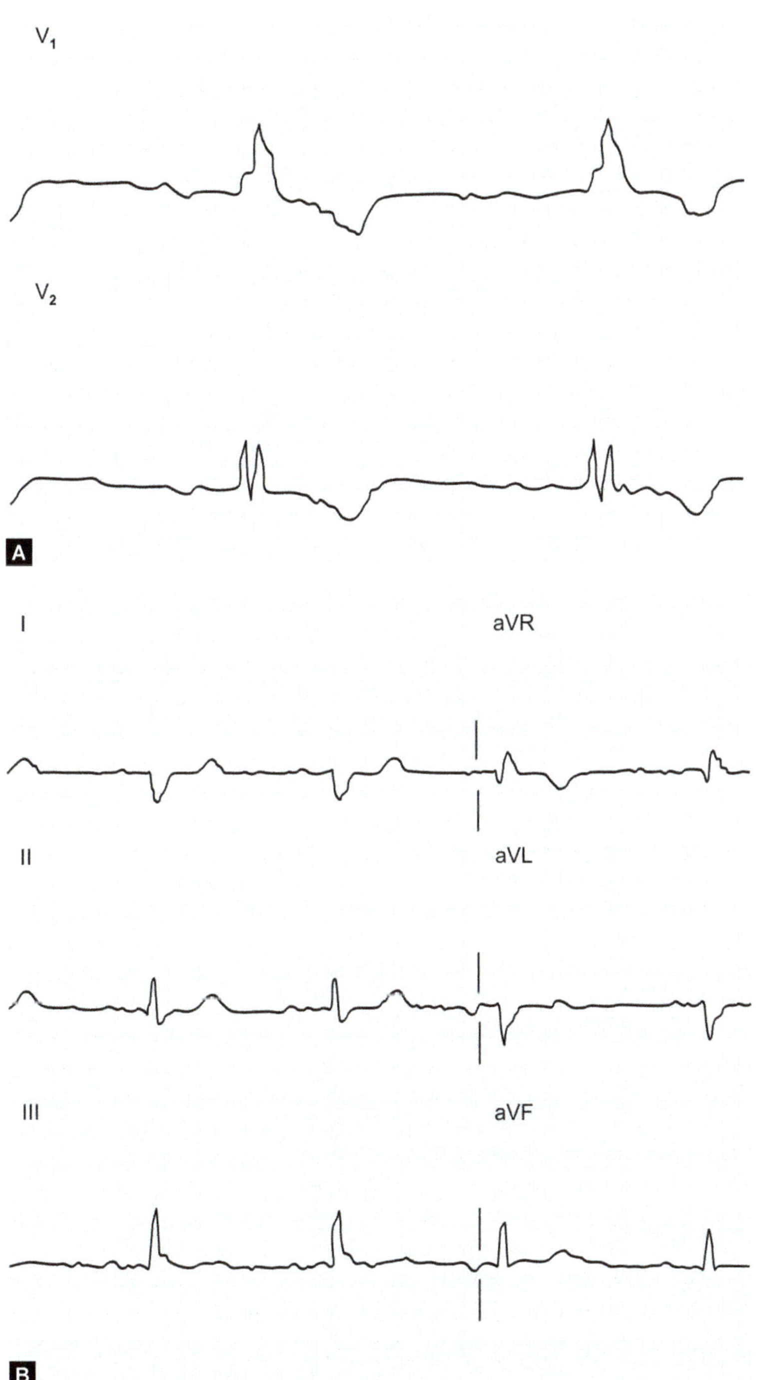

Figs. 9.9A and B: (A) Tracing of a patient with right bundle branch block and left posterior fascicular block: bifascicular block; (B) Left posterior fascicular block.

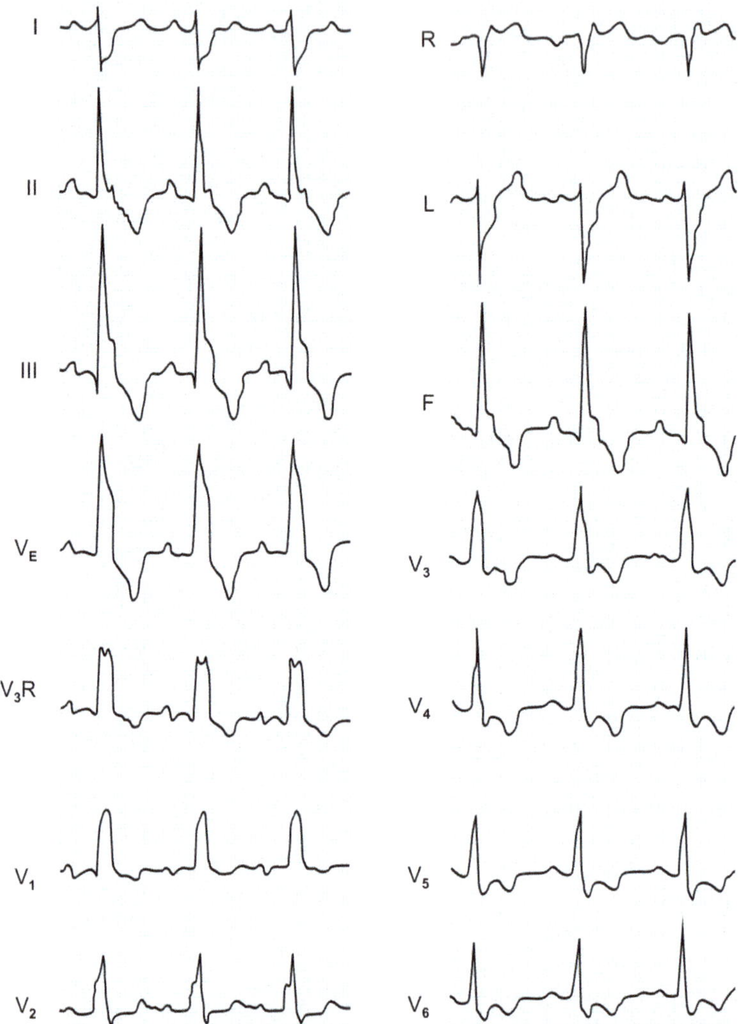

Fig. 9.10: Left posterior hemiblock. Note the right-axis deviation, the small r in leads I and aVL, and the small q in lead II. Complete right bundle branch block is also present in this patient.
Source: Adapted with permission from Wellens JJ, Conover MB. The ECG in Emergency Decision Making, Philadelphia: WB Saunders, Elsevier Science; 1992.

Bifascicular Block

- The combination of LAFB and RBBB occurs commonly (Figs. 9.8A and B), but rarely progresses to serious block; thus, pacing is rarely required.
- The combination of LPFB and RBBB occurs rarely. Figure 9.9A shows RBBB. Figure 9.9B shows a tiny initial R wave in leads I and aVL, and small q in lead II in keeping with left posterior hemiblock.
- Other examples of axis changes and hemiblock are given in Figure 9.10.

Miscellaneous Conditions

INTRODUCTION

After a methodical assessment of the P waves, the QRS duration for bundle branch blocks (left and right), the ST segment, Q waves, hypertrophy, and the electrical axis has been completed, an assessment for miscellaneous conditions is appropriate. A search for miscellaneous conditions is logically performed at Step 10 (Fig. 10.1).

The electrocardiogram (ECG) may reveal clues to the diagnosis of twelve or more miscellaneous conditions:

1. Atrial septal defect (ASD)
2. Acute pericarditis
3. Long QT interval
4. Hypokalemia
5. Hyperkalemia
6. Digitalis toxicity
7. Dextrocardia
8. Electrical alternans

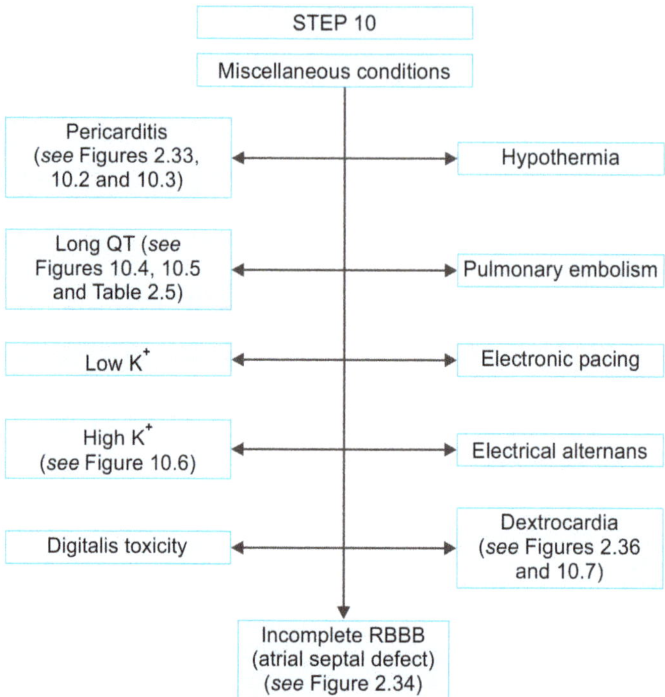

Fig. 10.1: Step-by-step method for accurate ECG interpretation. Step 10: assess for miscellaneous conditions. (RBBB, right bundle branch block)

9. Electronic pacing
10. Pulmonary embolism (PE) (the ECG is not diagnostic)
11. Hypothermia and hyperthermia
12. Hypercalcemia and hypocalcemia.

ATRIAL SEPTAL DEFECT

Incomplete right bundle branch block (RBBB) is a common and well-known finding in ASD (*see* Fig. 2.34).

A New Diagnostic Sign

Incomplete RBBB is a well-known finding in many patients with ASD. A characteristic "crochetage" on the R wave of leads II, III, and aVF has been reported. A "crochetage" was reported on the R wave tracing in inferior limb leads II, III, and aVF and the incomplete bundle branch block pattern in the V_1 lead on the ECG before operation (electro-cardiographic tracings from a 16-year-old girl with an ASD and partial anomalous venous return).

Three days after ASD surgical repair, the crochetage pattern disappeared, whereas the incomplete right bundle branch block pattern persisted.

PERICARDITIS

Diagnostic Criteria

- *Stage 1:* Widespread ST segment elevation, generally upwardly concave in all leads except aVR and occasionally V_1. ST segment elevation may persist for a few days (Figs. 10.2 and 10.3). Reciprocal ST segment depression occurs in aVR and sometimes in V_1 (*see* Figs. 10.2 and 10.3). The PR segment is elevated in aVR, and PR segment depression generally occurs in all leads except occasionally V_1.
- *Stage 2:* A few days later, the ST and PR segments become normal (isoelectric); the T wave remains normal or may be decreased in amplitude and may become flattened.
- *Stage 3:* After normalization of the ST segment, diffuse T wave inversion occurs.
- *Stage 4:* This stage lasts from days to weeks. The T waves normalize; rarely do they remain inverted.

Other Clues Suggestive of Acute Pericarditis

- Early PR segment depression, particularly in leads II, aVF, and V_4 through V_6, is suggestive of pericarditis.
- Sinus tachycardia may be the only finding if ST segment elevation has resolved and the T waves remain normal.

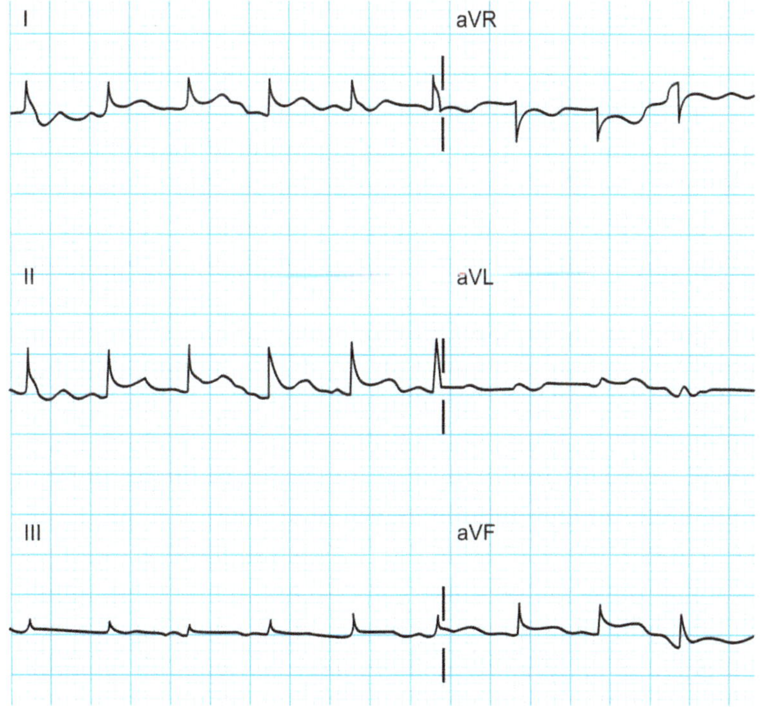

Fig. 10.2A

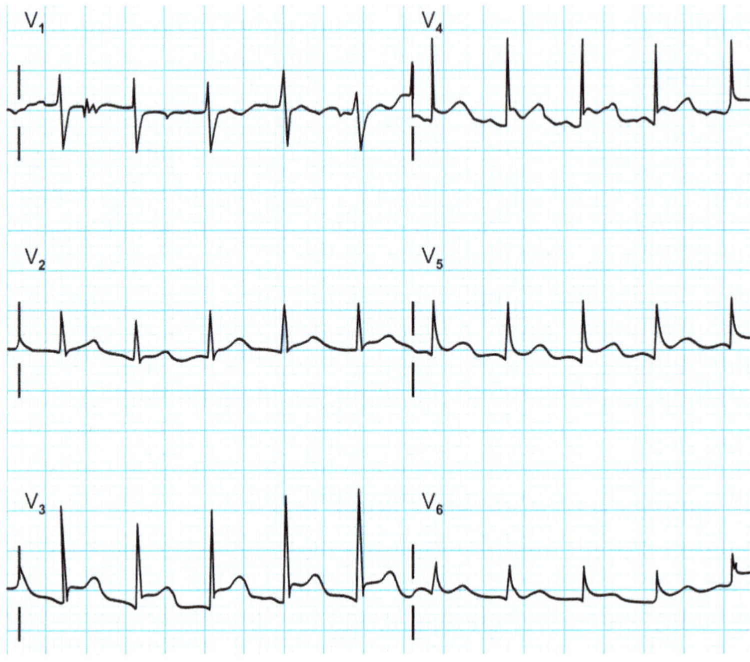

Figs. 10.2A and B: Widespread ST segment elevation, generally upwardly concave in all leads except aVR and V$_1$: acute pericarditis.

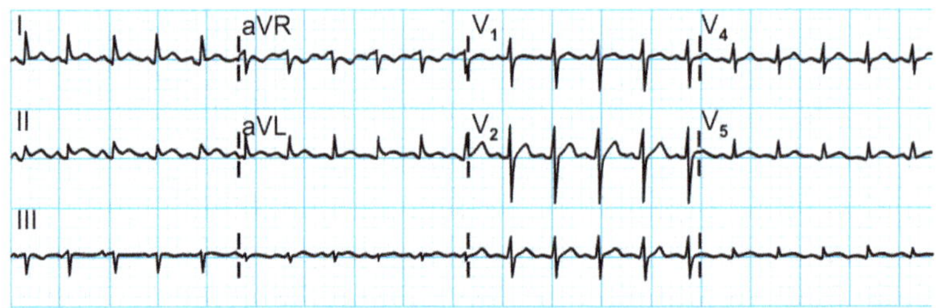

Fig. 10.3: Characteristic features of acute pericarditis: ST segment elevation in most leads: I, II, aVL, aVF, V$_5$, and V$_6$, with reciprocal ST depression and PR segment elevation in aVR. In addition, note sinus tachycardia commonly seen with acute pericarditis.

- Electrical alternans usually involves the QRS complex. Total alternans with involvement of the P, QRS, and T waves may occur with cardiac tamponade.
- Low-voltage QRS may occur when pericardial fluid accumulates.

LONG QT INTERVAL

The QT interval indicates the total duration of ventricular systole. A prolonged QT interval represents delayed repolarization of the ventricles and predisposes to re-entrant arrhythmias, such as torsades de pointes.

Diagnostic Criteria

- A rough guideline to remember is that the QT interval should be less than half the preceding RR interval at heart rates of 60–100 beats/minute.
- The QT interval varies with heart rate, and several formulas have been used to provide a corrected QT interval (QTc).
- The QTc also has limitations because of difficulties with obtaining exact measurements. Because it is difficult sometimes to define the end of the T wave, the measurement is often inaccurate, particularly when a U wave merges with the T. Thus, in clinical practice, the QT interval should be assessed mainly for excessive prolongation, using a lead that does not show a U wave (Figs. 10.4 and 10.5).
- See Table 2.5 for a clinically useful approximation of QT intervals.

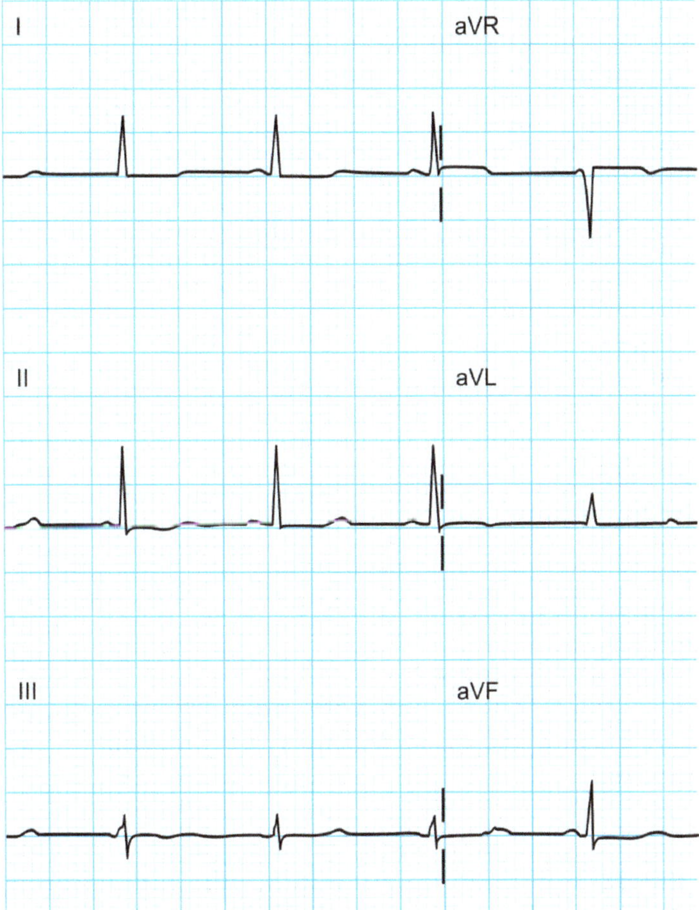

Fig. 10.4: QT interval 0.46 second; the heart rate is 67 bpm. The normal range of a QT interval at a heart rate of 67–100 bpm is 0.33–0.42 second (*see* Table 2.5).

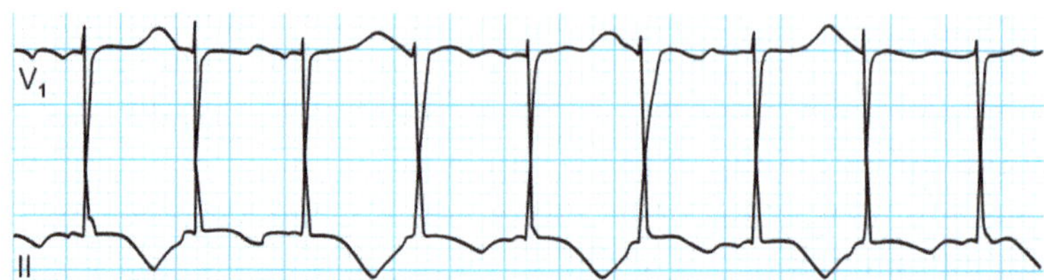

Fig. 10.5: The QT interval is prolonged, measuring approximately 600 milliseconds, with T wave alternans. The tracing was recorded in a patient with chronic renal disease shortly after dialysis.
Source: Adapted with permission from Braunwald E. Heart Disease: A Textbook of Cardiovascular Medicine, 5th edition. Philadelphia: WB Saunders, Elsevier Science, 1997.

Causes

A prolonged QT interval may be caused by the following:
- Drugs
  - Class 1 antiarrhythmics (e.g. disopyramide, procainamide, quinidine)
  - Class 3 antiarrhythmics (e.g. amiodarone, sotalol)
- Tricyclic antidepressants
  - Phenothiazines
  - Astemizole
  - Terfenadine
  - Adenosine
  - Antibiotics (e.g. erythromycin and other macrolides)
  - Antifungal agents
  - Pentamidine, chloroquine
- Ischemic heart disease
- Cerebrovascular disease
- Rheumatic fever
- Myocarditis
- Mitral valve prolapse
- Electrolyte abnormalities
- Hypocalcemia
- Hypothyroidism
- Liquid protein diets
- Organophosphate insecticides
- Congenital prolonged QT syndrome.
  A short QT interval is not of great concern and occurs rarely with the following:
- Hypercalcemia, a feature of malignancy and hyperparathyroidism
- Digitalis intoxication.

HYPOKALEMIA

Diagnostic Criteria

- *Progressive ST segment depression:* A small U wave normally has the same polarity as the T wave; when the serum potassium level falls to less than 3.5 mEq/L, the amplitude of the T wave decreases.

- A marked increase in U wave amplitude with potassium less than 3 mEq/L: the U wave becomes taller than the T wave: with serum potassium less than 1.5 mEq/ L, the T and the U wave may become fused. The changes are seen best in leads V_2 through V_5 (Figs. 10.4 and 10.5).
- K^+ *greater than 5.7 mEq/L:* Earliest signs are T wave peaked and narrow base (tented); PR interval may be prolonged.
- K^+ *greater than 7 mEq/L:* P wave flat or absent; QRS widens; prominent S wave.
- K^+ *greater than 8 mEq/L:* S wave becomes wider and deeper and moves steeply into the T wave; there is virtually no isoelectric ST segment; occasionally ST segment elevation.
- ST segment depression.
- An increase in the QRS duration.
- Slight prolongation of the PR interval.

HYPERKALEMIA

Diagnostic Criteria

- *Mild hyperkalemia:* At a serum potassium level of approximately 5.7–6.5 mEq/L, the P wave widens; tall, peaked, narrow-based, "tented" T waves appear in many leads; and first-degree atrioventricular (AV) block occurs (*see* Figs. 10.6A to C).
- *Severe hyperkalemia:* At a serum potassium level greater than 6.5 mEq/L, the second portion of the QRS complex shows significant widening, which may show notching or slurring, and thus the wide QRS merges with the tall, tented T waves. The ST segment may be elevated.
- *High-degree AV block:* P waves disappear.
- Ventricular tachycardia (VT), ventricular fibrillation (VF), or idioventricular rhythm.

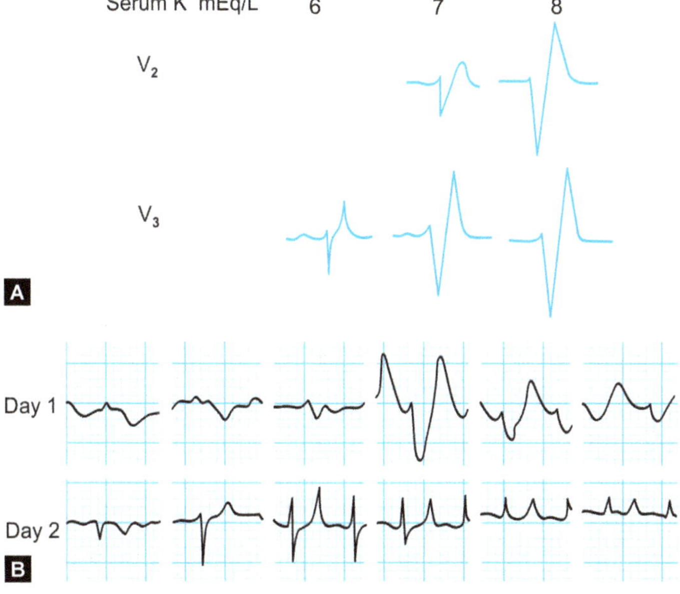

Figs. 10.6A and B

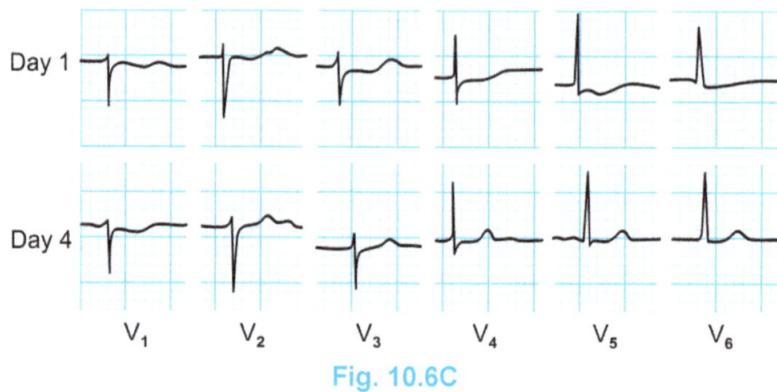

Fig. 10.6C

Figs. 10.6A to C: ECG signs of hyperkalemia.

DIGITALIS

Digitalis Effect

Digitalis effect revealed by the ECG does not imply toxicity and is suggested by the following:
- Sagging ST segment depression with upward concavity
- Decreased amplitude of T wave, which may be biphasic
- Shortening of the QT interval
- Prolonged PR interval; first-degree AV block
- Increased amplitude of the U wave.

Digitalis Toxicity

Digitalis toxicity is suggested by the occurrence of almost any type of arrhythmia or conduction defect, with the exception of bundle branch block.

Common arrhythmias include the following:
- Excitant disturbances such as ventricular premature beats (VPBs), especially bigeminy and multifocal VPBs; atrial tachycardia; AV junctional tachycardia; accelerated junctional rhythm; VT; bidirectional tachycardia; and VF.
- Suppressant disturbances such as sinus bradycardia, first-degree AV block, second-degree AV block, Mobitz type I (Wenckebach) block, and complete AV block.
- Combined disturbances such as atrial tachycardia with AV block [i.e. paroxysmal atrial tachycardia (PAT) with block] and regular, accelerated junctional rhythm in the presence of atrial fibrillation.

DEXTROCARDIA: TRUE DEXTROCARDIA (WITH SITUS INVERSUS)

Diagnostic Criteria

- In lead I, the P, QRS, and T waves are inverted or upside down (Figs. 10.7A and B).
- Leads aVR and aVL are reversed (aVL is now aVR); thus, prominent negative deflections are recorded in aVL with positive deflections in aVR.
- Lead II represents the usual lead III and vice versa.

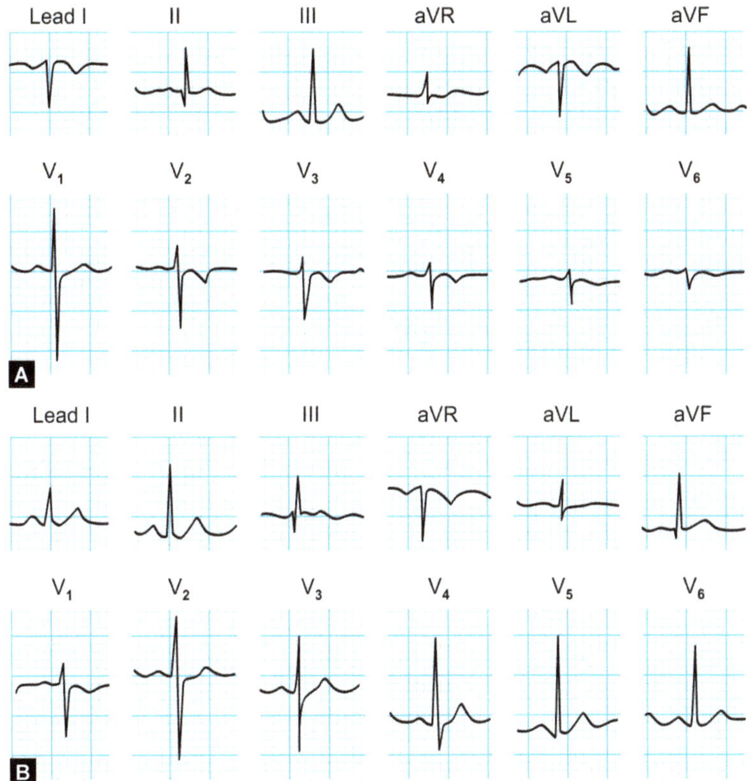

Figs. 10.7A and B: Mirror-image dextrocardia with situs inversus. The patient is a 15-year-old girl. There is no evidence of organic heart disease. (A) Tracing recorded with the conventional electrode placement; (B) Tracing obtained with the left and right arm electrodes reversed. The precordial lead electrodes also were relocated in the respective mirror-image positions on the chest. The tracing is within normal limits.
Source: Adapted with permission from Chou TC. Electrocardiography in Clinical Practice, 4th edition. Philadelphia: WB Saunders, Elsevier Science; 1996.

- Lead aVF is unaffected.
- There is decreasing R wave amplitude from leads V_1 through V_6. V_1 is the equivalent of the usual V_2 and vice versa.

Diagnostic Confirmation

The ECG should be repeated with the right and left arm leads reversed. Placing the V leads in the equivalent positions on the right side of the chest is necessary for accurate interpretation of the ECG.

Diagnostic Pitfalls

- *Incorrect arm lead placement:* Reversal of the arm leads can produce similar recordings in leads I, aVR, and aVL as observed with true dextrocardia but not in V_1 through V_6. A tip off to this error is the normal R wave progression in V_2 to V_6 and the marked dissimilarity of the record in leads I (negative complex) and V_6 with a normal amplitude R wave.

- Isolated dextrocardia without situs inversus invariably is associated with complicated cardiac malformations and is rarely seen in adults.
- In dextroposition, the heart is displaced to the right by lung disease. The ECG is normal, but R waves are prominent in V_1 through V_3 and decrease in amplitude from V_2 through V_6 (*See* Figs. 10.7A and B).
- *Dextroposition*: The heart and mediastinum are displaced to the right side of the chest usually because of a hypoplastic right lung case. In the ECG, the limb leads are normal except for a relatively large R wave in lead II and S wave in lead aVR. The precordial leads show:
  - Tall R waves in leads V_1 through V_3
  - The amplitude of the R waves decreases from V_2 through V_6.

ELECTRICAL ALTERNANS

- Electrical alternans refers to regular alternation in the amplitude, direction, or configuration of the QRS complexes in any or all leads. The RR intervals remain unchanged (regular).
- Total electrical alternans refers to involvement of the P, QRS, and T waves and occasionally the U wave.

Causes

- Alternans of the QRS complex is rare in patients with cardiac tamponade and occurs in some patients with a large pericardial effusion, particularly with malignancy.
- Total electrical alternans is almost diagnostic of cardiac tamponade, although it occurs in fewer than 10% of patients with tamponade and may be associated with a "swinging heart" on echocardiography.
- Severe coronary artery and hypertrophic heart disease is a rare cause of electrical alternans.
- Supraventricular tachycardia with a very rapid ventricular rate, mainly occurring in patients with Wolff-Parkinson-White syndrome (orthodromic) re-entrant tachycardia, is another cause.

ELECTRONIC PACING

Ventricular Pacing

- The pacemaker impulse, a sharp narrow spike, is followed by a QRS complex of different morphology than the intrinsic QRS. With right ventricular pacing, the QRS complex is similar to that of left bundle branch block.
- With left ventricular epicardial myocardial pacing, the QRS shows a RBBB morphology.
- Pacemakers in a "unipolar pacing mode" cause a larger amplitude spike than that of bipolar pacing.

Ventricular Demand Pacing (VVI)

Pacing output is inhibited by sensed ventricular signal.

Atrial Pacing

Pacemaker spike is followed by P wave and narrow paced QRS complexes in response to paced atrial beat (Fig. 10.8).

Atrial Demand Pacing (AAI)

Pacing output is inhibited by sensed atrial signal.

Atrioventricular Sequential Pacing

- Atrial followed by ventricular pacing.
- Could be pacing in both atrium and ventricle; senses R waves only (DVI pacing mode).
- Pacing in and senses both atrium and ventricle (DDD mode); synchronizes with atrial activity and paces ventricle after preset AV interval.
- Output inhibited by sensed atrial signal (AAI) and by sensed ventricular signal (VVI), but tracking of atrial rate by ventricular sensing does not occur (DDI pacing mode).

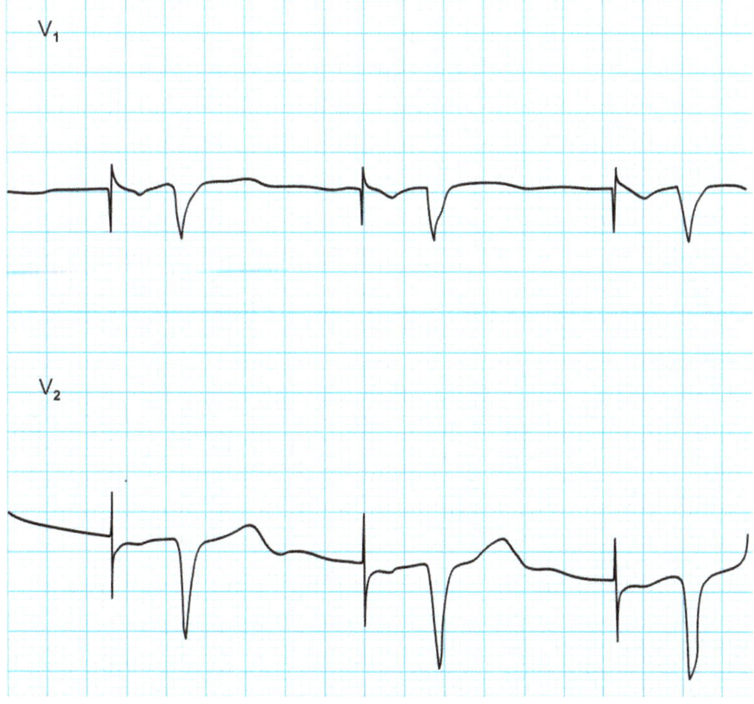

Fig. 10.8: Electronic pacemaker, atrial pacing; rate = 70 bpm.

- Fixed-rate (asynchronous) atrial and ventricular pacing at specific AV interval (DOO pacing mode).

Pacemaker Malfunction

Undersensing Malfunction

For a pacemaker in the inhibited mode, undersensing is diagnosed on ECG by a pacemaker spike at an inappropriately short interval after a spontaneous (intrinsic) event [i.e. a failure of the pacemaker to be inhibited by an appropriate intrinsic atrial or ventricular depolarization (QRS)]. Figure 10.9 shows accurate sensing. With sensing malfunction, the pacemaker operates like a fixed-rate pacemaker; the spontaneous intrinsic QRS complexes are not sensed.

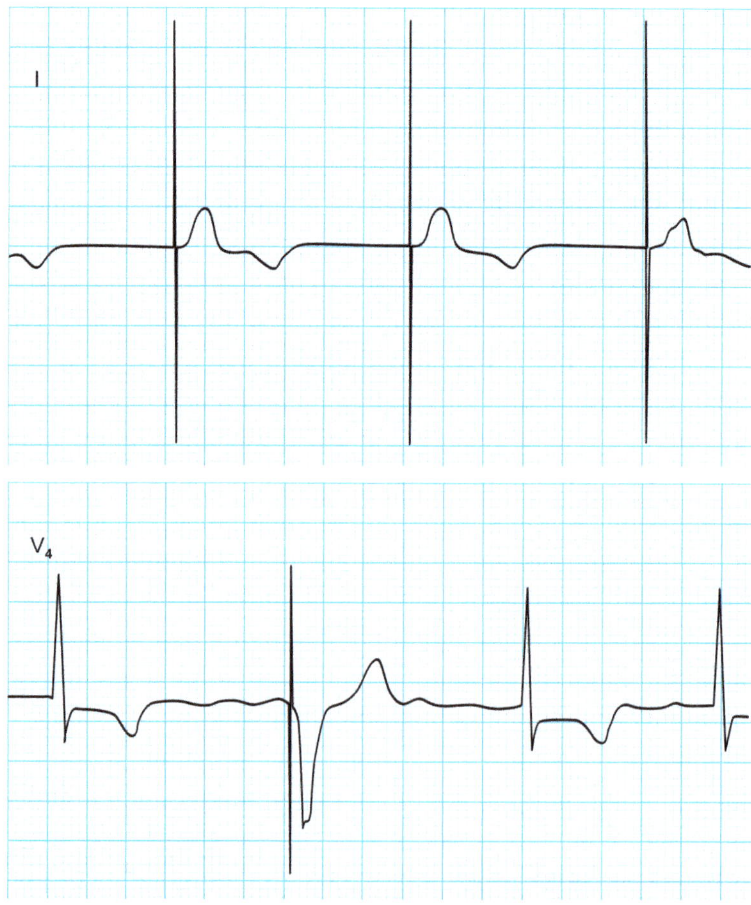

Fig. 10.9: Electronic pacemaker, demand mode; ventricular capture rate = 75 bpm. Note the spontaneous beat in V$_4$ is followed by sensing and pacemaker capture at the appropriate interval, which is equal to that shown in lead I. The pacemaker output is inhibited appropriately in response to the intrinsic QRS complex (the first beat in lead V$_4$).

Pacing Malfunction

- *Not firing:* Failure of appropriate pacemaker output, which may be caused by failure of the pacemaker impulse to depolarize the ventricle because of inadequate voltage output from the pulse generator, a broken lead wire, or electrode displacement.
- A ventricular demand pacemaker with sensing malfunction will show the pacemaker operates like a fixed-rate pacemaker. The spontaneous ventricular beats are not sensed.
- *Battery power failure:* Indicated by a decrease of the pacing rate.

PULMONARY EMBOLISM

The ECG findings are nonspecific; more importantly, the transient occurrence of the following should heighten clinical suspicion of PE:

- Sinus tachycardia
- Symmetrical T wave inversion; strain pattern in leads V_1 through V_3 or V_4
- ST depression in leads I, II, and V_3 through V_6
- S1Q3 or S1Q3T3 pattern
- Incomplete or complete RBBB pattern
- Q waves in leads V_1, III, and aVF but not in lead II
- QR in V_1
- ST segment elevation in leads V_1 through V_2 or V_3, aVR, and III may occur.
- ST segment depression in V_3 through V_5 or V_6 because of associated myocardial ischemia
- S1, S2, S3 pattern
- Arrhythmias that include premature beats, atrial flutter or atrial fibrillation, and VF
- Right atrial enlargement
- Right-axis deviation.

In the presence of submassive PE, the ECG may show no significant abnormality. With massive PE causing syncope, cardiogenic shock, or acute right-sided heart failure, at least two of the preceding ECG changes usually occur.

BIBLIOGRAPHY

1. Heller J, Hagege AA, Besse B, et al. "Crochetage" (notch) on R wave in inferior limb leads: a new independent electrocardiographic sign of atrial septal defect. J Am Coll Cardiol. 1996;27(4):877-82.

Arrhythmias

ATRIAL PREMATURE BEATS

ECG Diagnostic Points

- The morphology of an atrial premature P wave is different from that of the sinus P wave (Fig. 11.1).
- The premature P wave is usually followed by a QRS complex similar to that with the normally conducted sinus beat. The premature P wave may be unrecognizable because it is hidden in the preceding T wave, hence the admonition "search the T for the P" (Figs. 11.2 and 11.3).
- The PR interval of an atrial premature beat (APB) is more than 0.11 second; if the P wave is inverted in leads II, III, and aVF, the PR should be more than 0.11 second to distinguish an APB from a junctional premature beat.
- Early occurring APBs may trigger atrial tachycardia (*see* Fig. 11.2), atrial flutter, or atrial fibrillation.
- Atrial premature beats that follow every sinus beat cause atrial bigeminy (*see* Fig. 11.1).
- The atrial premature P wave may not be conducted, resulting in a pause.
  Nonconducted APBs are the most common causes of pauses. If the premature P waves are not identified, the rhythm may be misinterpreted as sinus bradycardia.
- If the APB traverses the atrioventricular (AV) junction at a time when one of the bundle branches is still refractory, aberrant ventricular conduction may occur. The QRS is wide and

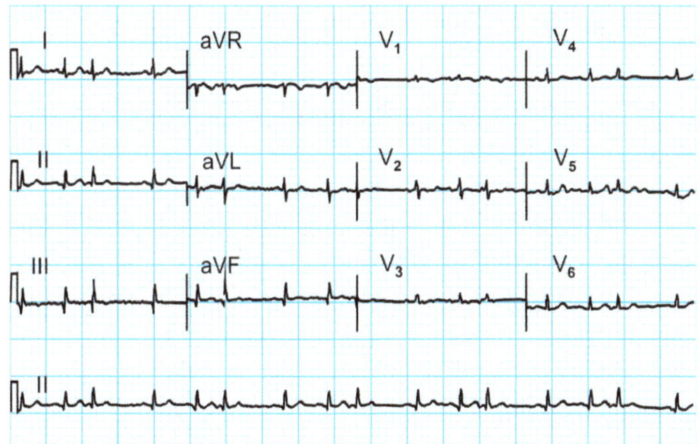

Fig. 11.1: Atrial trigeminy: each sinus beat is followed by a pair of atrial premature beats (APBs): this is true atrial trigeminy. If every third beat is an APB but not a pair of APBs the condition should not be termed atrial trigeminy. Nondiagnostic inferior Q waves noted.

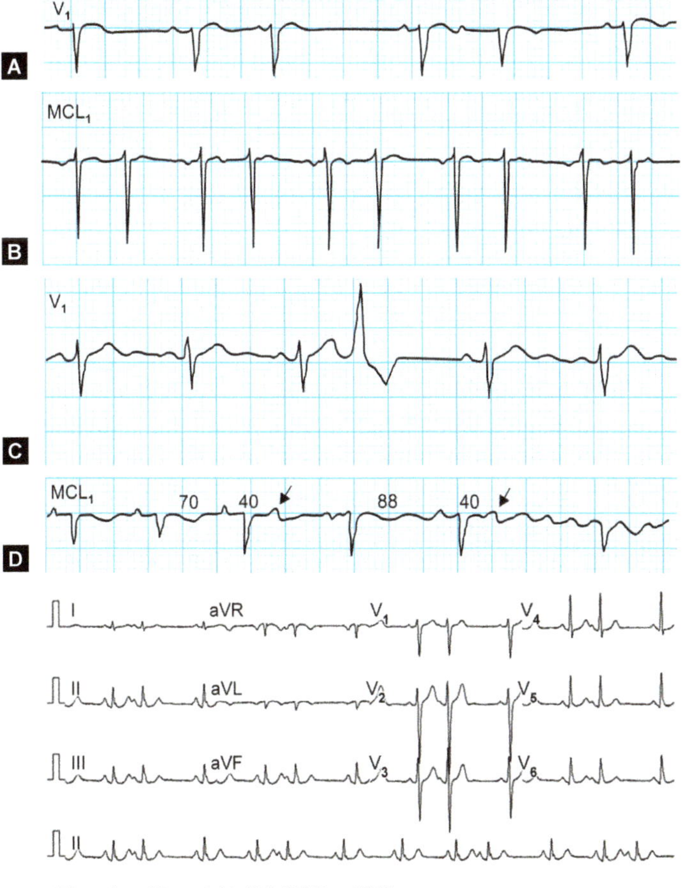

Figs. 11.2A to D: Search the P wave for the T, clearly seen in lead 11: atrial premature beats.

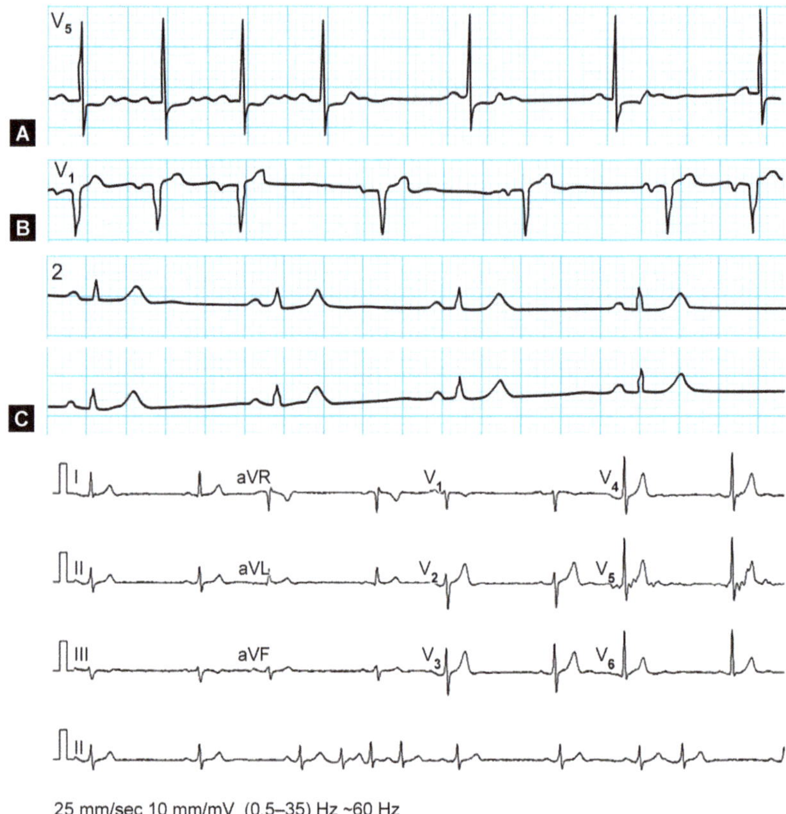

25 mm/sec 10 mm/mV (0.5–35) Hz ~60 Hz

Figs. 11.3A to C: Lead 11; after 3 sinus beats a run of 3 atrial premature beats (APBs)

resembles a ventricular premature beat (VPB) (*see* Fig. 11.2C). Examination of the preceding T wave may reveal a deformity caused by a P wave stuck on the T wave, as shown in Figure 11.2C. In addition, a postectopic cycle that is less than compensatory points to atrial ectopy with aberration.

- Multiple APBs may cause an irregularly irregular pulse.

JUNCTIONAL OR NODAL PREMATURE BEATS

ECG Diagnostic Points

- Junctional P waves may activate the atria retrogradely, and the retrograde P wave may precede the QRS complex. Retrograde conduction may not be observed, and the P wave may become lost in the QRS complex. Occasionally, the P wave follows the QRS complex.
- The P wave, when visible, is inverted in leads II, III, aVF, V_1, V_5, and V_6 and is upright in leads I, aVR, and aVL.
- The P wave may precede the QRS complex by less than 0.11 second.
- The terms upper-, mid-, or lower-nodal rhythm have been replaced by the term junctional rhythm.

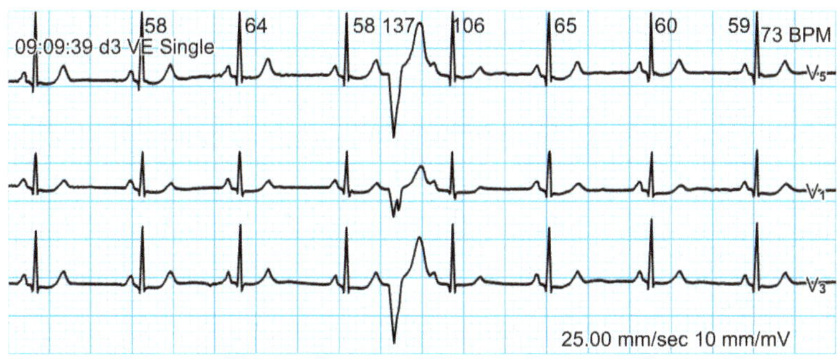

Fig. 11.4: A VPB early in the cycle close to the T wave is clinically important as may trigger VT.

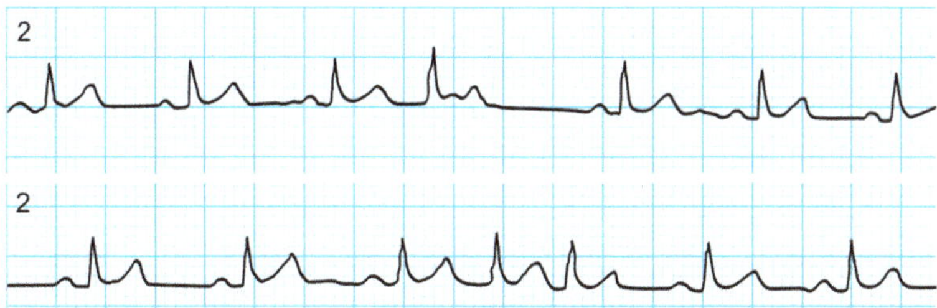

Fig. 11.5: Ventricular premature beats.

VENTRICULAR PREMATURE BEATS

ECG Diagnostic Points

- There is a wide, bizarre, premature QRST complex, with ST segment sloping off in the direction opposite the abnormal QRS complex (Figs. 11.4 to 11.6).
- There have been no preceding premature P waves. Retrograde conduction of ectopic ventricular impulses occurs often. The retrograde P wave is usually hidden in the ventricular complex but occasionally can cause retrograde capture of the atria, and the inverted P wave may be observed following the VPB.
- A VPB usually is followed by a fully compensatory pause, but this rule is often broken, and pauses may be less than compensatory.
- VPB duration generally is greater than 0.11 second, but occasionally, VPBs can be as short as 0.1 second in duration.
- If in V_1 the abnormal-looking QRS shows a left "rabbit ear" larger than the right "rabbit ear" (Figs. 11.7A to C), a diagnosis of VPB is certain. If the left "rabbit ear" is smaller than the right, no firm conclusion can be made from the morphology alone.
- Figure 11.8 shows ventricular bigeminy.
- A run of two beats is called a couplet; of three consecutive beats, a triplet or a salvo of three (Fig. 11.9); more than three consecutive VPBs is called ventricular tachycardia (VT) (Fig. 11.10).

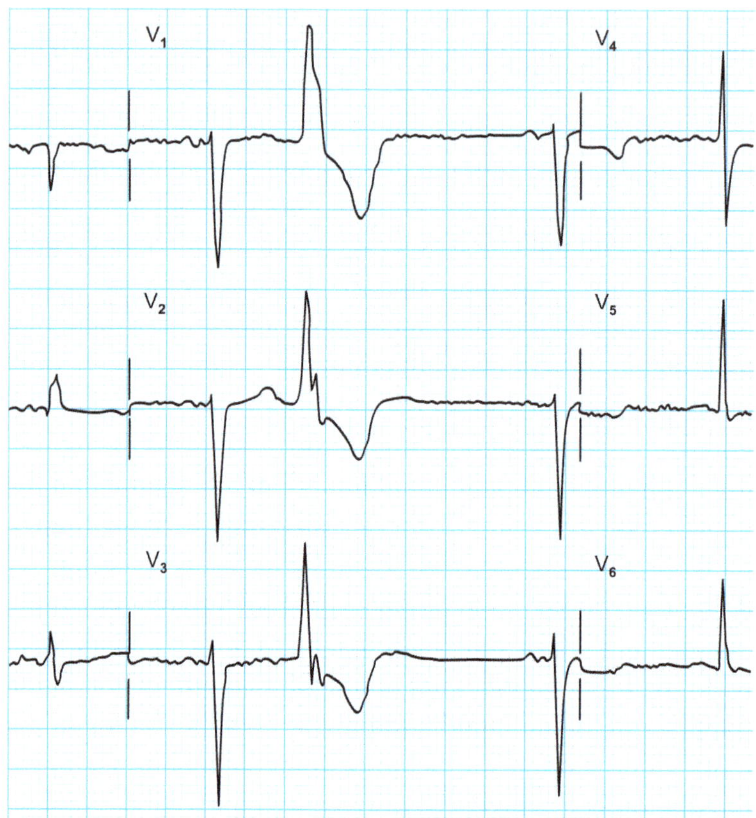

Fig. 11.6: A ventricular premature beat: The ST segment slopes in the direction opposite the slope of the abnormal QRS complex; V_1 shows a peaked "r" wave with the left limb taller than the right = a left "rabbit ear" larger than the right "rabbit ear."

With multifocal VPBs, the coupling intervals vary; with unifocal VPBs, the coupling intervals are equal. Unifocal VPBs are of little consequence. VPBs that occur early, close to the T wave or R on T, and that are multifocal or multiform, occurring as couplets or triplets, may trigger VT (Figs. 11.7 and 11.11).

Ventricular premature beats occur commonly in normal and abnormal hearts. The word *beat* denotes an electrical and mechanical event and is preferred to the word *contraction*, which implies a mechanical event. This text uses the terms VPBs and APBs, not VPCs and APCs.

BRADYARRHYTHMIAS

First-degree Atrioventricular Block

ECG Diagnostic Points

- PR interval is longer than 0.2 second; usually 0.22 to 0.48 second, but can be as long as 0.8 second (Fig. 11.12). Some normal individuals have intervals up to 0.22 second.

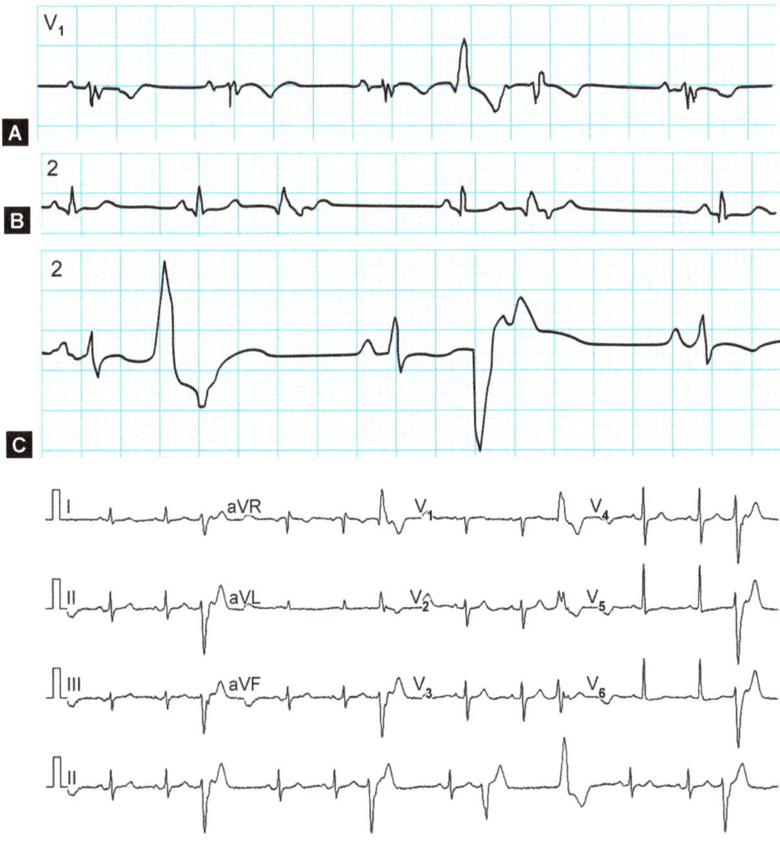

Figs. 11.7A to C: VPBs: note in lead V_1 tip of the R wave, left rabbit ear taller than the right is diagnostic for VPB and if a run of > 3 beats = VT. Rhythm strip 11 shows VPBs of different shapes = multifocal beats, and two in a row interpreted as a couplet or a pair.

- The PR interval should be constant.
- Each P wave should be followed by a QRS complex.

Second-degree Atrioventricular Block: Mobitz Type I (Wenckebach) Block

ECG Diagnostic Criteria

- There is progressive prolongation of the PR interval until the P wave is blocked, the impulse fails to conduct to the ventricles, and the QRS beat is dropped.
- After the dropped QRS beat, the PR interval reverts to near normal; the PR interval that follows the blocked P wave is always short (Figs. 11.13 and 11.14). Because there is usually a progressive shortening of the RR interval before a P wave is blocked, beats often are grouped in pairs (bigeminy) or trios (trigeminy). This group pattern is a hallmark of Wenckebach but is not necessary for the diagnosis.

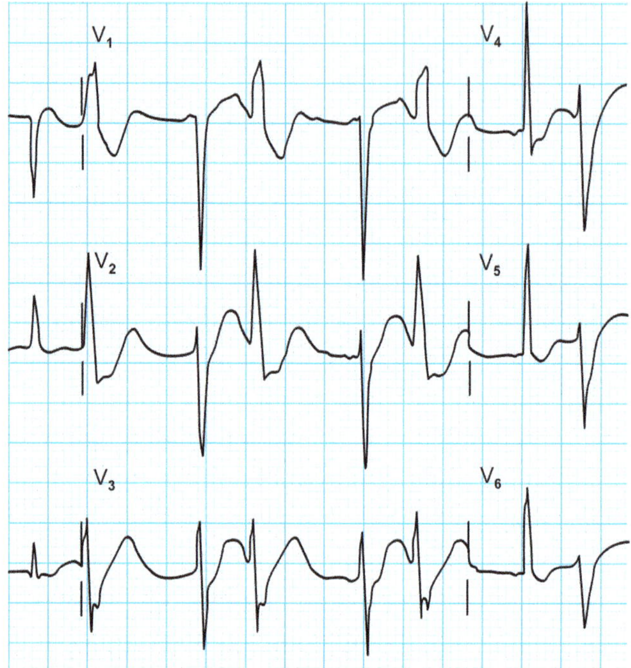

Fig. 11.8: Ventricular bigeminy.

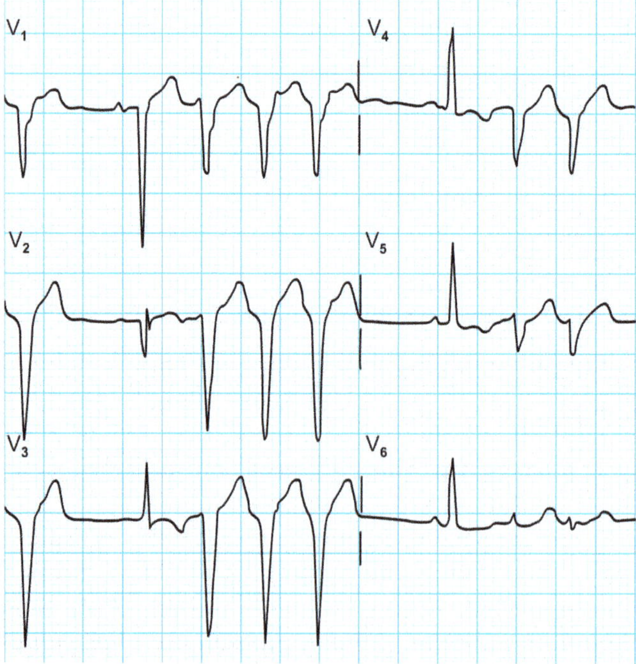

Fig. 11.9: Ventricular premature beats occur in pairs (couplets) and in salvos of three (triplets).

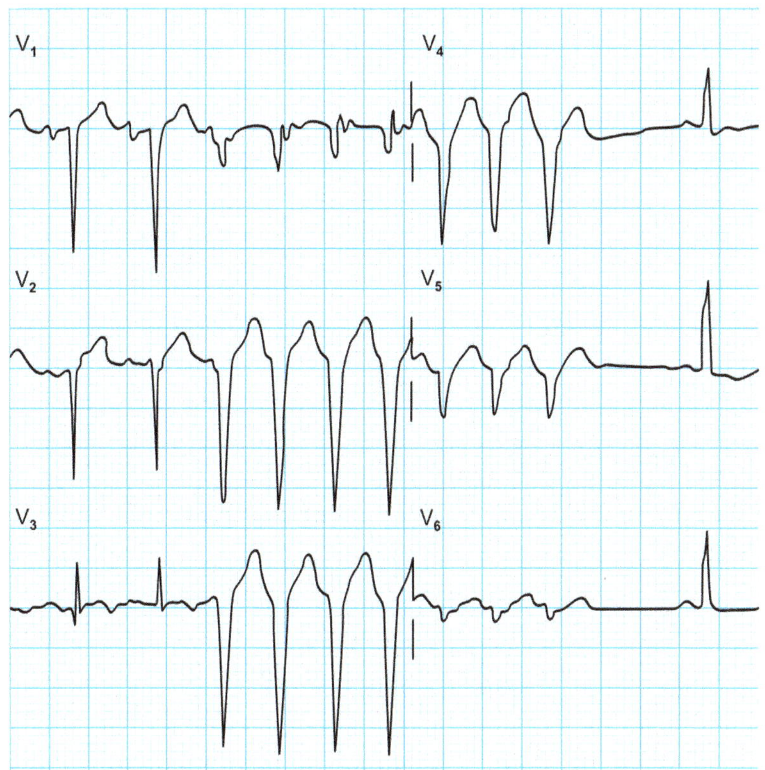

Fig. 11.10: Short run of nonsustained ventricular tachycardia.

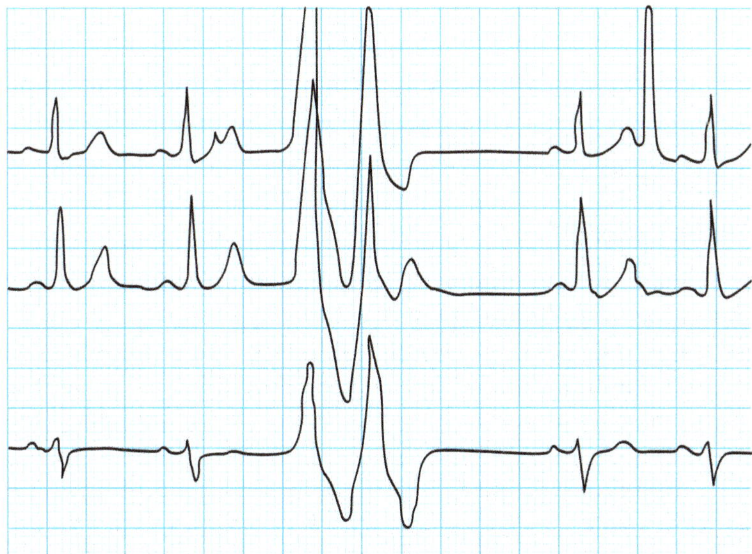

Fig. 11.11A

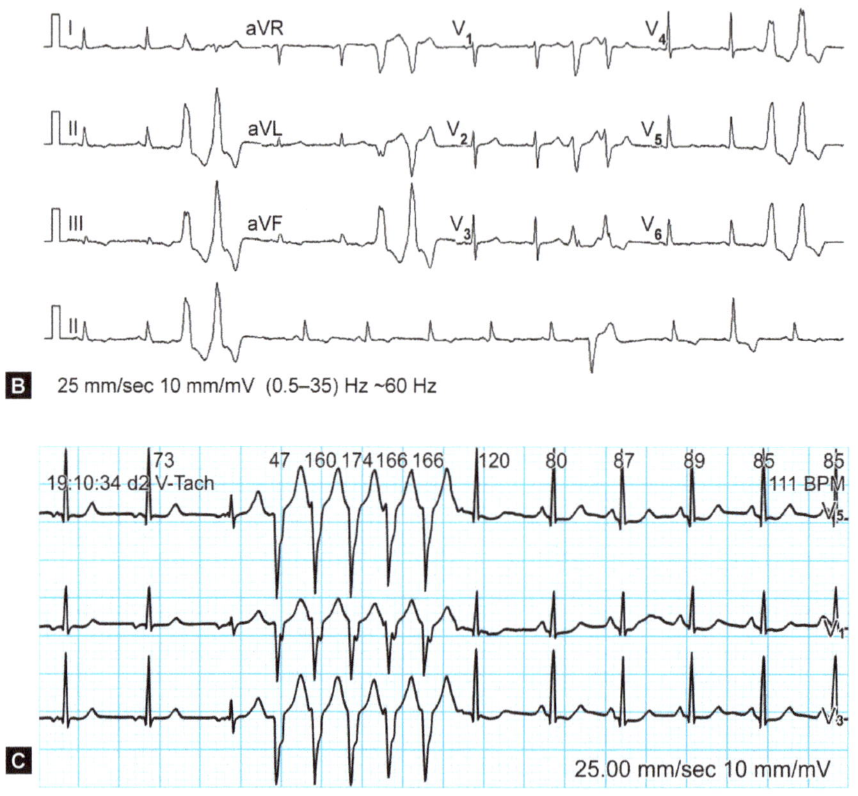

Figs. 11.11A to C: (A) Holter monitor showing multifocal ventricular premature beats: couplet, salvos of three, nonsustained ventricular tachycardia; (B) Couplets (pairs) VPBs/multifocal; (C) Run of 5 VPBs: VT.

Second-degree Atrioventricular Block
Mobitz Type II Block

ECG Diagnostic Criteria

- At least **two regular and consecutive atrial impulses are conducted with the same PR interval before the dropped beat** (Figs. 11.15A and B).
- Mobitz type II second-degree atrioventricular (AV) block. **Two consecutive PR intervals are unchanged before the dropped beat** (Fig. 11.15A and B). With type II, high-grade second-degree AV block (Fig. 11.15B), two or more consecutive atrial impulses fail to be conducted because of the block itself. The diagnosis is strengthened if the atrial rate is slow [less than 135 beats/min (bpm)] in the absence of interference by an escaping subsidiary pacemaker that may prevent conduction.
- Intermittent nonconducted P waves are observed, but with no evidence for atrial prematurity.
- The RR interval containing the nonconducted P wave is equal to two PP intervals.

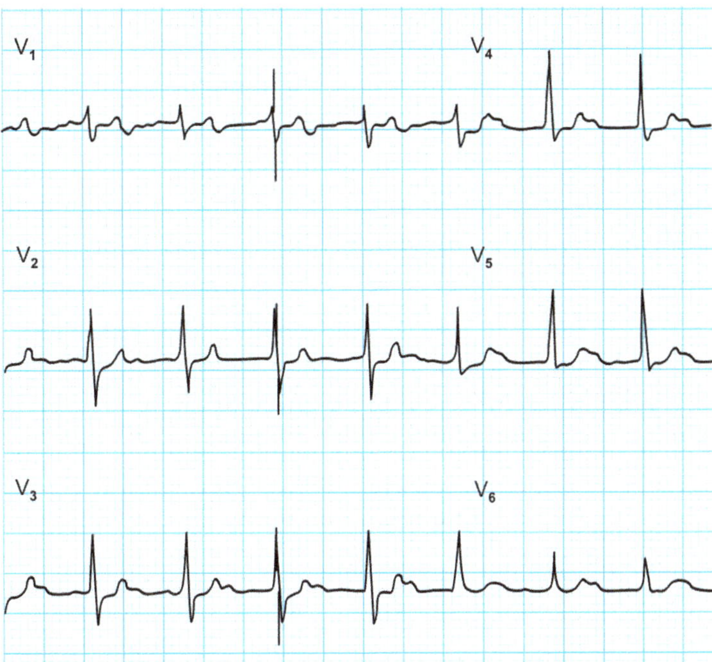

Fig. 11.12: Sinus tachycardia: rate, 118 bpm; PR is prolonged to 0.28 second: first-degree atrioventricular block.

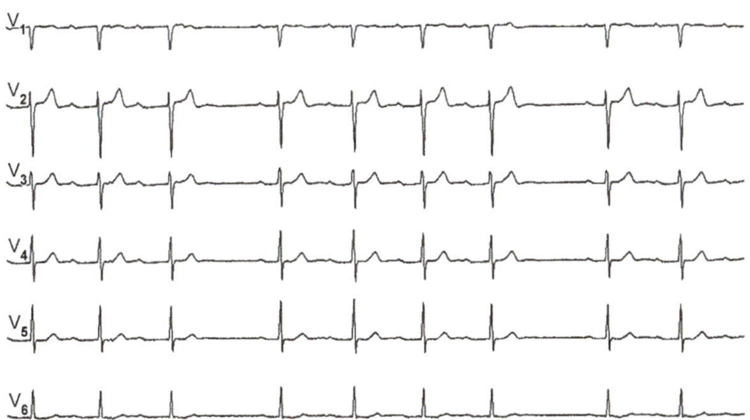

Fig. 11.13: Type 1 AV block. Typical Wenckebach phenomenon: Note in lead V_2 and V_3, in beat 3 the PR is markedly prolonged, and the QRS complex is followed by a dropped beat (the P wave may deform the T wave, then a long pause, as there is failure to conduct this P wave). After this pause the PR following is the shortest (4th QRS). The PR interval is shortest after the pause. Beat 7 is followed by a pause. The QRS are grouped in pairs or trios, a clue to the presence of Wenckebach.
Note: Not all type 1 AV blocks reveal a Wenckebach pattern.

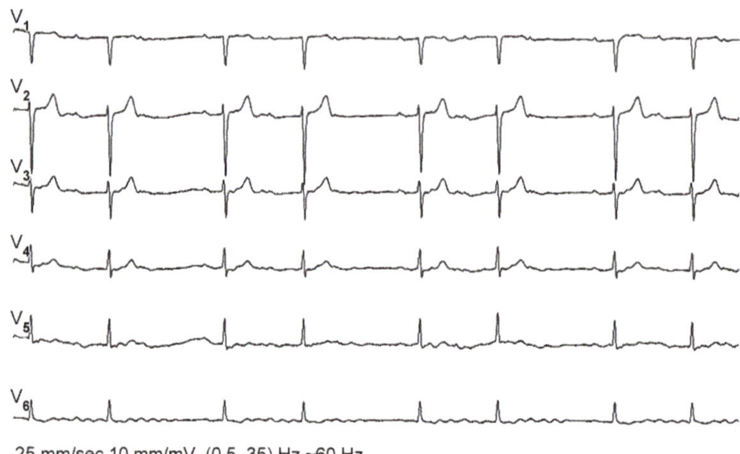

Fig. 11.14: Type 1 second-degree AV block; Typical Wenckebach phenomenon; P waves best seen in V_1–V_2–V_3.

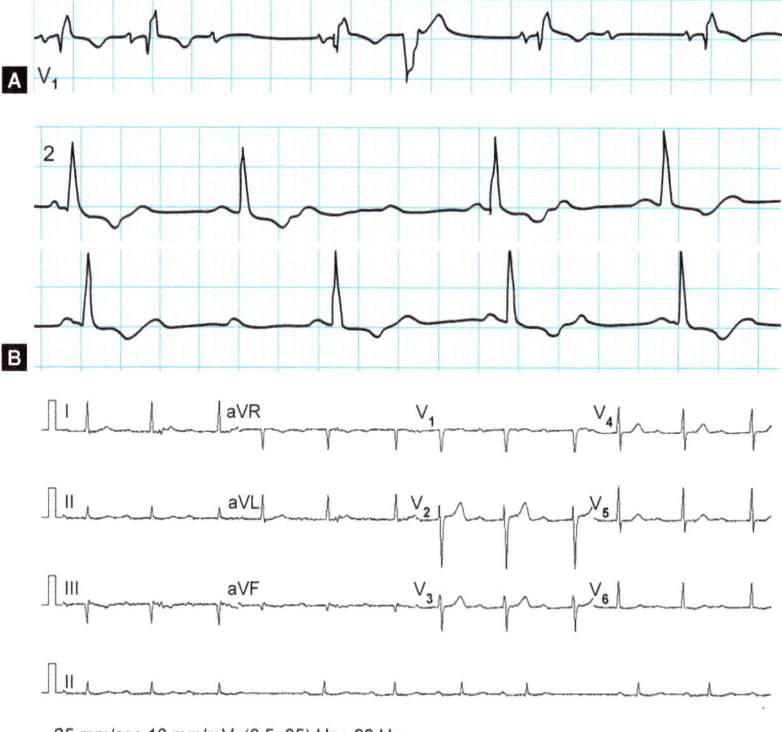

Figs. 11.15A and B: Mobitz type II second-degree atrioventricular (AV) block. *Rhythm strip, lead 11:* Two or more consecutive PR intervals are unchanged before the dropped beat. To be certain of the diagnosis at least two consecutive atrial beats (= P waves) with constant PR interval must be conducted before the dropped beat. The diagnosis may be faulty if this criterion is not used. The PR interval may be normal or slightly prolonged but remains constant, without prolongation.

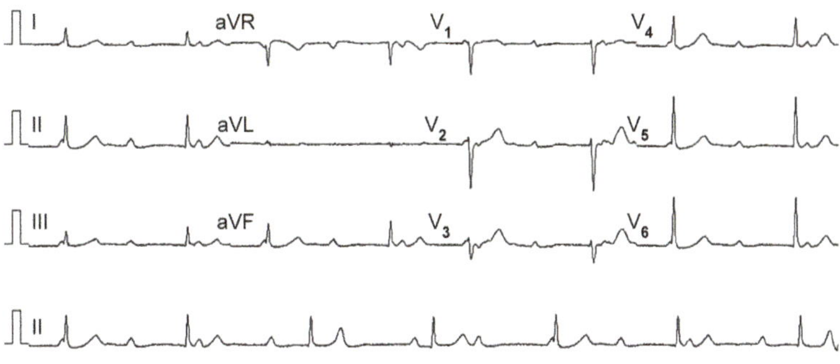

Fig. 11.16: Complete heart block. Note few QRS complexes and abundance of P waves, with constant P-P and RR intervals, but the PR intervals are not constant because the P waves bear no relation to the QRS complexes, and both P waves and QRS beat regularly, but are independent of each other, simply not married to each other; complete AV dissociation. The atrial rate is virtually always faster than the ventricular rate. The PR intervals are completely variable. P waves may fall on T waves (second QRS in lead 11) or QRS complexes distorting them, or distort the QRS: (first and fifth QRS in lead 11, see bottom rhythm strip). QRS complexes are narrow indicating that the ventricles are paced from the atrioventricular junction. When pacing is below the junction the QRS complexes are wide > 120 ms with a very slow rate ~30–40/min.

- *The PR interval remains constant and is normal or slightly prolonged.*
- The ventricular rhythm is irregular because of nonconducted beats.
- If the conduction problem is in the bundle of His, the QRS complex remains narrow, but it will be longer than 0.12 second if the lesion is below the bundle of His.

Complete (Third-degree) Atrioventricular Block

ECG Diagnostic Criteria

- P waves are sinus and plentiful with few QRS complexes.
- There is AV dissociation: no relationship between P waves and QRS complexes: complete absence of AV conduction (Figs. 11.16 and 11.17).
  Note that AV dissociation may occur in the absence of third-degree AV block; the clue here is that the ventricular rate is faster than the atrial rate.
- The RR intervals are regular. The QRS complex is narrow if the site of block is in the AV node with an escape rhythm originating in the AV junction. The QRS is wide if the escaped rhythm originates from the ventricle or in the AV junction in the presence of bundle branch block.
- The atrial rate is faster than the ventricular rate.
- The ventricular rate usually is very slow (less than 45 bpm), but with congenital AV block, rates may be 40–60 bpm.
- With complete AV block, anterograde conduction never occurs, but in less than 20% of complete AV blocks, retrograde conduction to the atria occurs.
  Note that AV dissociation may occur in the absence of third-degree AV block.

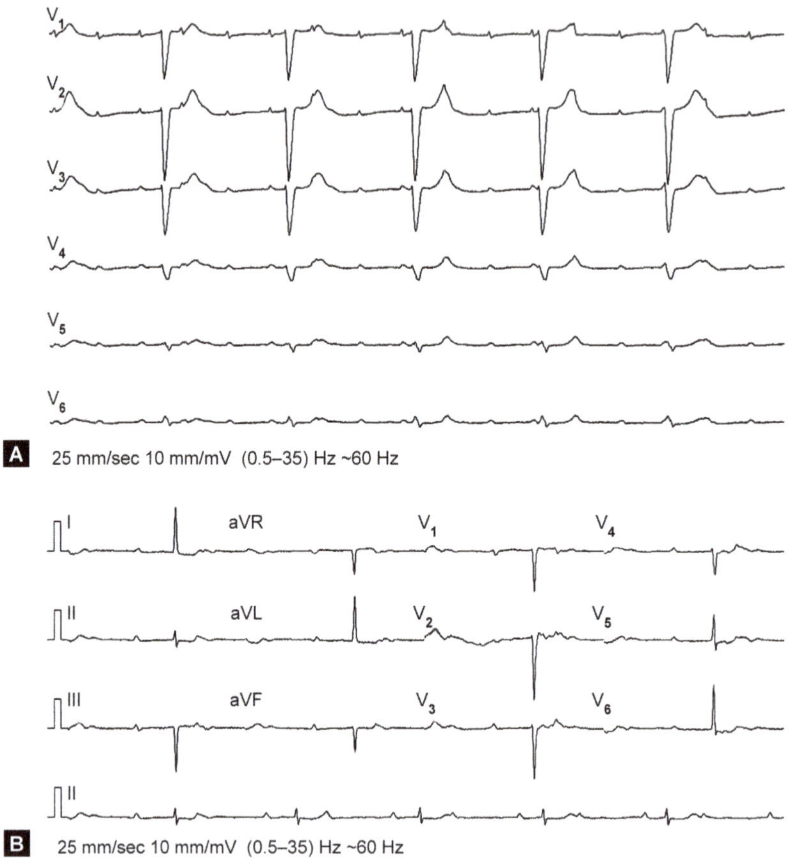

A   25 mm/sec 10 mm/mV (0.5–35) Hz ~60 Hz

B   25 mm/sec 10 mm/mV (0.5–35) Hz ~60 Hz

Fig. 11.17A and B: (A) Complete AV block; plentiful P waves with few QRS complexes. There is AV dissociation: no relationship between P waves and QRS complexes: complete absence of AV conduction. The narrow QRS complexes suggest that the escape pacemaker is junctional in origin. P waves best seen in V1. (B) Typical features of complete AV block.

NARROW QRS TACHYCARDIAS

Tachycardias should be differentiated as narrow QRS or wide QRS, then as regular or irregular (Figs. 11.18A and B). Some may prefer regular/irregular, narrow or wide.

Narrow QRS Tachycardia

A comparison of the entire 12-lead ECG during tachycardia with the ECG in sinus rhythm is most helpful for clarifying the diagnosis. Careful assessment of leads II, III, aVF, V_1, and V_6 should reveal clues to the diagnosis.

Sinus Tachycardia

Sinus tachycardia always should be considered if the rate is 100–130 bpm because it is the most common cause of narrow QRS tachycardia (Figs. 11.19A and B). With faster rates, the sinus P

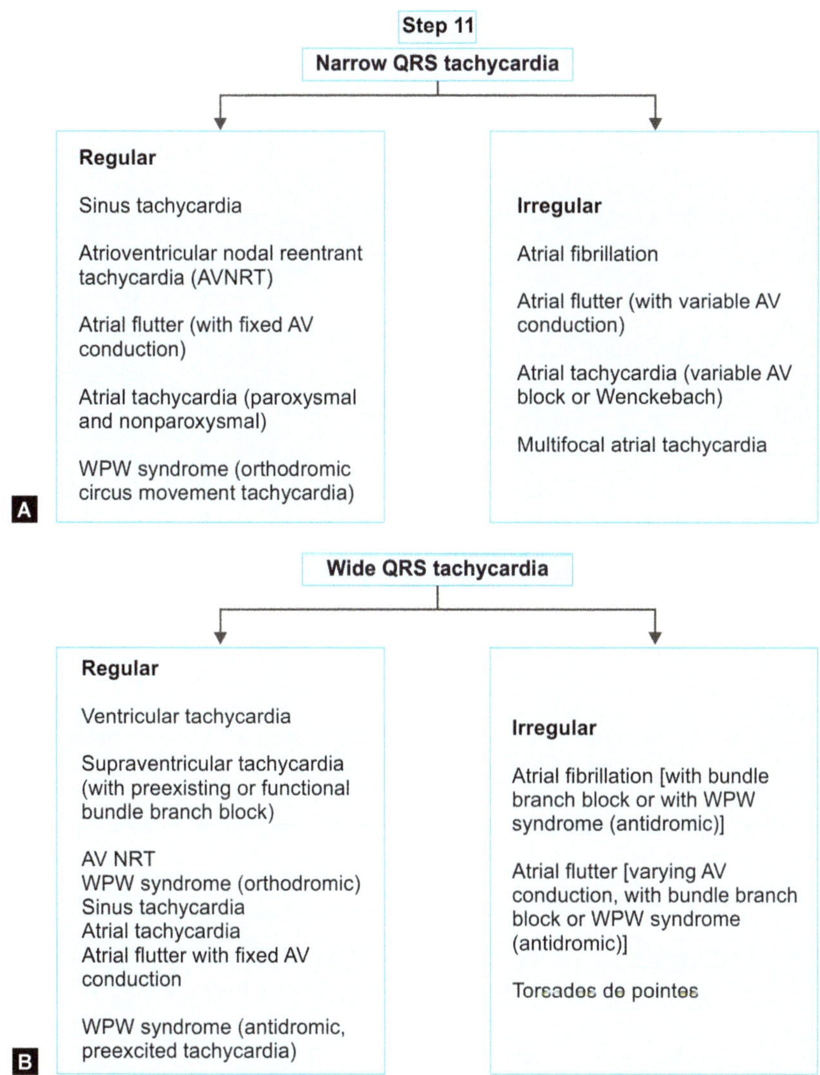

Figs. 11.18A and B: Step-by-step method for accurate ECG interpretation. Step 11: Assess arrhythmias: differential diagnosis of narrow QRS tachycardia (A) and wide QRS tachycardia (B). AV, atrioventricular; WPW, Wolff-Parkinson-White.

wave may be hidden in the T waves and mimic supraventricular tachycardia (SVT), AVNRT or atrial flutter. The sinus P wave can be revealed by carotid massage.

Atrioventricular Nodal Reentrant Tachycardia

Atrioventricular nodal reentrant tachycardia (AVNRT) is the most common cause of a paroxysmal, narrow, regular QRS tachycardia. The ventricles are activated from the anterograde path of the circuit, with activation of the atrium by the retrograde path.

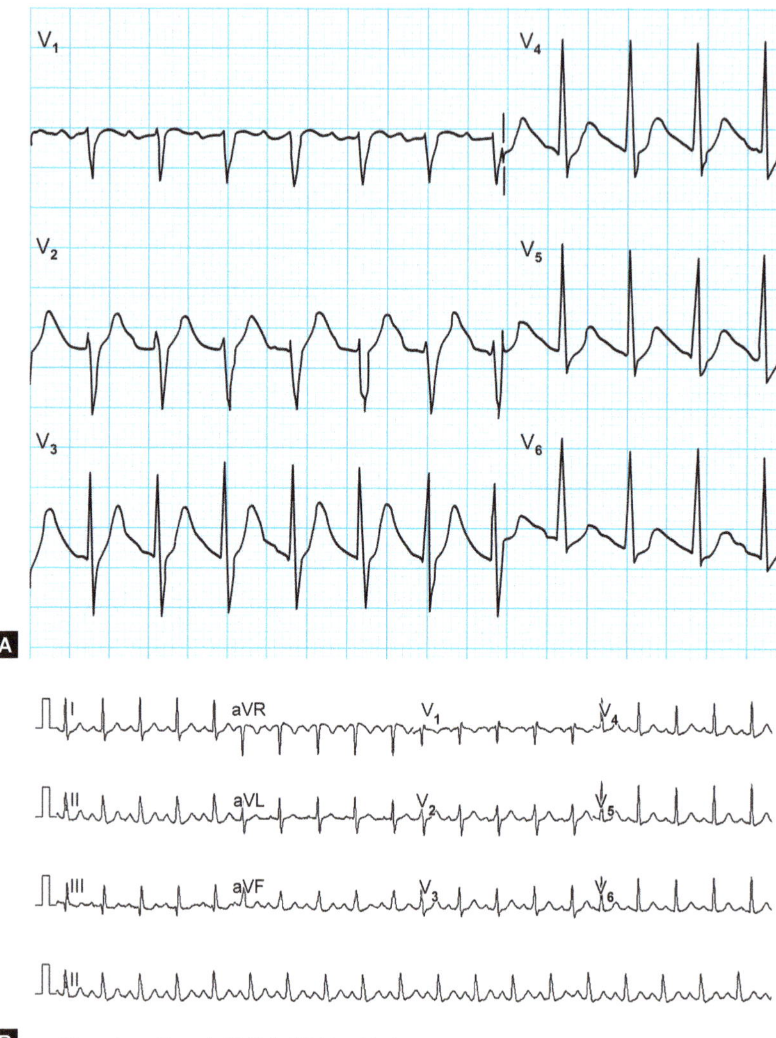

Figs. 11.19A and B: (A) Sinus tachycardia; rate, 165 bpm; (B) Sinus tachycardia; RSR' in V$_1$; IRBBB: incomplete right bundle branch block.

ECG Diagnostic Points

- A rapid, regular rhythm, usually 150–225 bpm, is present. A rate greater than 230 bpm should prompt the search for Wolff-Parkinson-White (WPW) syndrome.
- QRS is less than 0.12 second.
- In more than 50% of cases, P waves are hidden within the QRS complex and are not visible; the QRS complex is identical to that of a tracing during sinus rhythm.
- In approximately 45% of cases, P waves appear hidden, but on careful scrutiny they are visible at the end of the QRS in leads II, III, and aVF as they distort the terminal forces of the QRS complex, resulting in pseudo–S waves in leads II, III, and aVF (Figs. 11.20 and 11.21).

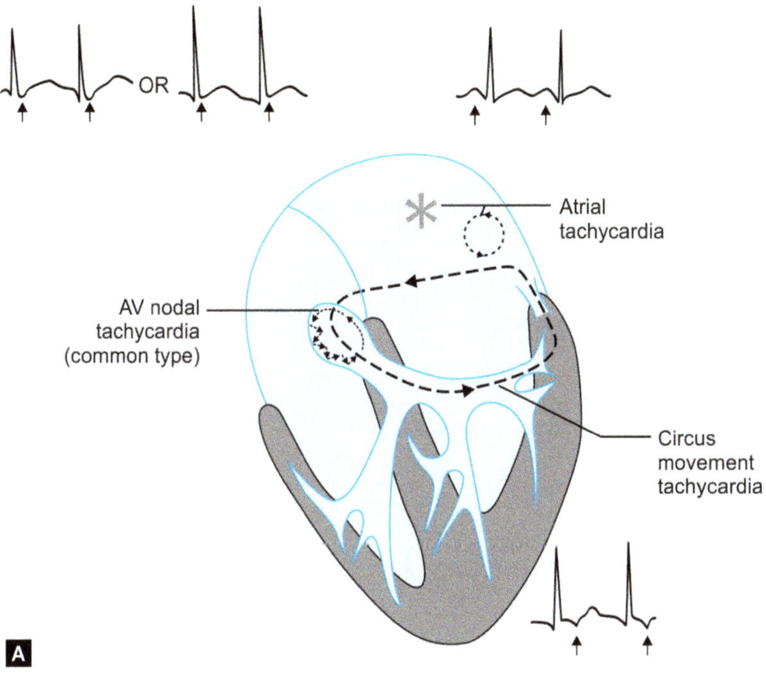

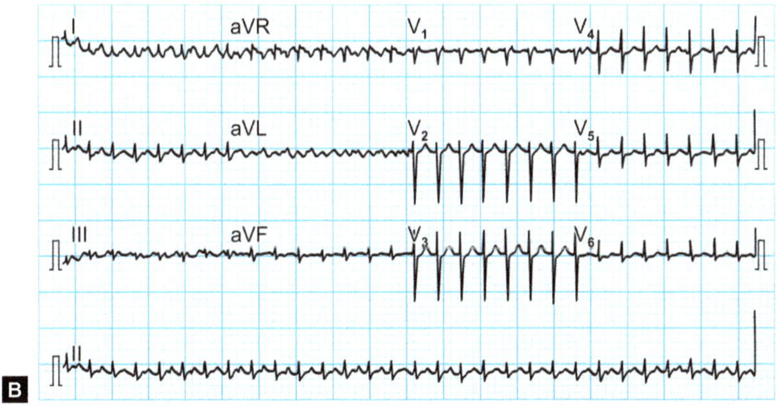

Figs. 11.20A and B: AV nodal reentrant tachycardia; rate 180 beats/min (a fairly common rate 170–190 beats/min). Assess lead V_1: in the most common variety of AVNRT the P waves cause a distortion of the terminal forces in V_1, forming pseudo-r waves (a pseudo I RBBB pattern with QRS duration <120 ms). The P wave may deform the terminal forces in II, III, and aVF, forming a pseudo-S wave; this subtle terminal deformity is shown in Figures 11.21 and 11.22. The diagnosis depends on detecting that P waves are:

- Distorting the terminal forces of the QRS
- Totally hidden within the QRS
- Rarely P waves may be seen at the junction or the QRS causing pseudo-Q waves in II, III, aVF.

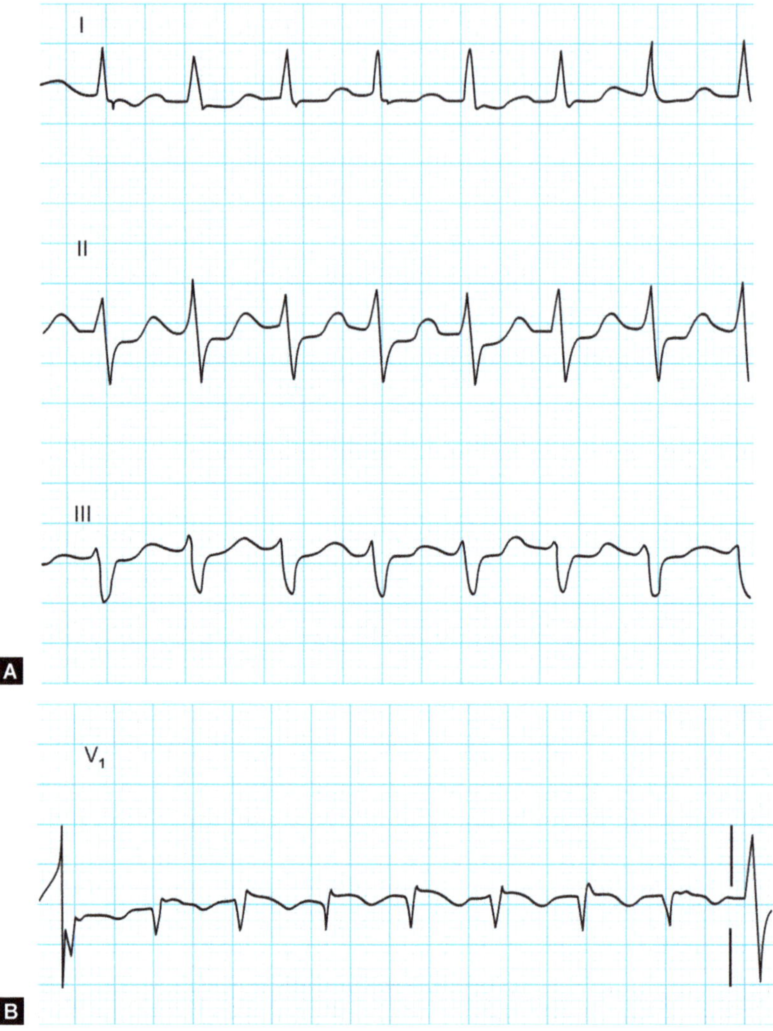

Figs. 11.21A and B: The limb leads of a patient with supraventricular tachycardia: rate, 184 bpm. (A) Note the distortion of the terminal QRS in lead III, a pseudo-S wave: typical features of the common form of atrioventricular nodal reentrant tachycardia (AVNRT); (B) The V_1 lead in the same patient. Note the distortion of the terminal QRS resulting in a pseudo–r' wave: typical feature of the common form of AVNRT (*see* Fig. 11.20).

The distortion causes a pseudo r' wave in lead V_1 that mimics RSr' or incomplete right bundle branch block (RBBB) (Figs. 11.20 to 11.22).

- In fewer than 5% of cases, P waves are discernible at the beginning of the QRS and cause pseudo–Q waves in leads II, III, and aVF.
- In a rare form of AVNRT, P waves are negative in leads II, III, and aVF but follow the QRS after a prolonged duration such that the RP interval is greater than the PR interval. It is impossible to distinguish this rare form of AVNRT from the rare type of WPW circus movement tachycardia

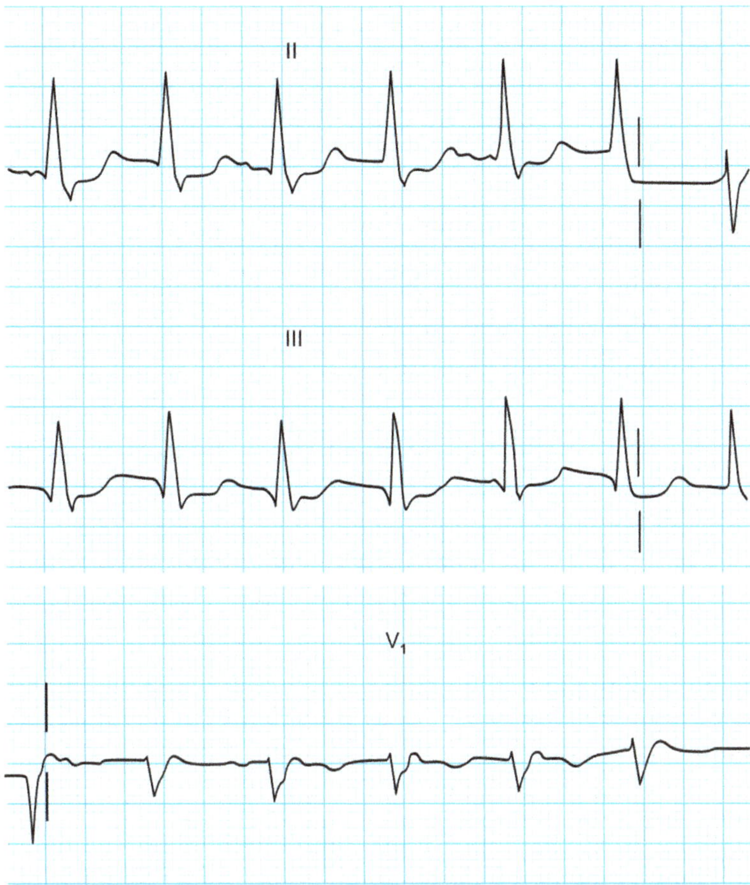

Fig. 11.22: Atrioventricular nodal reentrant tachycardia (AVNRT): rate, 140 bpm. Note pseudo-R' wave in V₁, typical of the common type of AVNRT.

using the retrograde, slow accessory pathway to activate the atria (see subsequent section on Wolff-Parkinson-White syndrome).

Paroxysmal Atrial Tachycardia with or without Atrioventricular Block

ECG Diagnostic Points

- The P wave precedes the QRS, and its contour is different from that of the sinus P wave. P waves are often small, are not easily identified, and may be hidden in the T wave or QRS; the arrhythmia may be mistaken for sinus tachycardia or AV junctional tachycardia. The PR interval is normal or prolonged.
- The morphology of the P waves depends on the location of the ectopic atrial pacemaker (Fig. 11.23). The RR intervals are equal except for a warm-up period in the automatic type.
- The atrial rate may range from 110 bpm to 260 bpm. If the atrial rate is not rapid and AV conduction is not depressed, each P wave may conduct to the ventricle. With digitalis excess,

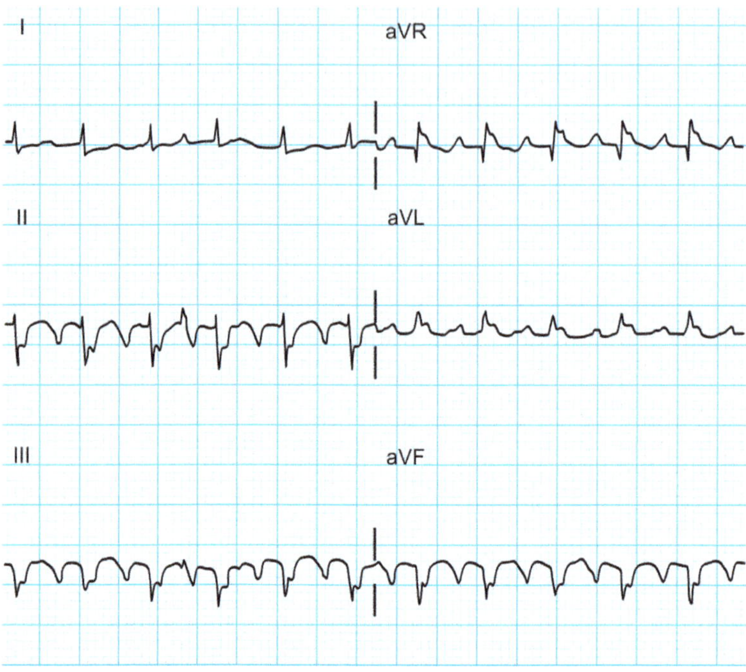

Fig. 11.23: Atrial tachycardia. The P waves are barely discernible in lead I and are inverted in II, III, and aVF. There is 2:1 atrioventricular block. The atrial rate is 264 bpm; ventricular rate is 132 bpm. Note the isoelectric baseline between the P wave and the QRS complex.

AV conduction may be delayed, resulting in paroxysmal atrial tachycardia with block, but digitalis toxicity is not the only cause of this arrhythmia.

- Variable AV conduction occurs: a 2:1 conduction is common; a 3:1 conduction or Wenckebach phenomenon may occur, causing an irregular rhythm. At times, the varying AV block may result in an irregular ventricular rhythm that may be mistaken for atrial fibrillation.
- An isoelectric baseline exists between the P wave and the QRS complex (Fig. 11.23).
- The differentiation of atrial tachycardia and atrial flutter may be difficult if the atrial rate is rapid; carotid sinus massage or adenosine brings out the flutter waves if atrial flutter is present.
- Atrial tachycardia persists despite the development of AV block, and this feature excludes WPW syndrome.

Persistent (Incessant) Atrial Tachycardia

The incessant nature of atrial tachycardia, a rare tachycardia, may cause dilated (congestive) cardiomyopathy.

ECG Diagnostic Points

- The rhythm is regular (Fig. 11.24).
- The P wave precedes the QRS complex. The P wave polarity depends on the site of origin in the atrium.

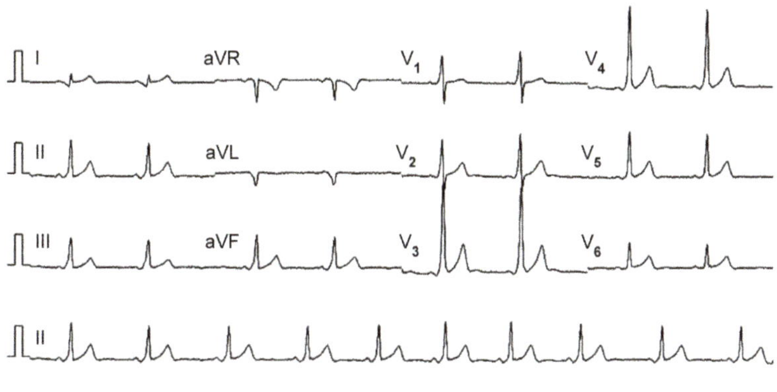

25 mm/sec 10 mm/mV (0.5–35) Hz ~60 Hz

Fig. 11.24: WPW: Tall R waves V_1–V_3. Delta waves variable in some leads.

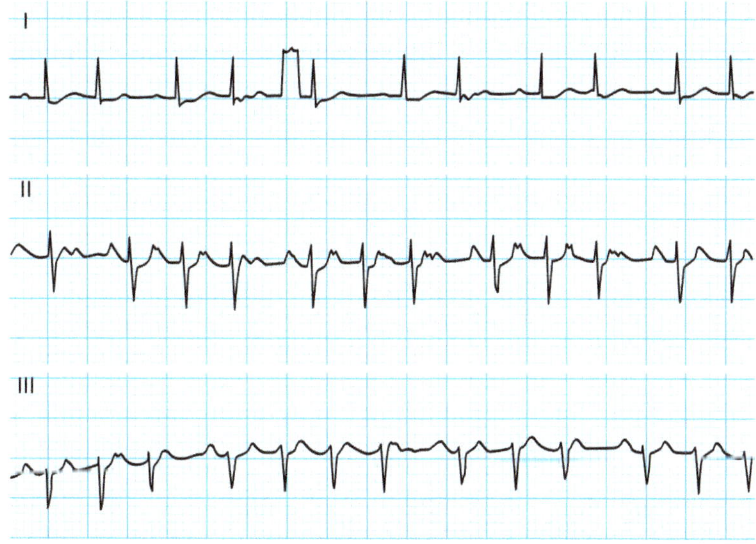

Fig. 11.25: Short PR, with delta wave prominent in V_2–V_6; inferior leads II, III aVF may mimic old inferior MI.

- There is variable AV conduction of 1:1 and 2:1, including Wenckebach phenomenon (Fig. 11.25).
- Carotid sinus massage or adenosine increases AV block and facilitates the diagnosis.

Multifocal Atrial Tachycardia (Chaotic Atrial Tachycardia)

ECG Diagnostic Points

- Atrial rate is 100–140 bpm.

- There are frequent multifocal premature beats, at least three different P wave morphologies with changing PR intervals in one lead, and isoelectric baseline between P waves.
- The rhythm is completely irregular; PR, RR, and RP intervals are variable.
- One dominant atrial pacemaker, such as sinus rhythm, is absent, and multifocal APBs are present.
- Causes of multifocal atrial tachycardia include chronic obstructive pulmonary disease, theophylline, and digitalis (rarely).

Wolff-Parkinson-White Syndrome

ECG Diagnostic Criteria

- The QRS complex duration is ≥0.11 second; in approximately 20% of individuals, the QRS complex may not be >0.1 second. PR is <0.12 second.
- A delta wave is prominent, often in V_3 through V_6, and is a subtle finding (Fig. 11.24) in some leads (Figs. 11.26A and B). In type A WPW syndrome, a tall R wave present in V_1 and V_2 can mimic right ventricular hypertrophy, RBBB, or posterior infarction (Fig. 11.27).
- Pseudo–Q waves in inferior leads may mimic inferior myocardial infarction (*see* Figs. 11.24 to 11.28). In type B WPW pattern, the QRS complex is predominately negative in V_1 through V_3 and upright in V_5 and V_6. The pattern may resemble left bundle branch block (Fig. 11.28).

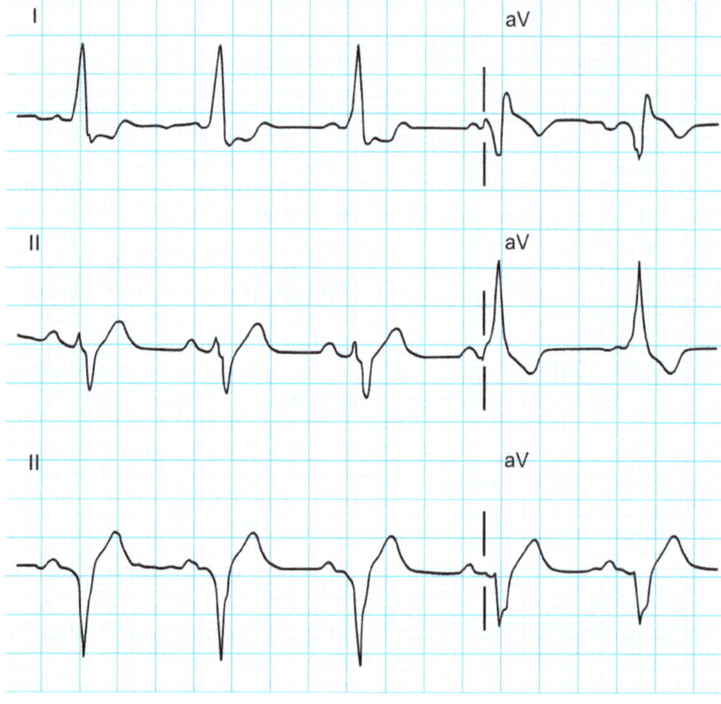

Fig. 11.26A

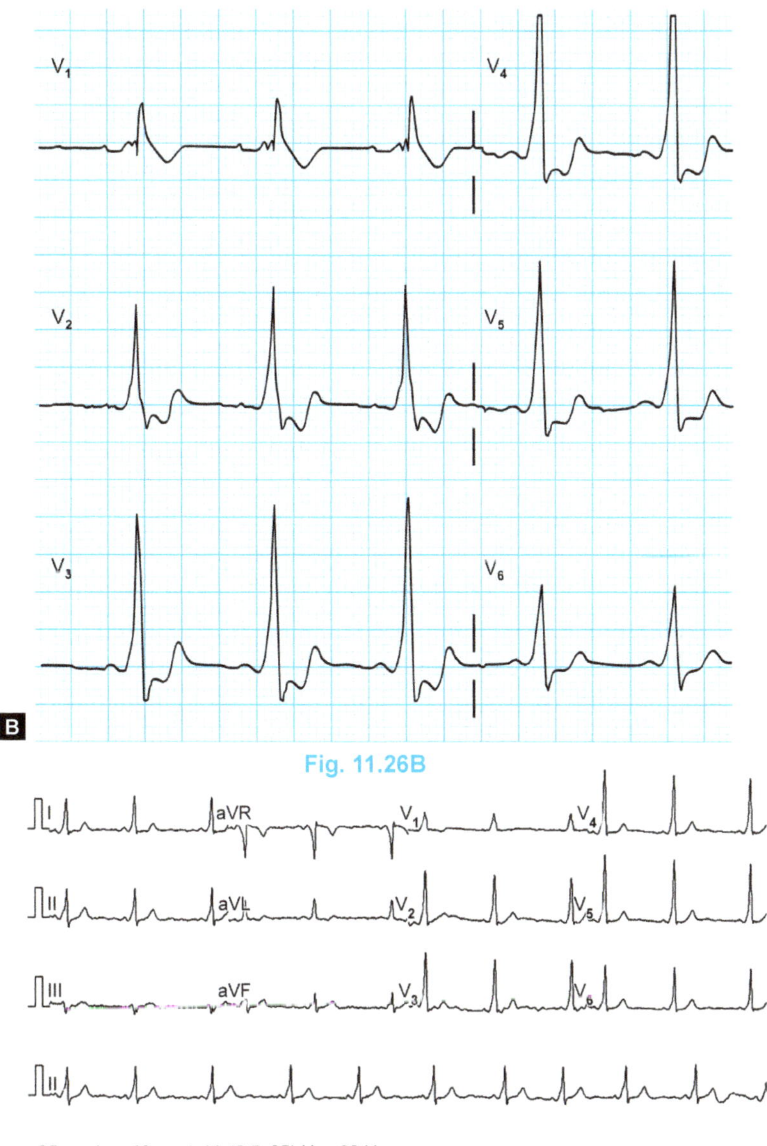

Fig. 11.26B

25 mm/sec 10 mm/mV (0.5–35) Hz ~60 Hz

Figs. 11.26A and B: Features of Wolff-Parkinson-White syndrome. Prominent delta waves seen in this figure and very short PR interval. Lead III AVF pattern mimics inferior infarction. WPW, mimic RBBB.

CLUES DURING TACHYCARDIA

- There is narrow QRS complex tachycardia, with regular rhythm.
- P waves follow the QRS at a distance; shape depends on the location of the accessory pathway. With a left lateral accessory pathway, the P wave is negative in lead I. If the location is posteroseptal, P waves are negative in leads II, III, and aVF and positive in aVR and aVL.

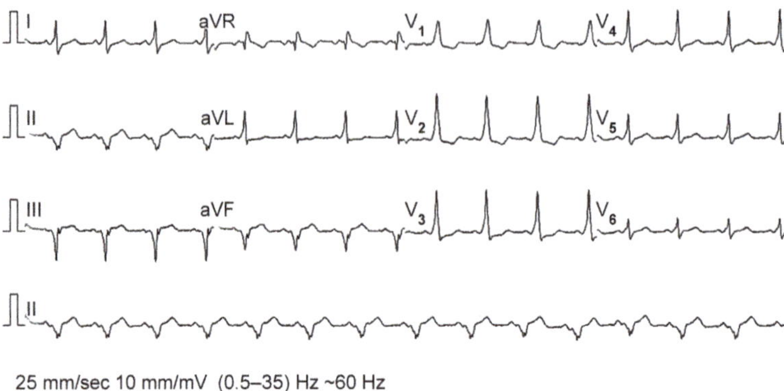

25 mm/sec 10 mm/mV (0.5–35) Hz ~60 Hz

Fig. 11.27: Mimic RBBB and inferior MI.

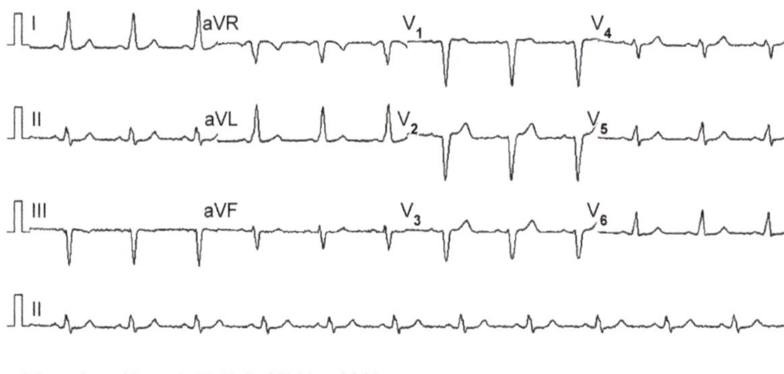

25 mm/sec 10 mm/mV (0.5–35) Hz ~60 Hz

Fig. 11.28: Limb leads in patient with Wolff-Parkinson-White syndrome mimic inferior infarction. WPW mimic LBBB.

- In the common orthodromic circus movement tachycardia, the RP interval is shorter than the PR interval because of retrograde use of the fast accessory pathway to activate the atria
- Mimic RBBB (Fig. 11.30).
- In a rare form of orthodromic circus movement tachycardia with retrograde activation of the atria through a slowly conducting accessory pathway, the P wave occurs late retrogradely. Thus, the RP interval is longer than or equal to the PR interval and the P wave is negative in leads II, III, aVF, and V_4 through V_6. This arrhythmia pattern is similar to the rare form of AVNRT described previously. This rare type of WPW syndrome may manifest as a persistent (incessant) orthodromic circus movement tachycardia and cause a dilated cardiomyopathy with congestive heart failure.
- Electrical alternans sometimes occurs during orthodromic circus movement tachycardia but rarely occurs with other narrow QRS tachycardias.

Summary Differential Diagnosis of Narrow QRS Regular Tachycardia

- If AV block is present or can be produced by carotid sinus massage or adenosine, WPW syndrome can be ruled out; atrial flutter and atrial tachycardia persist despite AV block.
- If the P wave is hidden within the QRS or is distorting the terminal QRS, causing a pseudo-S in leads II, III, and aVF or a pseudo-r' in V_1, the diagnosis is the common form of AVNRT (*see* Figs. 11.20 to 11.22).
- A negative P wave in lead I suggests WPW syndrome or left atrial tachycardia.
- A P wave following the QRS complex distinctly with an RP interval shorter than the PR interval is diagnostic of the most common type of WPW syndrome, orthodromic circus movement tachycardia.
- An RP interval that is greater than the PR interval indicates the rare WPW orthodromic type, the rare type of AVNRT, or atrial tachycardia.
- Positive P waves in leads II, III, and aVF with atrial tachycardia rule out AVNRT or WPW syndrome tachycardia.
- P waves negative in leads II, III, and aVF suggest AVNRT or WPW syndrome.
- A ventricular rate greater than 220 bpm with QRS alternans usually indicates WPW syndrome.
- A ventricular rate greater than 250 bpm with RR intervals less than 240 milliseconds (six small squares) suggests WPW syndrome.

FOUR TYPES OF WOLFF-PARKINSON-WHITE SYNDROME TACHYCARDIA

1. *Orthodromic circus movement tachycardia*: This is the most common tachycardia. The ventricles are activated via the AV node and bundle of His, and the impulse retrogradely uses the fast accessory tract to activate the atria; thus the P wave is close to the preceding QRS complex, and the RP interval is shorter than the PR interval.
2. *Rare orthodromic tachycardia*: The activation of the ventricles via the AV node and His bundle is similar to that in circus movement tachycardia, but the impulse returns to the atria via the slow accessory tract. Therefore, the P wave follows the QRS at a distance, making the RP interval greater than the PR interval. This arrhythmia mimics the rare form of AVNRT.
3. *Rare antidromic tachycardia*: The ventricle is activated by anterograde (preexcited tachycardia) use of the bypass tract, causing tachycardia similar to VT, atrial flutter, or atrial fibrillation with a wide QRS complex (see discussion of wide QRS tachycardia).
4. *Rare antidromic anterograde conduction*: The ventricle is activated by two or more accessory pathways, resulting in wide QRS tachycardia.

DIAGNOSIS BASED ON CAROTID SINUS MASSAGE OR INTRAVENOUS ADENOSINE

- AVNRT converts to sinus rhythm or no effect.
- Circus movement tachycardia reverts to sinus rhythm or no effect.
- *Persistent atrial tachycardia*: Increased AV block facilitates recognition of the atrial origin, temporary slowing of heart rate with AV block, or no effect.

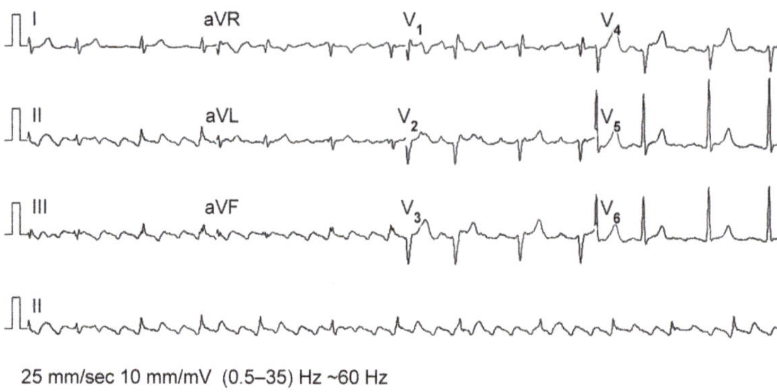

25 mm/sec 10 mm/mV (0.5–35) Hz ~60 Hz

Fig. 11.29: A sawtooth pattern is seen in leads II, III, and aVF.

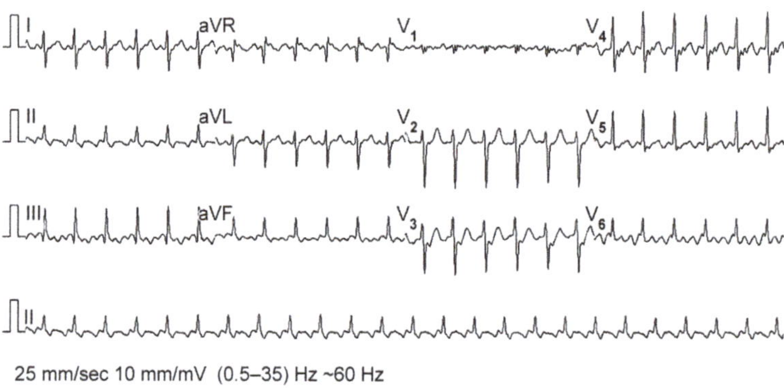

25 mm/sec 10 mm/mV (0.5–35) Hz ~60 Hz

Fig. 11.30: Atrial flutter rapid ventricular rate; note absence of flutter waves in lead I, a typical finding.

- *Atrial flutter*: Temporary slowing of the ventricular rate reveals flutter waves if not previously visible, or no effect.

Atrial Flutter

- A sawtooth pattern is seen in leads II, III, and aVF (Figs. 11.29 to 11.33). The downward deflection of the F waves has a gradual slope followed by an abrupt upward deflection. This results in the typical sharp spikes of the sawtooth pattern: There are positive, "spiky" P-like waves in lead V_1 and negative P-like waves in leads V_5 and V_6. There is almost no atrial activity in lead I, and leads V_5 and V_6 often show negligible atrial activity (*see* Figs. 11.32 to 11.34).
- A ventricular response of 150 bpm is typical of atrial flutter. The atrial rate is often 300 bpm. With 2:1 AV conduction, the ventricular response is 150 bpm. This 2:1 ratio may not be apparent because an F wave may be partially obscured by the QRS complex and the second F wave is hidden in the T wave (Figs. 11.34A and B). This pattern mimics sinus tachycardia or reentrant junctional tachycardia. Carotid sinus massage should reveal sinus P waves or F

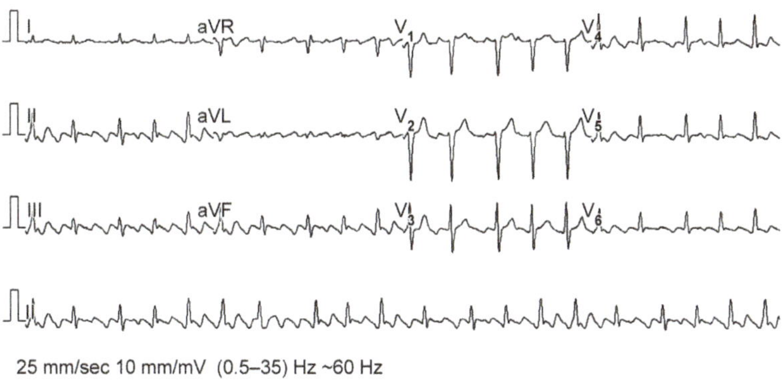

Fig. 11.31: Atrial flutter rapid ventricular rate.

waves. Conduction ratios of 2:1 and 4:1 may occur. The ventricular rate may vary from 100 bpm to 230 bpm. A ventricular response of greater than 250 bpm suggests WPW syndrome.

- The rhythm is regular but becomes irregular when there is variable AV conduction.
- The atrial rate varies from 250 bpm to 400 bpm but can be less than 200 bpm in patients taking quinidine.

Atrial Fibrillation

ECG Diagnostic Points

- RR intervals are completely irregular (irregularly irregular) (Figs. 11.35 and 11.36).
- Irregular undulations of the baseline are usually most prominent in V_1; these may be gross (Figs. 11.37A to D) or barely perceptible, described as coarse and fine fibrillation, respectively. Occasionally, there may be no recognizable undulations of the baseline, and careful measurement of the RR interval is necessary to detect slight irregularities.
- The atrial rate ranges from 400 bpm to 700 bpm; there is variable AV conduction, resulting in a chaotic ventricular response.
- QRS complexes often vary in amplitude.
- Further examples of atrial fibrillation are given in Figure 11.38.
- The heart rate is commonly 100–180 bpm but can accelerate to more than 200 bpm. Rates of more than 240 bpm with the QRS complex more than or equal to 0.10 second should suggest WPW syndrome. With WPW antidromic tachycardia, wide QRS tachycardia with rates of 250–320 bpm may occur.

Figure 11.38 gives clues that assist with the diagnosis of supraventricular arrhythmias.

WIDE QRS TACHYCARDIA

ECG Diagnostic Steps

- Define the QRS duration as ≥0.12 second.
- Define the tachycardia as regular or irregular (*see* Fig. 11.18B).

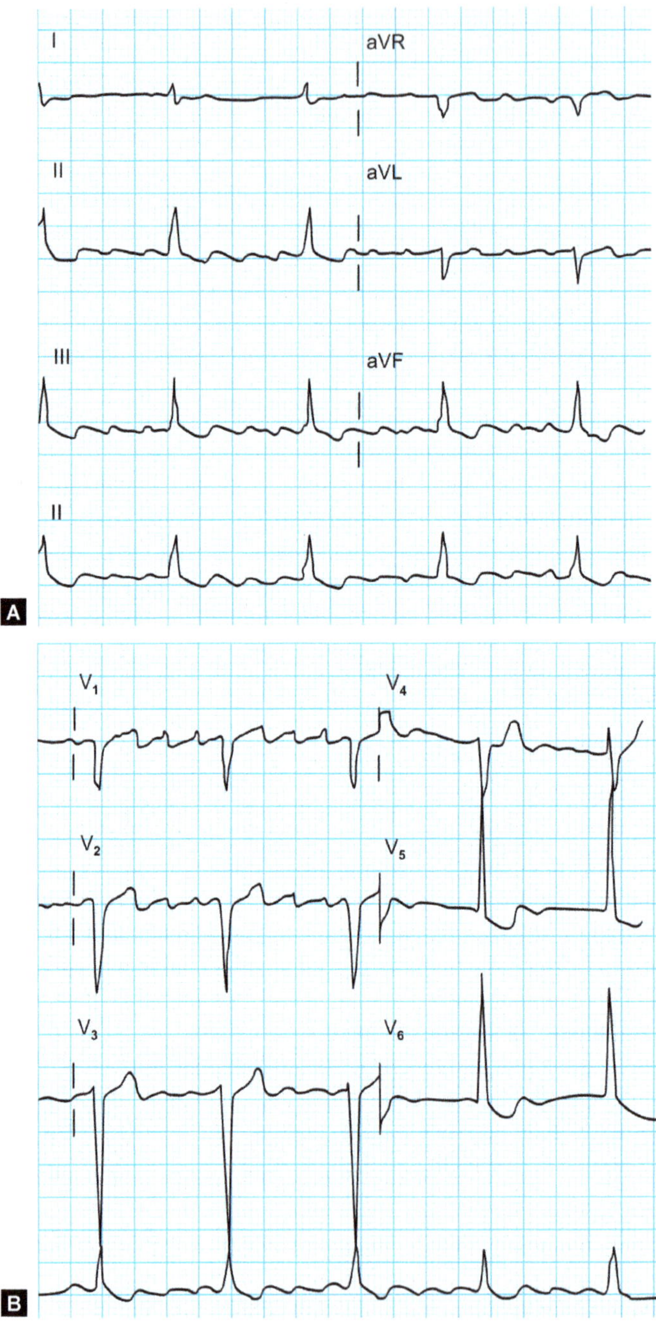

Figs. 11.32A and B: Atrial flutter. Note no flutter waves in lead I is a clue to confirm the diagnosis.

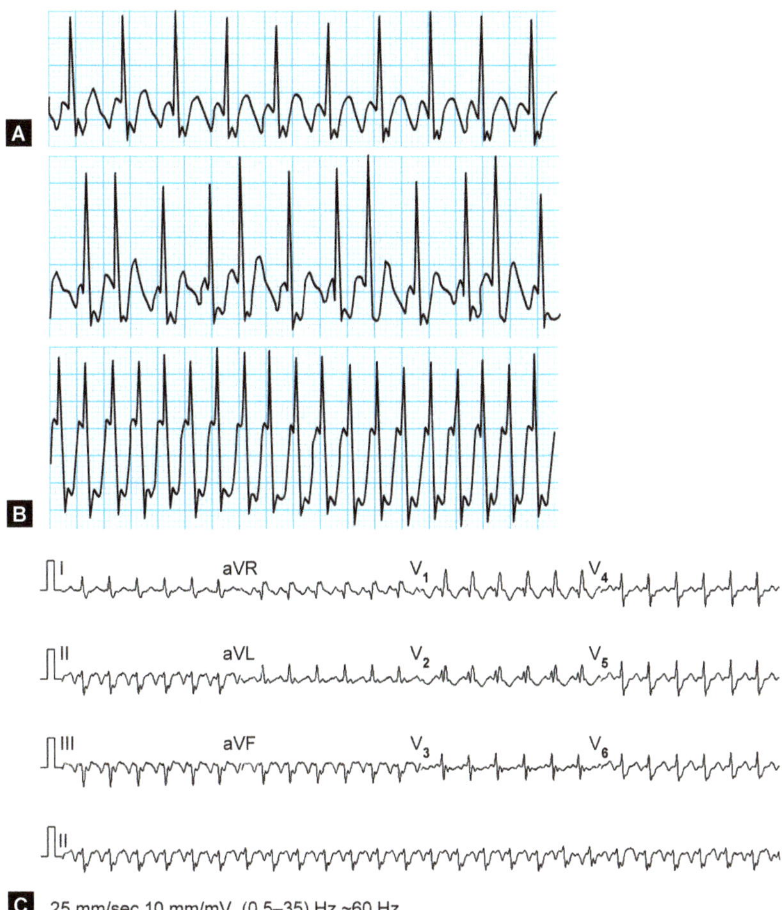

Figs. 11.33A to C: (A and B) Atrial flutter. (C) Atrial flutter rapid ventricular response; not clue in lead I no flutter waves.

REGULAR WIDE QRS TACHYCARDIA

Regular wide QRS tachycardia includes the following:
- *Ventricular tachycardia*: Consider all wide QRS regular tachycardias as VT until proven otherwise.
- *SVT with preexisting or functional bundle branch block*: These tachycardias include AVNRT, orthodromic circus movement tachycardia (WPW), atrial tachycardia, and atrial flutter with fixed AV conduction.
- Antidromic circus movement tachycardia or preexcited tachycardia (WPW) is usually exhibited by a very rapid rate >250 beats/min and may be irregular due to atrial fibrillation.

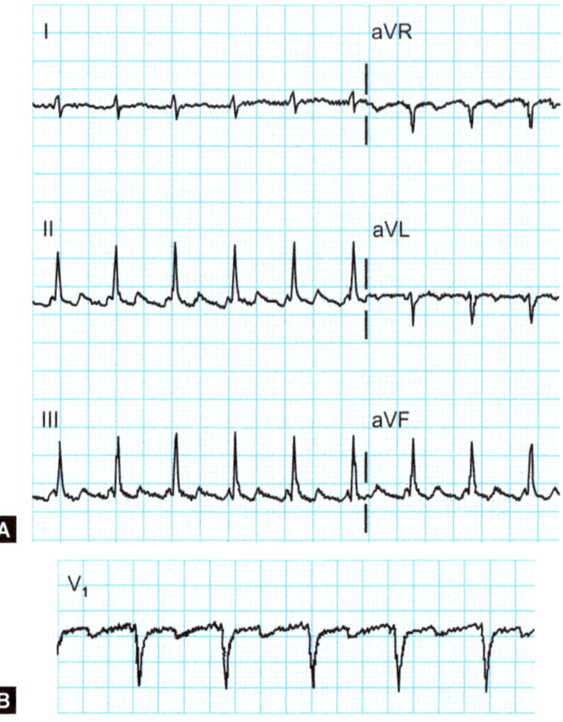

Figs. 11.34A and B: Atrial flutter: atrial rate, 270 bpm; ventricular rate, 135 bpm. Note the downward deflection of F waves in leads II, III, and aVF has a gradual slope followed by an abrupt upward deflection. This causes the sawtooth pattern. Alternate F waves coincide with the QRS complex, and the diagnosis may be missed.

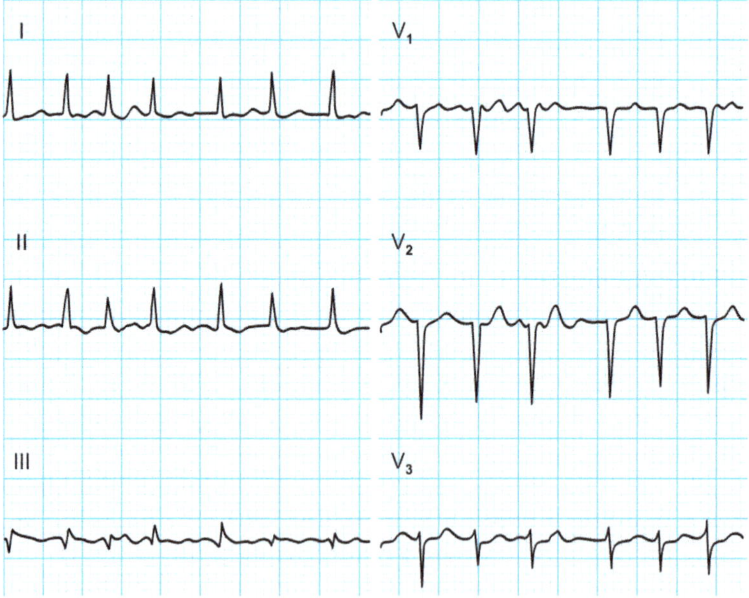

Fig. 11.35A

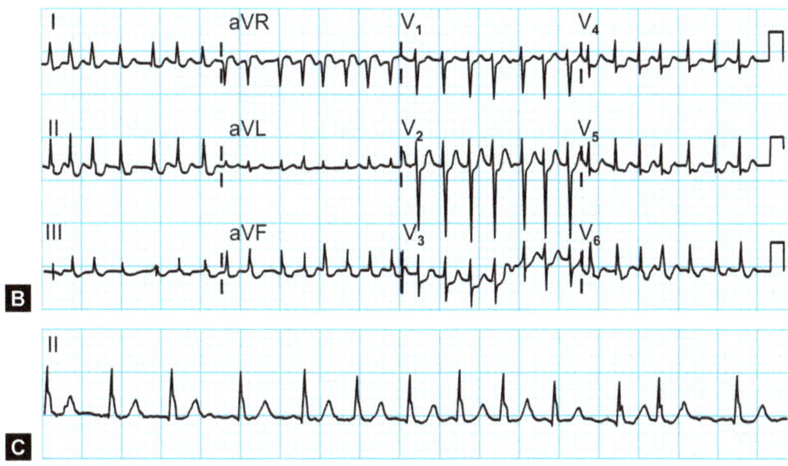

Figs. 11.35A to C: (A) Atrial fibrillation with a ventricular response of 156 bpm; (B) Atrial fibrillation with a rapid ventricular rate of 175 bpm; (C) Atrial fibrillation, same patient as in (B); controlled ventricular rate of 108 bpm.

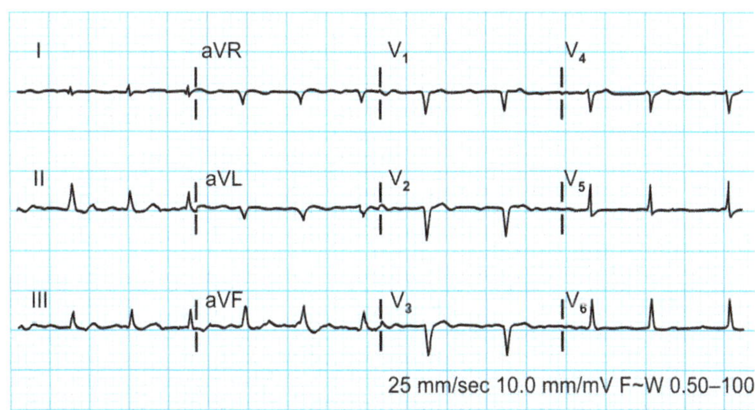

Fig. 11.36: Atrial fibrillation with slow ventricular response; rate, 70 bpm. Patient is 80 years old and is not taking digoxin or a β-blocker. Rates < 70 bpm commonly seen in older adults who are not taking cardiac medications should raise suspicion of sick sinus syndrome.

Ventricular Tachycardia

The ECG diagnosis of VT requires the assessment of all 12 ECG leads. The precordial leads are more diagnostic than lead II or other limb leads.

The diagnosis of VT can be confidently made by careful scrutiny of the morphologic pattern of the QRS complexes in V_1 through V_6.

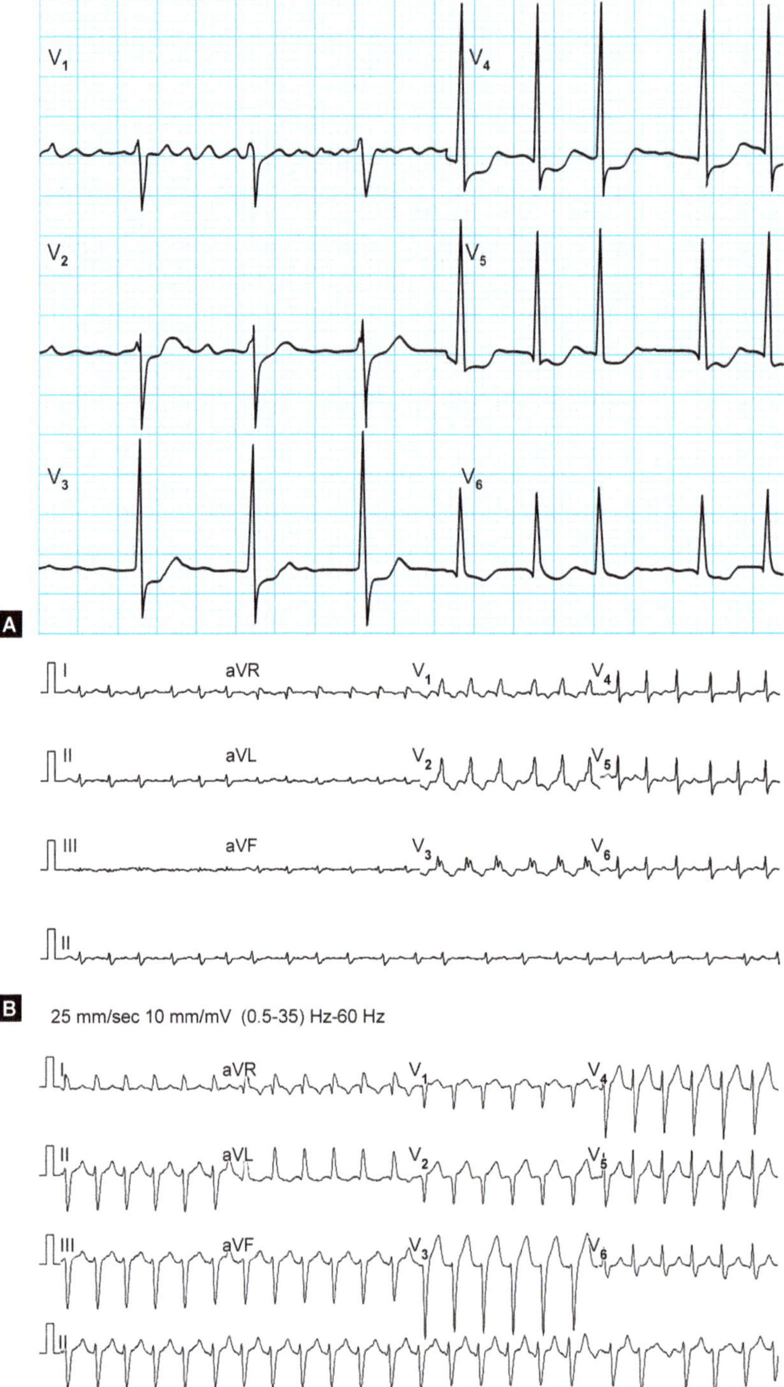

Figs. 11.37A to C

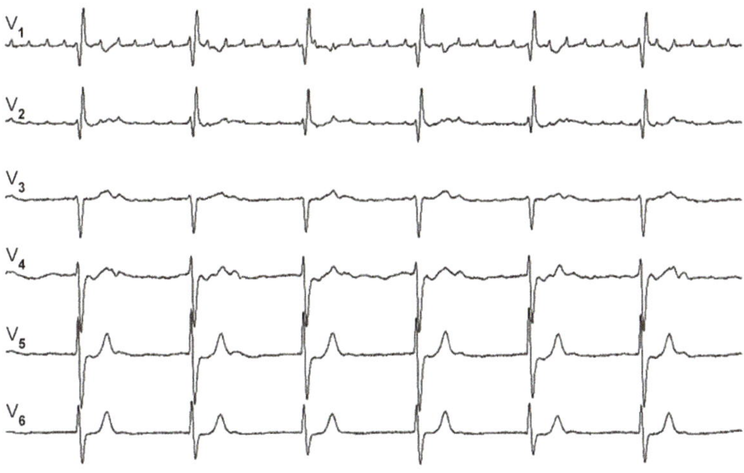

Fig. 11.37D

Figs. 11.37A to D: (A) Atrial fibrillation with a ventricular response rate of 104 bpm. Note the coarse atrial fibrillation in V_1; (B) Atrial fibrillation with rapid mean ventricular response 140 beats/min. RBBB; (C) Atrial fibrillation rapid ventricular response, and IVCD; (D) Atrial fibrillation fibrillatory waves V_1.

- If the QRS complexes are all negative in V_1 through V_6 (i.e. negative precordial concordance), the diagnosis of VT is certain (*see* Figs. 11.39 and 11.40). Negative precordial concordance excludes WPW regular wide complex tachycardia during anterograde conduction over an accessory pathway.
- Finding of predominately negative QRS complexes in V_4 through V_6 is diagnostic of VT (*see* Figs. 11.39 to 11.41)
- The presence of a QR complex in one or more of precordial leads V_2 through V_6 is diagnostic of VT (Figs. 11.39 and 11.40).
- Note that negative precordial concordance is diagnostic of VT but that positive concordance (all complexes positive in V_1 through V_6) can result from VT or circus movement antidromic tachycardia WPW syndrome.
  Findings in V_6 are most useful clues:
- A QS or rS in V_6 (net negative complex) (*see* Figs. 11.39 and 11.40).
  Findings in V_1 are useful clues:
- A wide small r wave more than 0.03 second (*see* Fig. 11.39).
- An RS interval longer than 0.1 second, measured from the R wave to the nadir of the S wave in any precordial lead.
- A steeper R wave upstroke than downstroke in V_1 (taller left "rabbit ear"). The morphology in V_1 may be helpful: If the left "rabbit ear" is taller than the right in lead V_1, VT is the most likely diagnosis (Fig. 11.39). Note that the rabbit ear may be subtle.

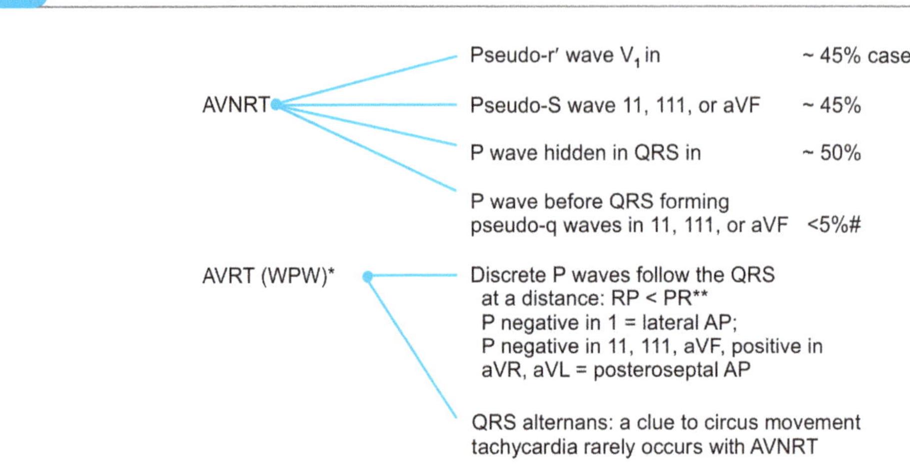

Fig. 11.38: Supraventricular arrhythmias: Key diagnostic clues.
*Common circus movement tachycardia uses the fast accessory pathway (AP); rare form uses the slow AP and the RP is > PR
** May occur with atrial tachycardia
#Rare form; negative Ps follow the QRS with RP > PR

Other helpful features include:

- *AV dissociation*: The presence of more QRS complexes than P waves supports the diagnosis of VT, but P wave identification may be difficult. The terminal portion of the T wave or initial parts of the QRS may resemble P waves, leading to an incorrect diagnosis of SVT. In addition, in some cases of VT, 1:1 ventricular/atrial conduction may be observed because retrograde impulse conduction to the atria from the ventricular focus often occurs. AV dissociation is not a reliable diagnostic point and is observed in less than 45% of VTs.
- With VT, the axis is commonly −90° to ±180°. However, the axis may be normal in patients with idiopathic VT and other varieties of VT.
- *Positive concordance*: A positive QRS complex in V_1 through V_6 is suggestive of VT, but this pattern can be seen with WPW syndrome. Negative precordial concordance is diagnostic of VT because this pattern does not occur during antidromic circus movement tachycardia (WPW syndrome) in which conduction is anterograde over the bypass tract (Fig. 11.42).

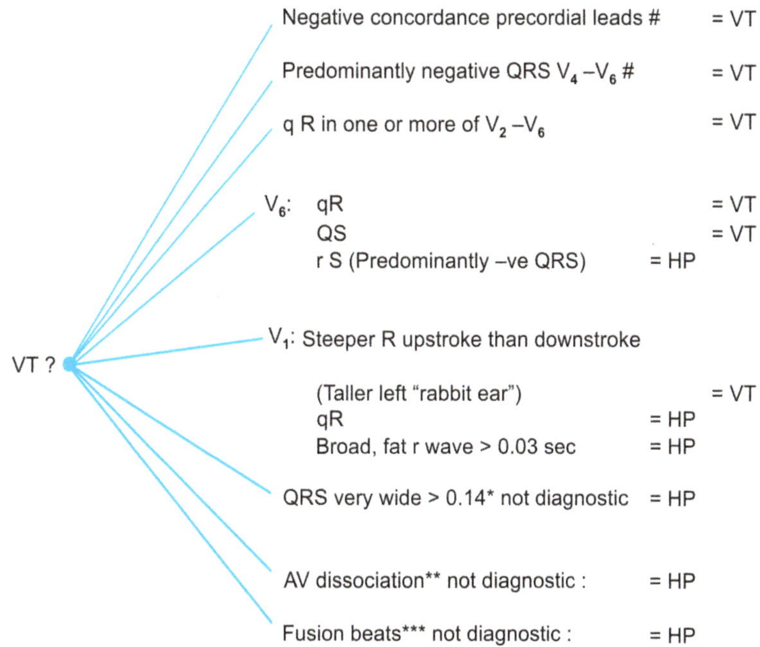

Fig. 11.39: Ventricular tachycardia: Key Diagnostic Clues.

*HP = High probability VT
#Excludes a preexcited WPW antidromic techycardia
*QRS: if known in recent past to be normal duration
** Only observed in < 45% VT. and can occur with junctional tachycardia with LBBB
***Observed in only ~ 15% of VT and fusion of aberrantly conducted junctional impulses with simultaneous sinus impulses do occur

IRREGULAR WIDE QRS TACHYCARDIA

Irregular wide QRS tachycardias include the following:

- Torsades de pointes.
- Atrial fibrillation with bundle branch block or with the antidromic variety of WPW, anterograde conduction over the bypass tract (Figs. 11.43 and 11.44).
- Atrial flutter with varying AV conduction and bundle branch block or atrial flutter and varying AV conduction in the WPW syndrome with anterograde conduction (antidromic) over the bypass tract (Fig. 11.45).

Torsades de Pointes

- Torsades is a polymorphic VT that usually occurs in the presence of a prolonged QT interval.
- The RR interval is irregular; the QRS complexes show a typical twisting of the points (Figs. 11.46A and B).
- The amplitudes of the complexes vary and appear alternately above and below the baseline.
- The ventricular rate varies from 200 bpm to 300 bpm, but can reach 400 bpm, and is usually not sustained (lasting 30 seconds to 1 minute).

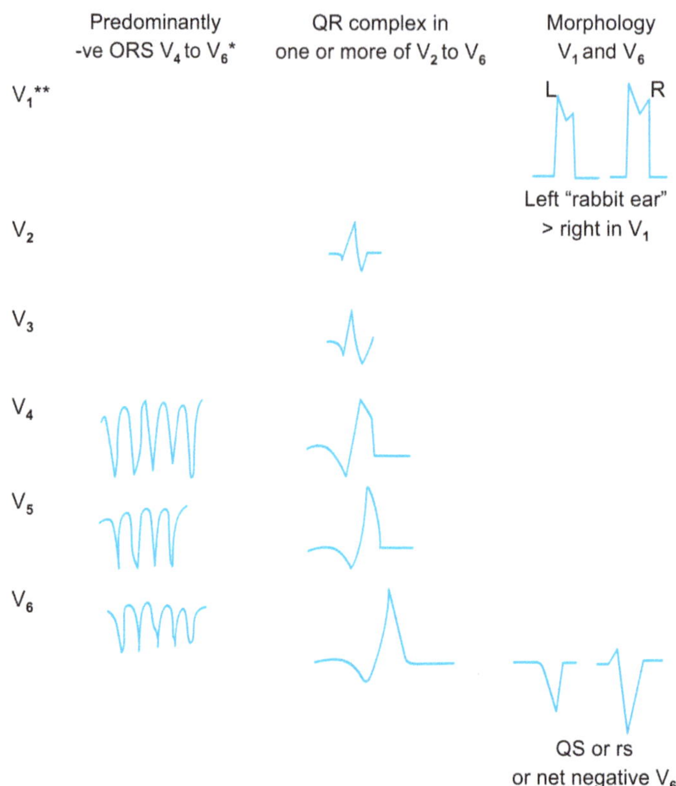

Fig. 11.40: Electrocardiographic hallmarks of ventricular tachycardia (VT).
* = or concordant negativity in leads V$_1$ through V$_4$ Positive concordance in leads V$_1$ through V$_6$ can be caused by VT or Wolff-Parkinson-White antidromic (preexcited) tachycardia
** = it is necessary to study the entire 12-lead tracing with particular emphasis on leads V$_1$ through V$_6$ lead II may be useful for assessment of P wave and AV dissociation

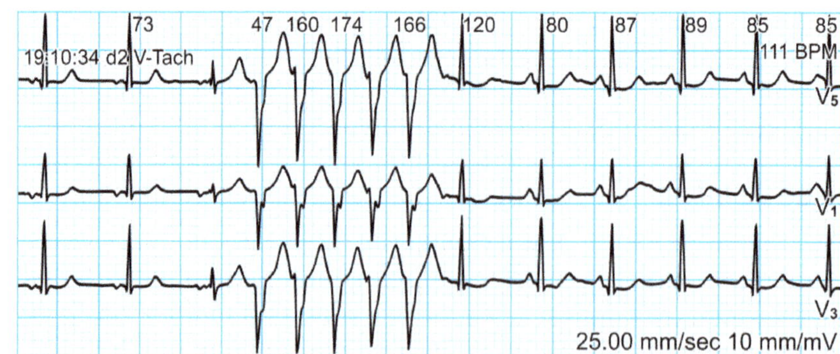

Fig. 11.41: Onset of a wide regular QRS tachycardia with negative precordial concordance in V$_1$–V$_3$, V$_6$, also Figure 11.40 indicates ventricular tachycardia. Negative precordial concordance indicates VT because such a pattern does not occur during anterograde conduction over an accessorWy pathway.

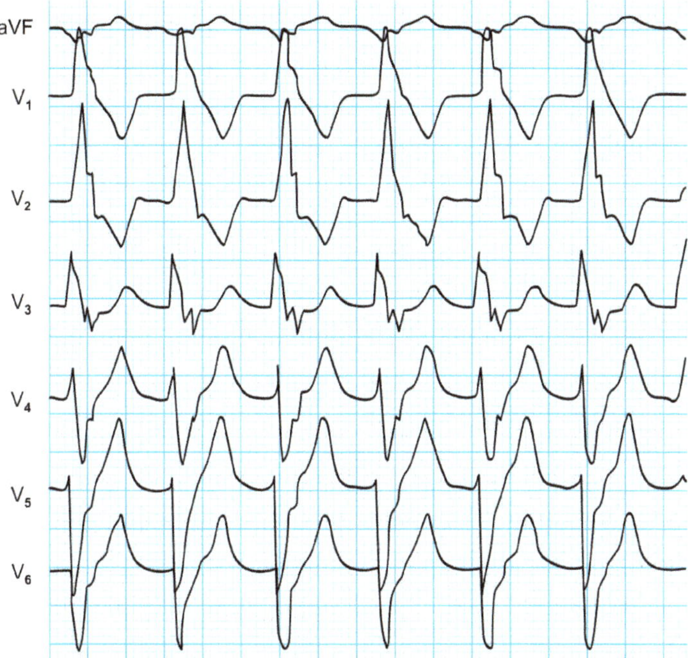

Fig. 11.42: Ventricular tachycardia. Note the steep monophasic R wave in lead V₁ (left "rabbit ear") and the deep S in lead V₆, signs of ventricular tachycardia. The northwest axis is also a helpful clue.

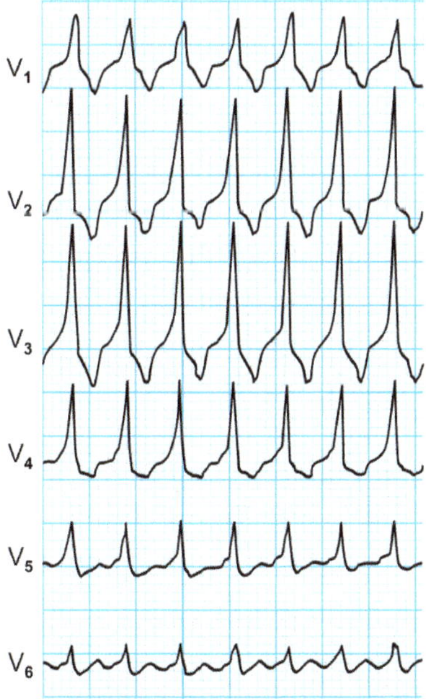

Fig. 11.43: Broad QRS tachycardia with positive precordial concordance. The mechanism is atrial flutter with 2:1 conduction over a left-sided accessory pathway.

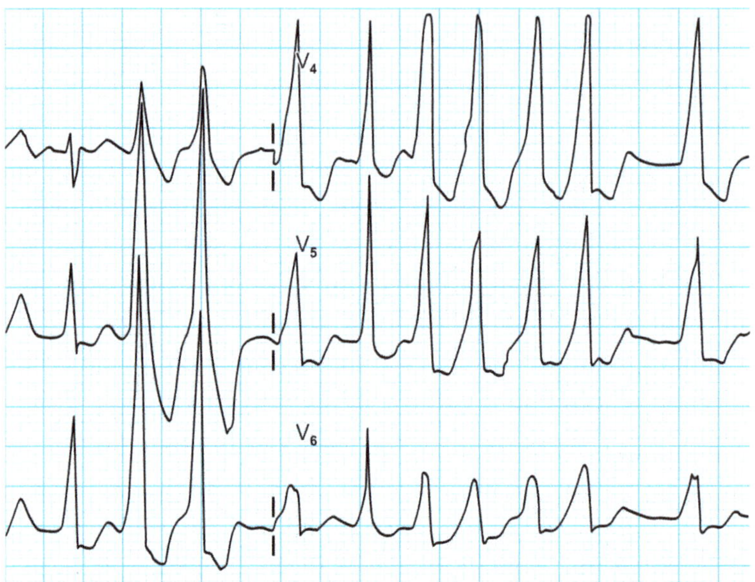

Fig. 11.44: Atrial fibrillation with wide QRS tachycardia in a patient with Wolff-Parkinson-White syndrome: antidromic tachycardia.

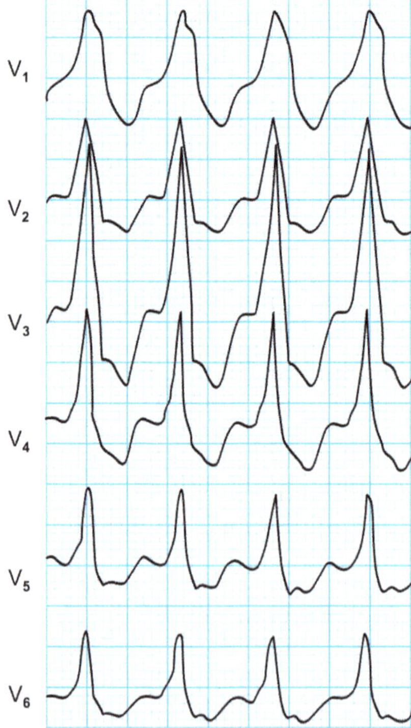

Fig. 11.45: A 12-lead ECG from a patient with antidromic circus movement tachycardia.

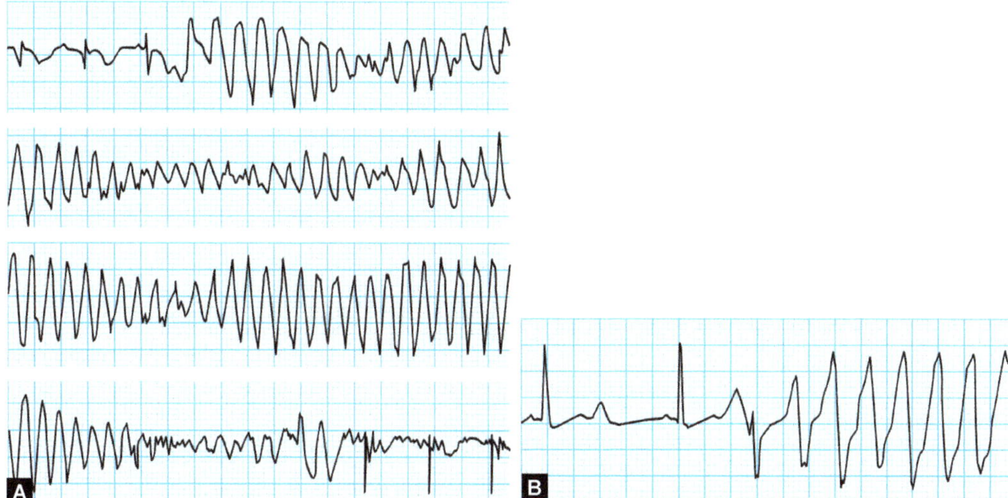

Figs. 11.46A and B: Torsades de pointes. (A) Continuous recording monitor lead. A demand ventricular pacemaker (VVI) has been implanted because of Mobitz type II second degree AV block. After treatment with amiodarone for recurrent ventricular tachycardia (VT), the QT interval became prolonged (approximately 640 milliseconds during paced beats), and the patient developed episodes of torsades de pointes. In this recording, the tachycardia spontaneously terminates, and a paced ventricular rhythm is restored. Motion artifact is noted at the end of the recording as the patient lost consciousness; (B) Tracing from a young boy with a congenital long QT syndrome. The QTU interval in the sinus beats is at least 600 milliseconds. Note TU wave alternans in the first and second complexes. A late premature complex occurring in the downslope of the TU wave initiates an episode of VT.

- Longer episodes degenerate into ventricular fibrillation.
  Drugs and conditions that may precipitate torsades include the following:
- Antiarrhythmics known to increase the QT interval (e.g. quinidine, procainamide, amiodarone, disopyramide, sotalol)
- Tricyclic antidepressants and phenothiazines
- Histamine (H1) antagonists (e.g. astemizole, terfenadine)
- Antiviral and antifungal agents and antibiotics
- Hypokalemia, hypomagnesemia
- Insecticide poisoning
- Bradyarrhythmias
- Congenital long QT syndrome
- Subarachnoid hemorrhage
- Chloroquine, pentamidine
- Cocaine abuse.

ECG Board Self-Assessment Quiz

CONTENTS

ECG Board Self-Assessment Quiz
Answers to ECG Board Self-Assessment Quiz

(Note: See pages 337–345 for answers)

Source: From *Contemporary Cardiology: Rapid ECG Interpretation, 3e* by: M. Gabriel Khan ©
Humana Press, a part of Springer Science+Business Media, LLC 2008.

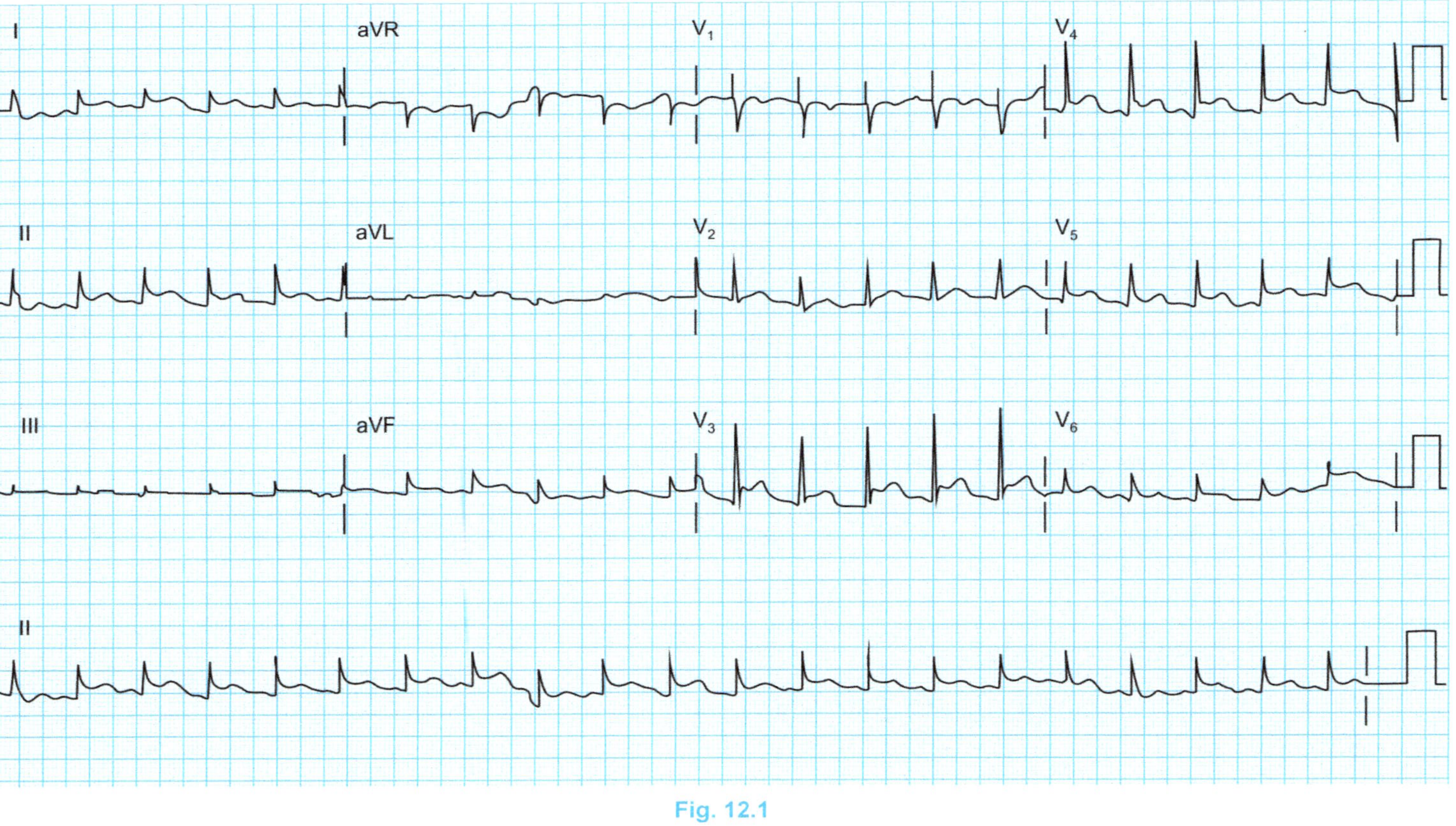

Fig. 12.1

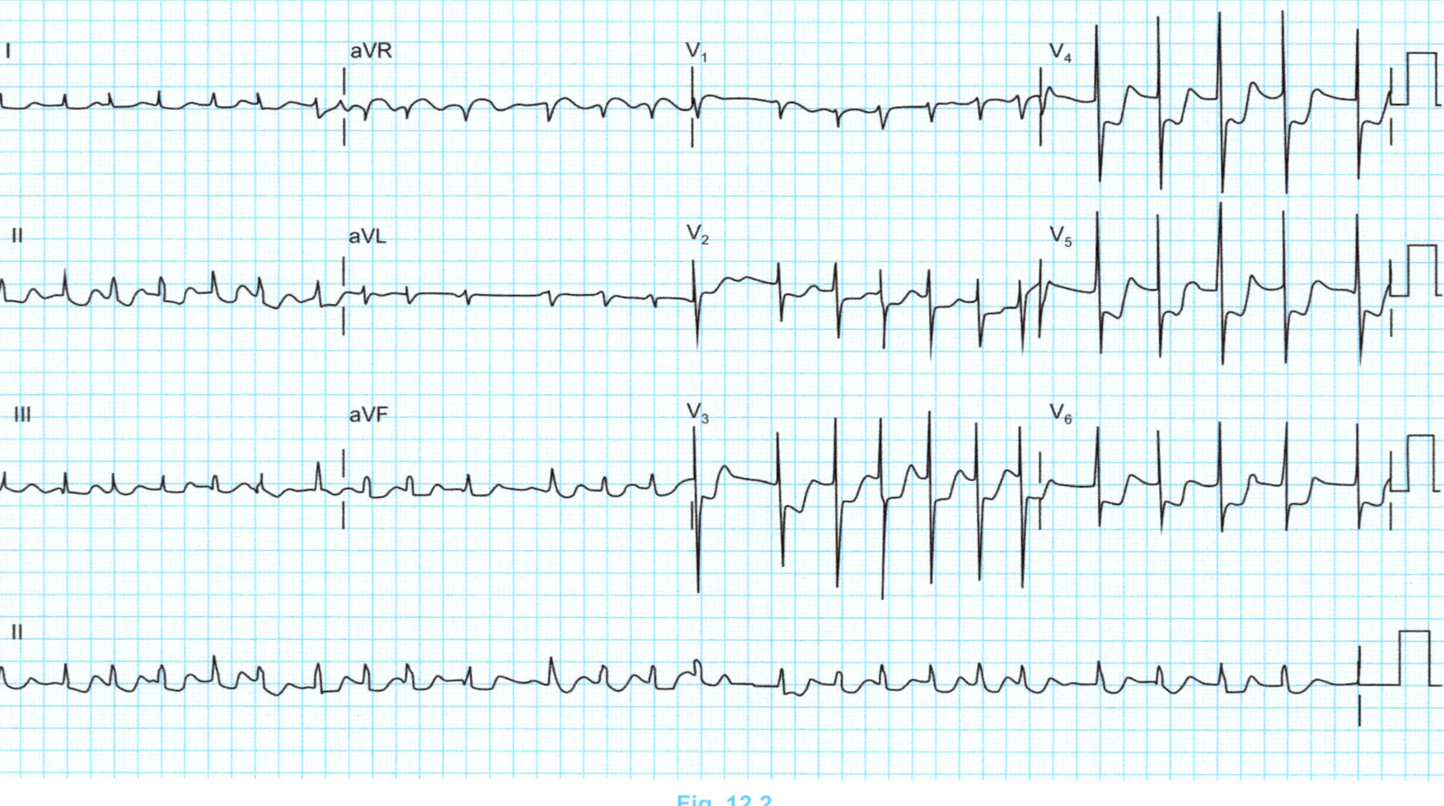

Fig. 12.2

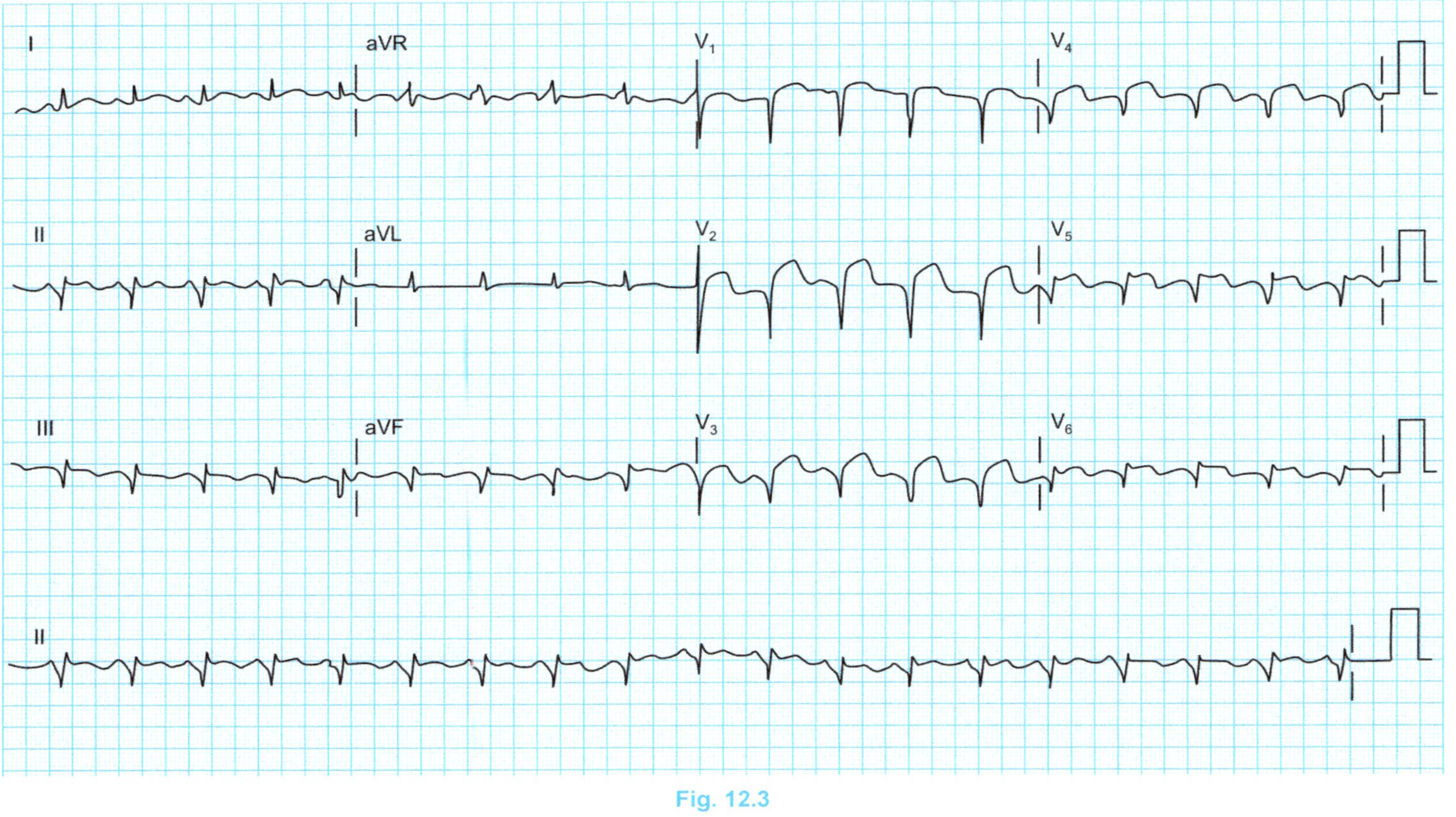

Fig. 12.3

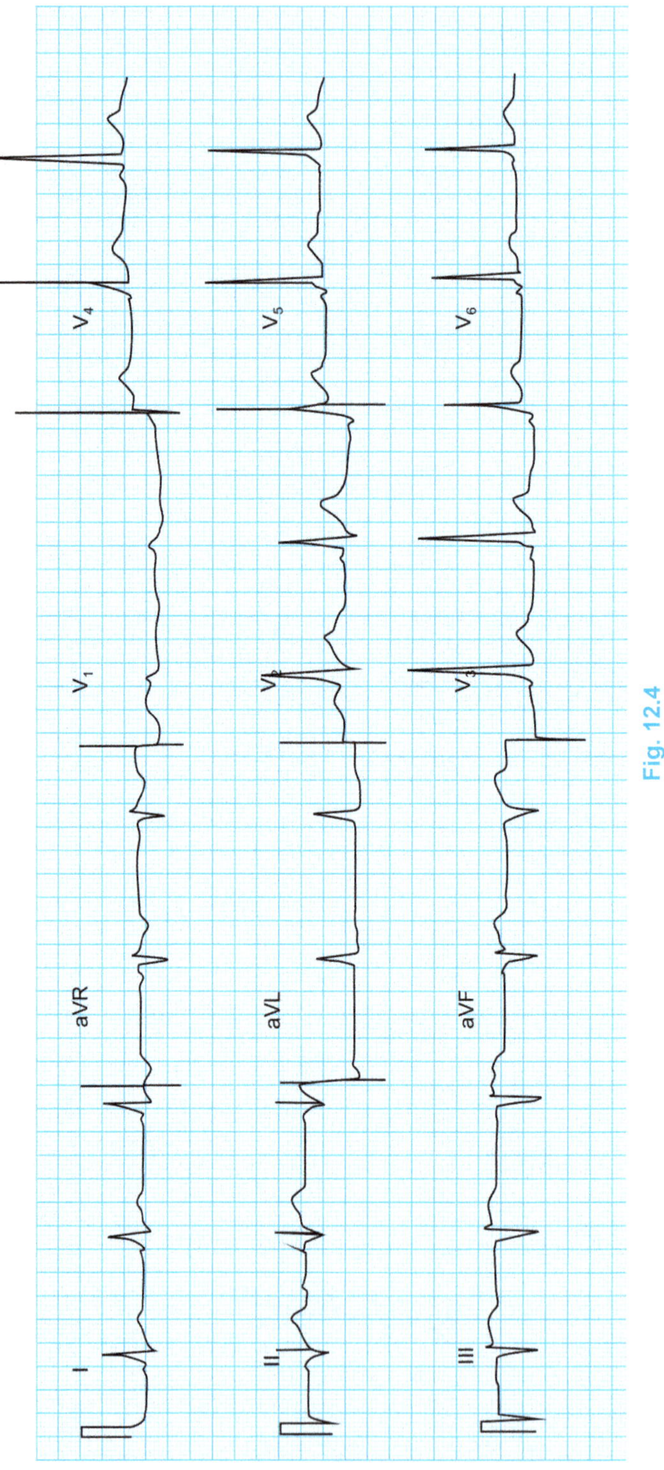

Fig. 12.4

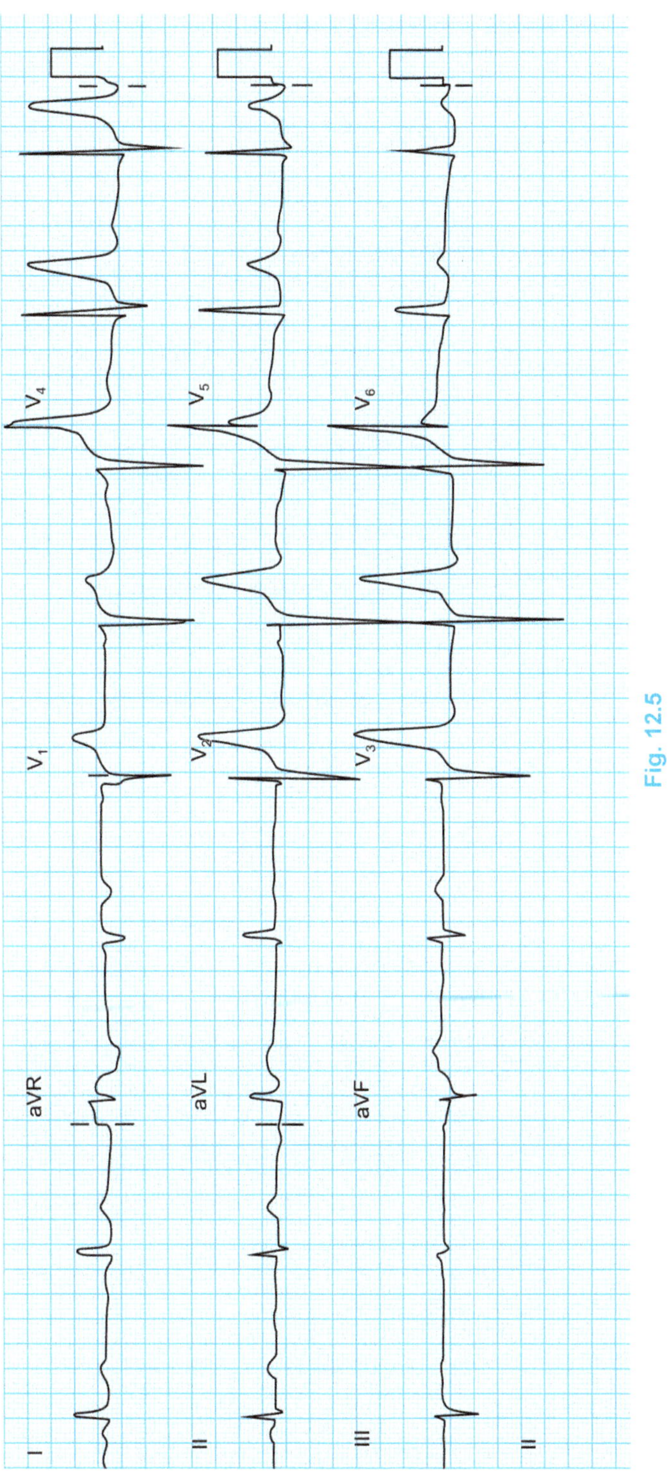

Fig. 12.5

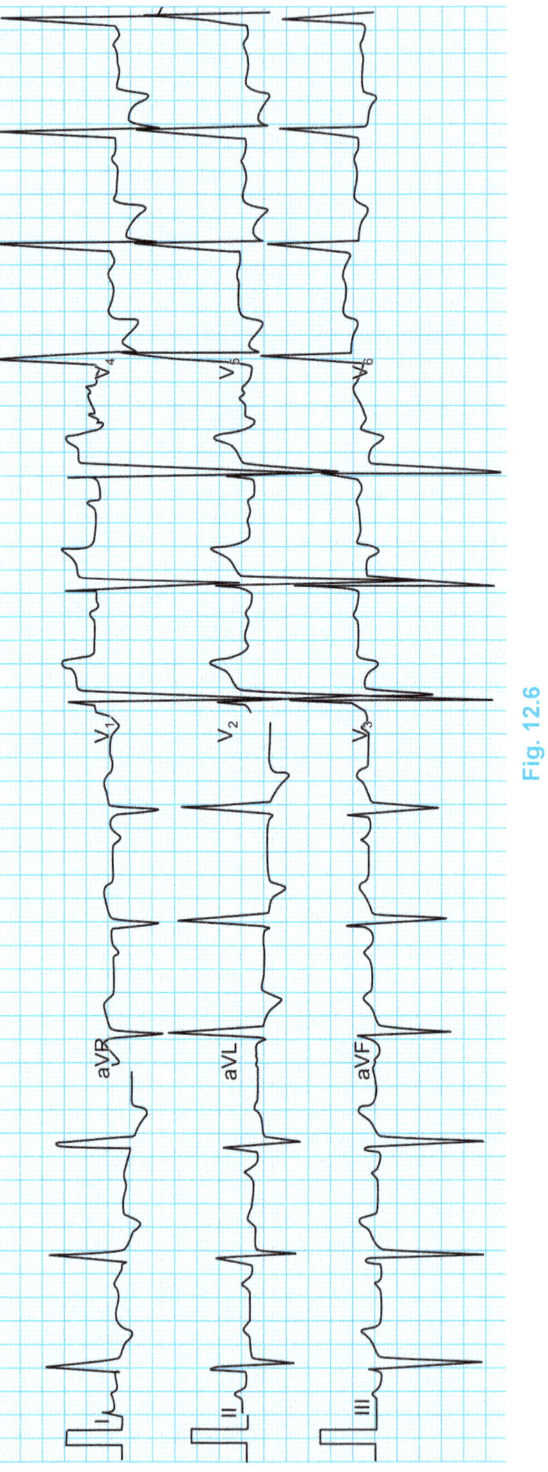

Fig. 12.6

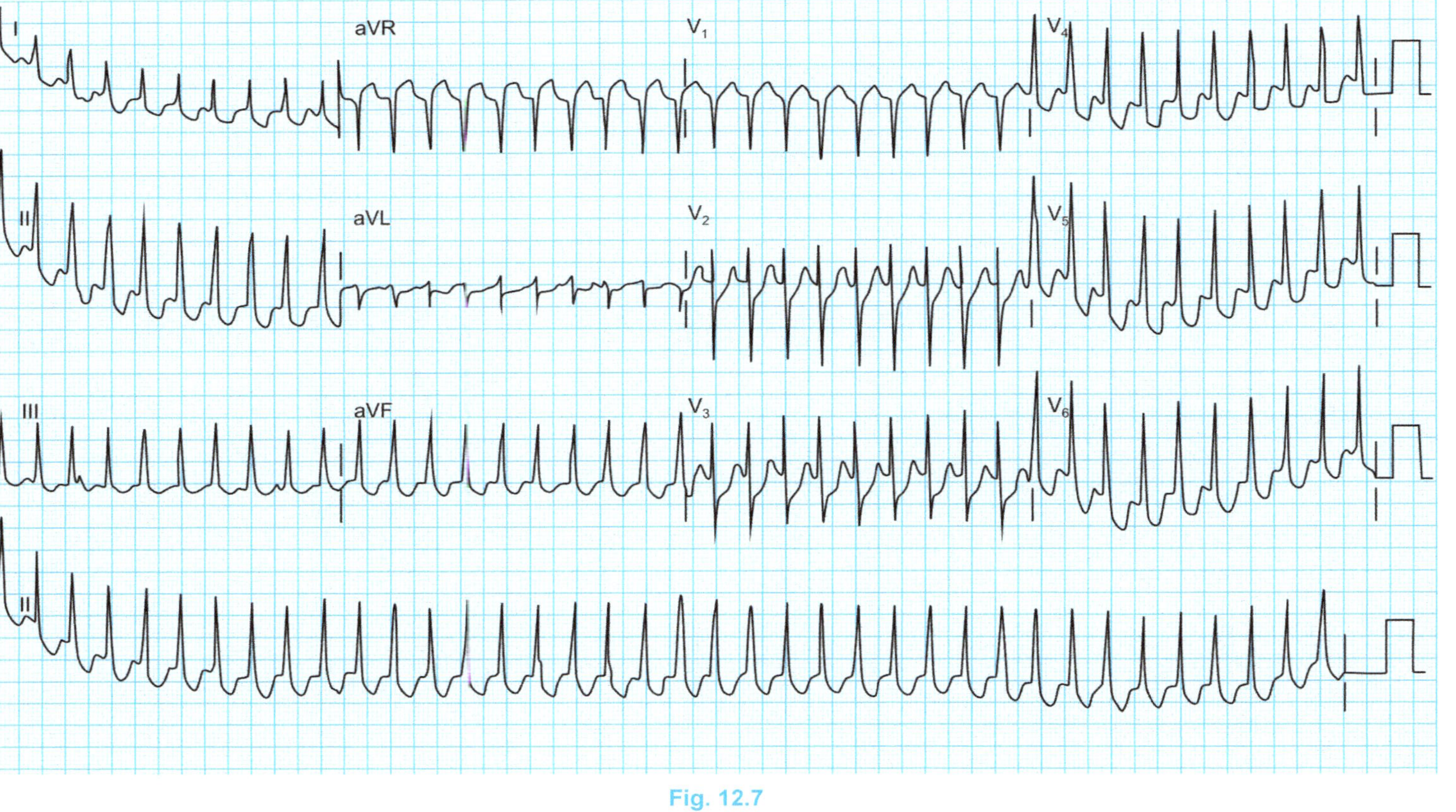

Fig. 12.7

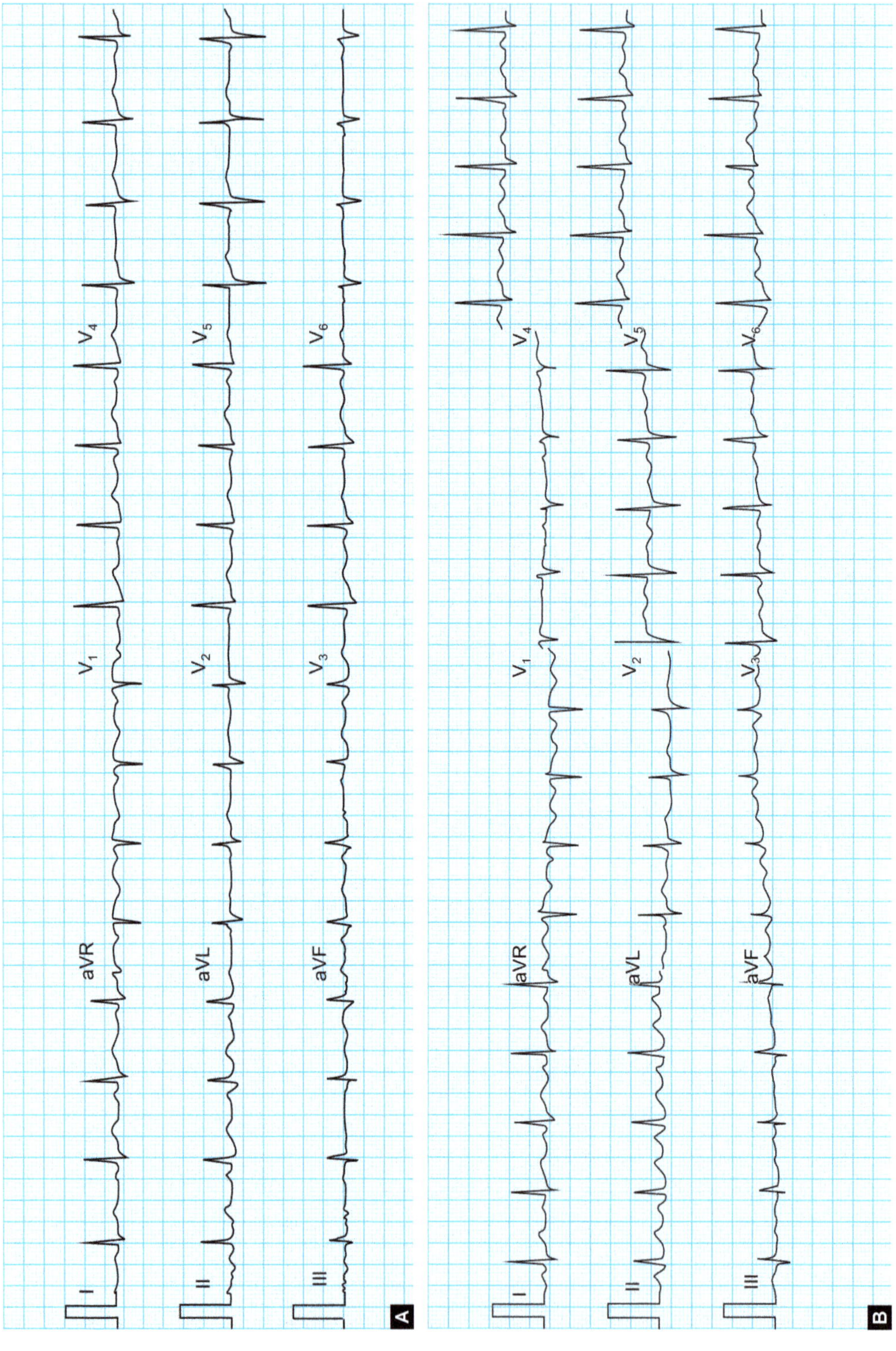

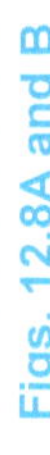

Figs. 12.8A and B

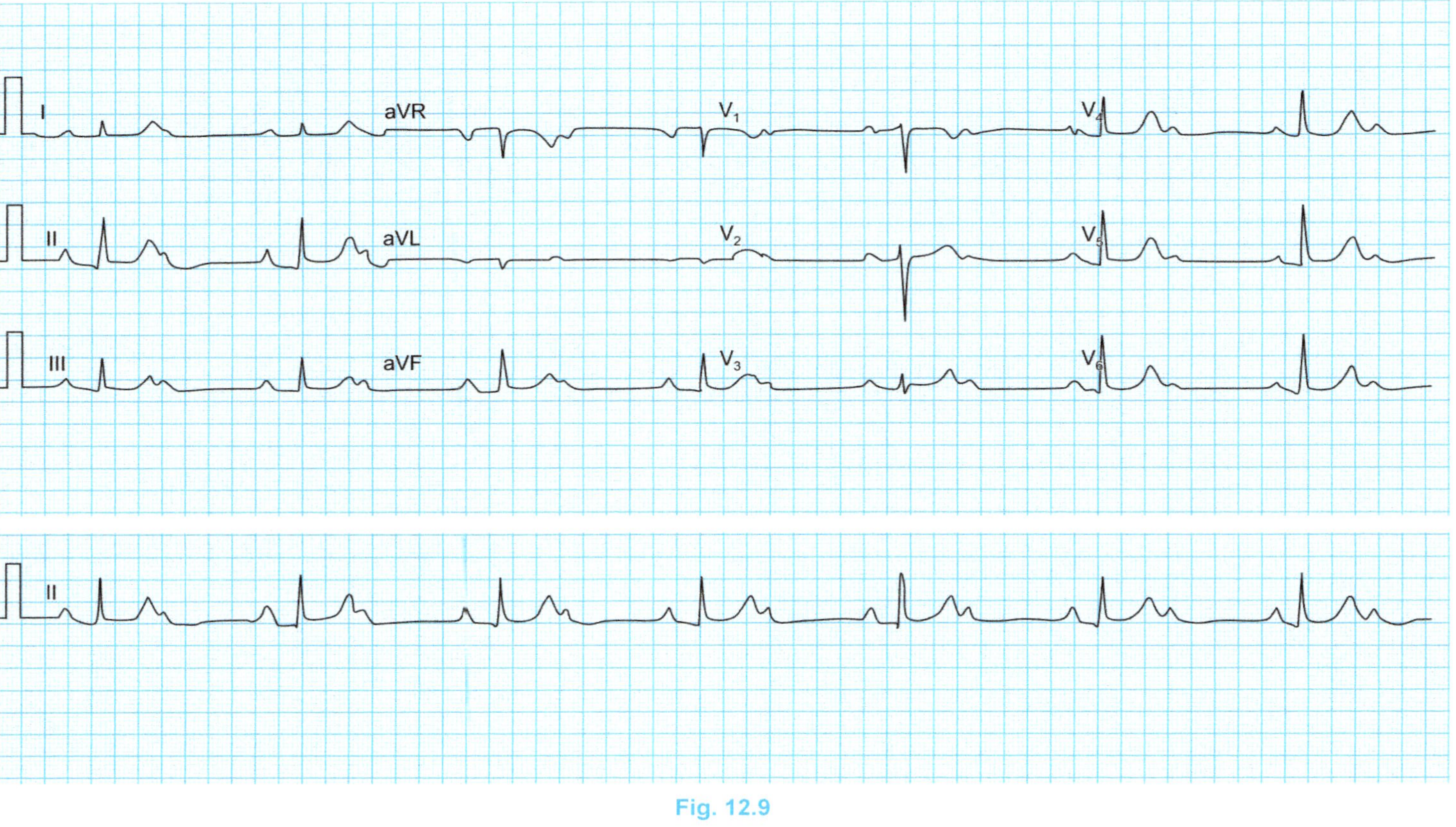

Fig. 12.9

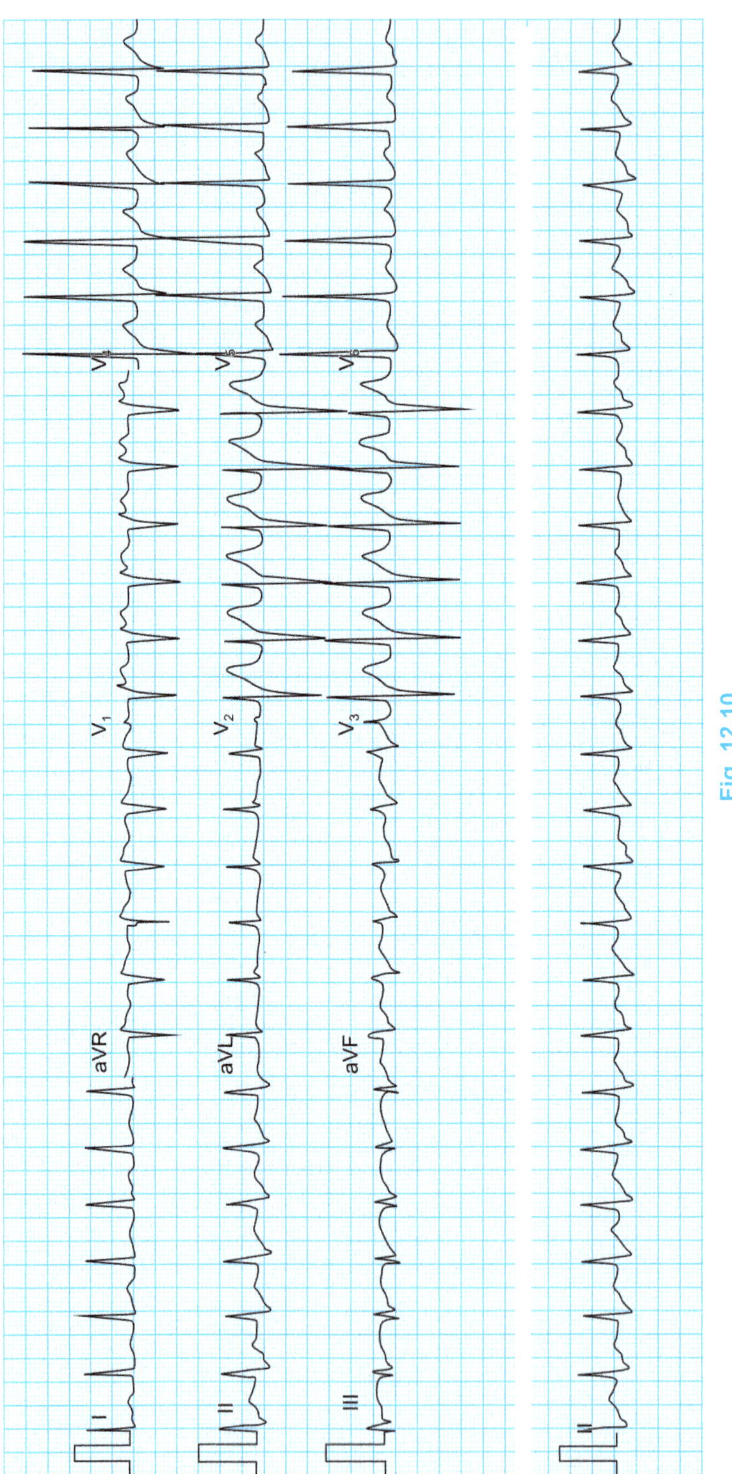

Fig. 12.10

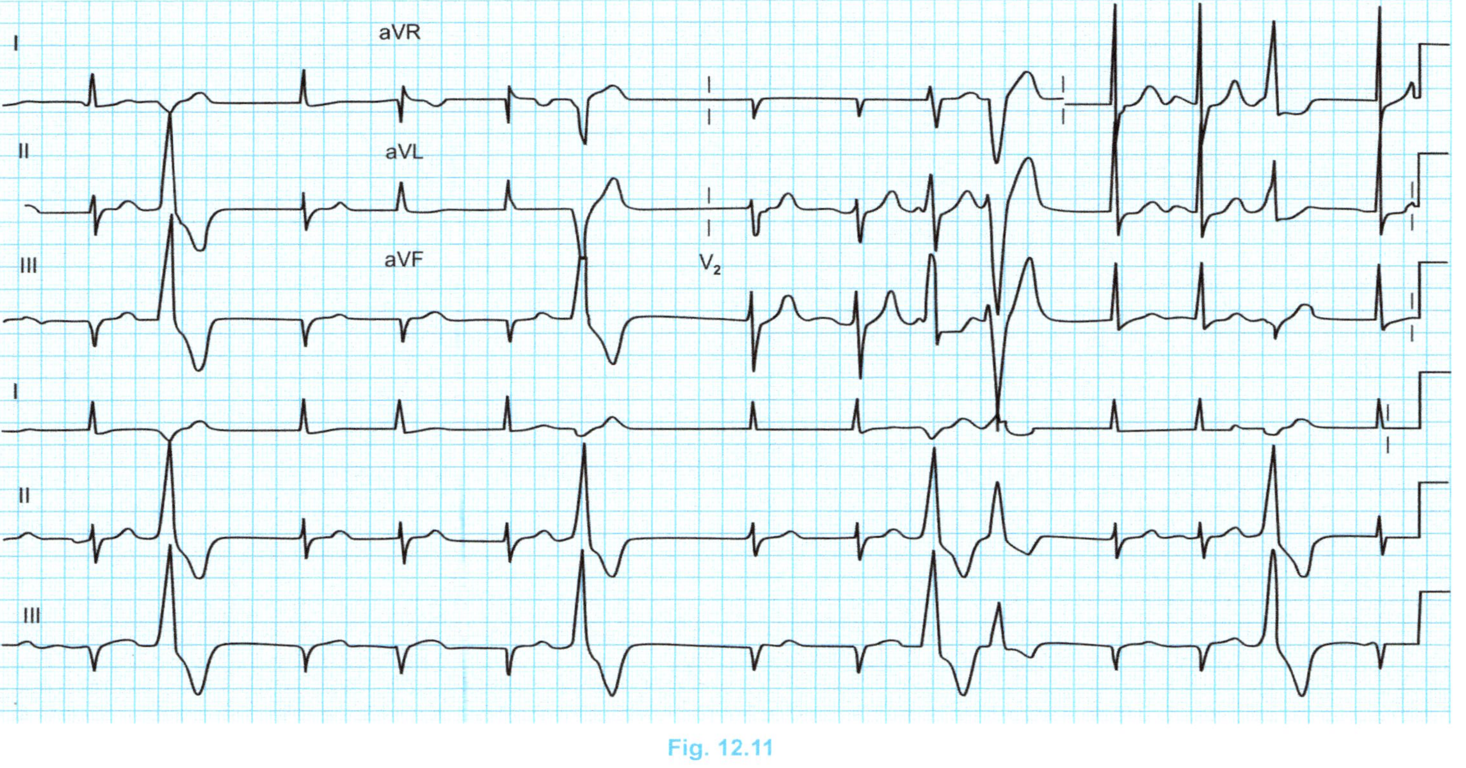

Fig. 12.11

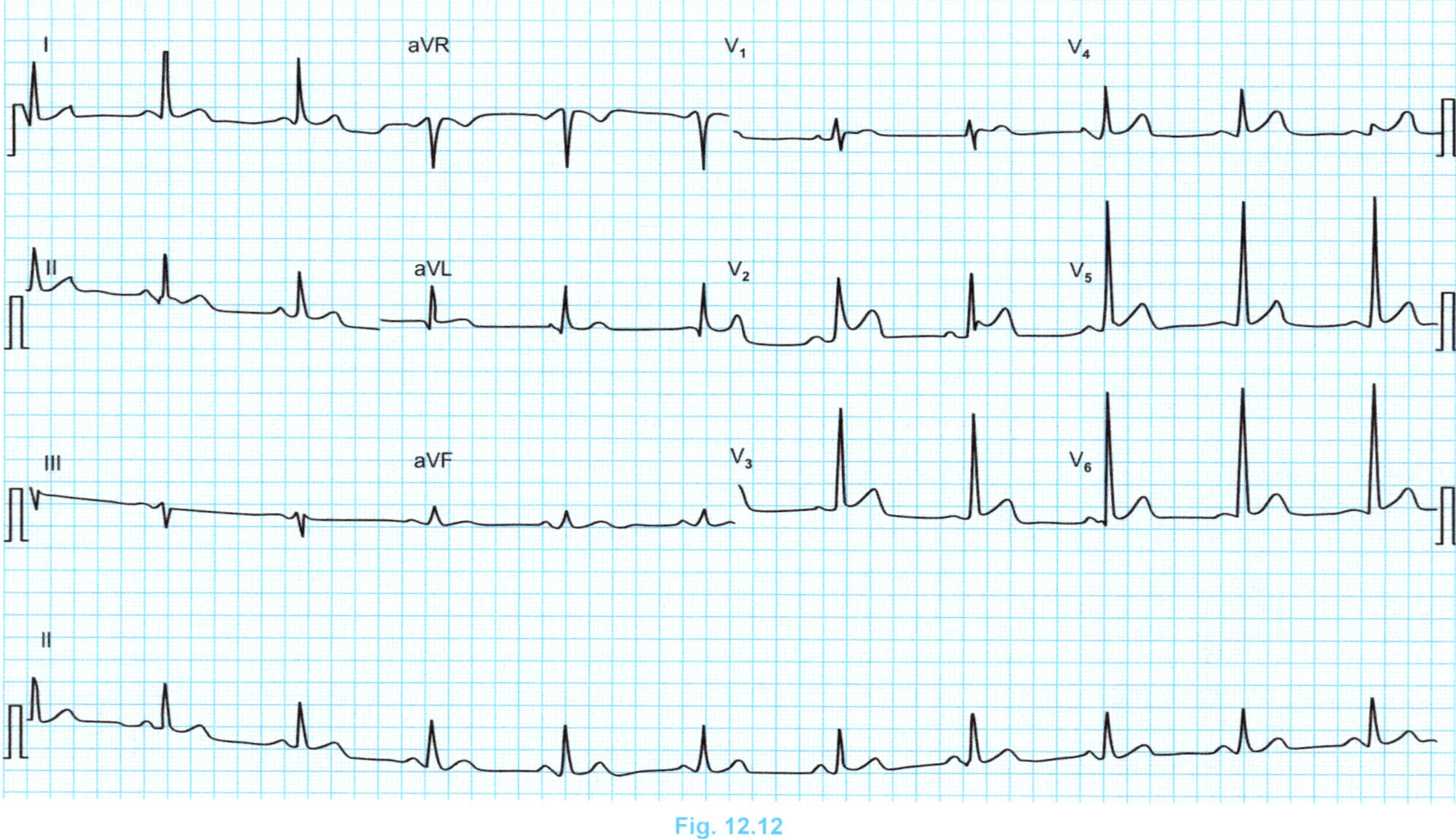

Fig. 12.12

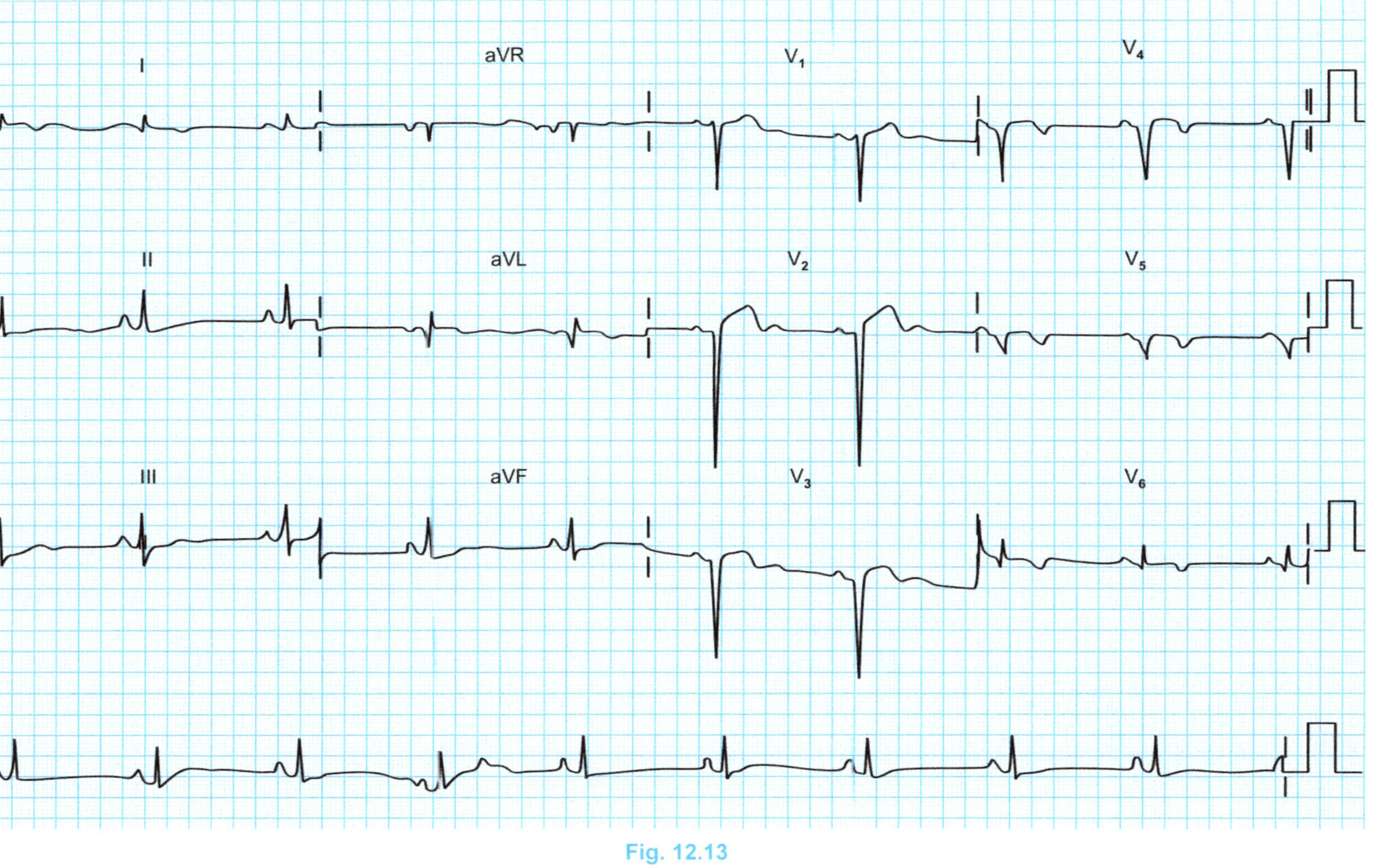

Fig. 12.13

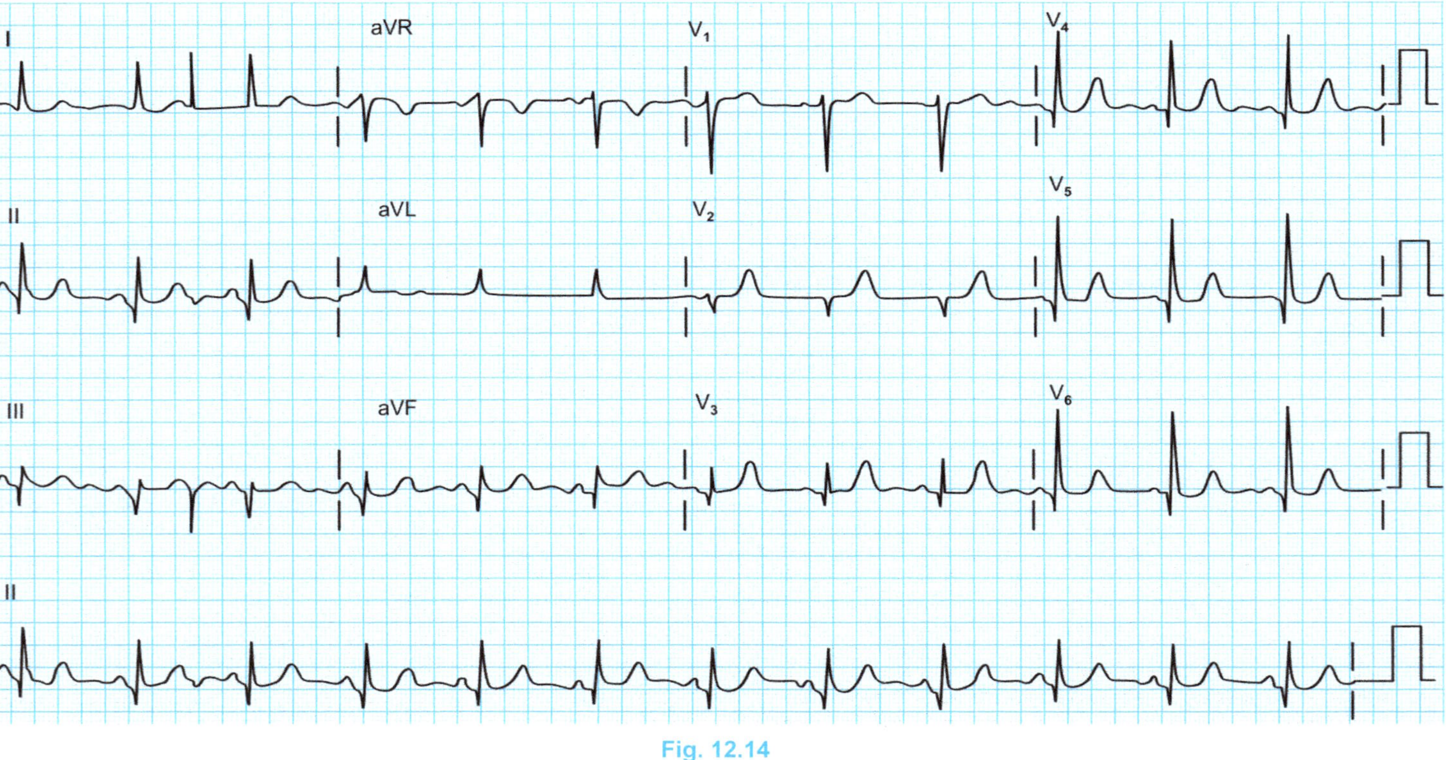

Fig. 12.14

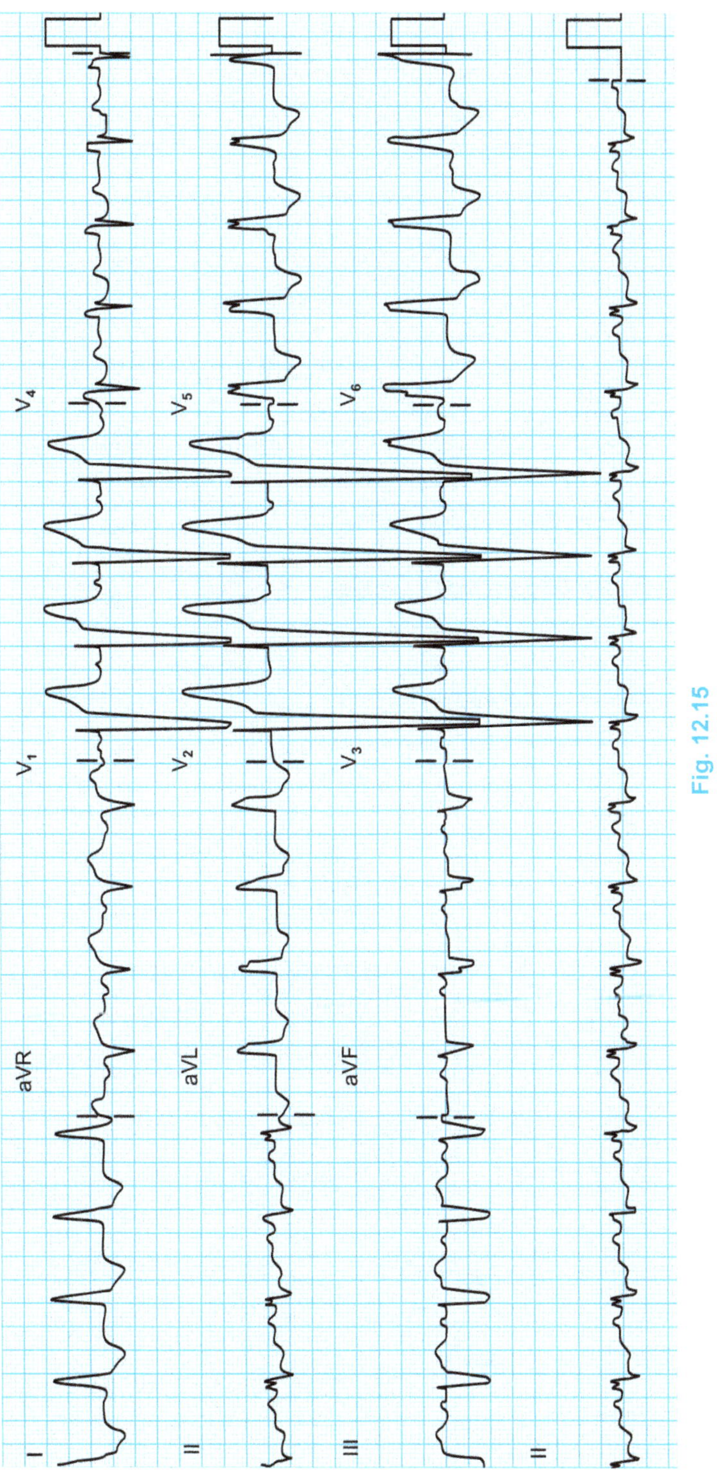

Fig. 12.15

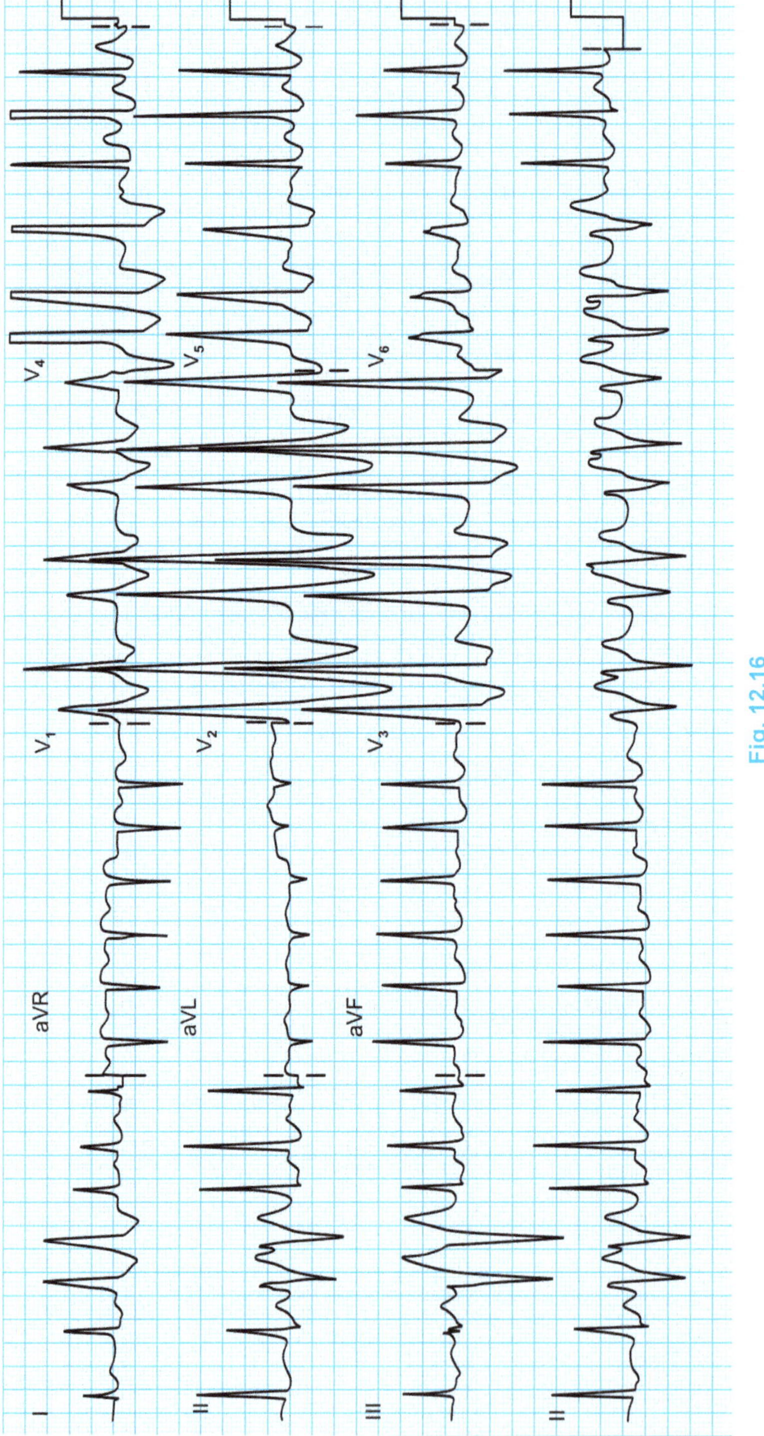

Fig. 12.16

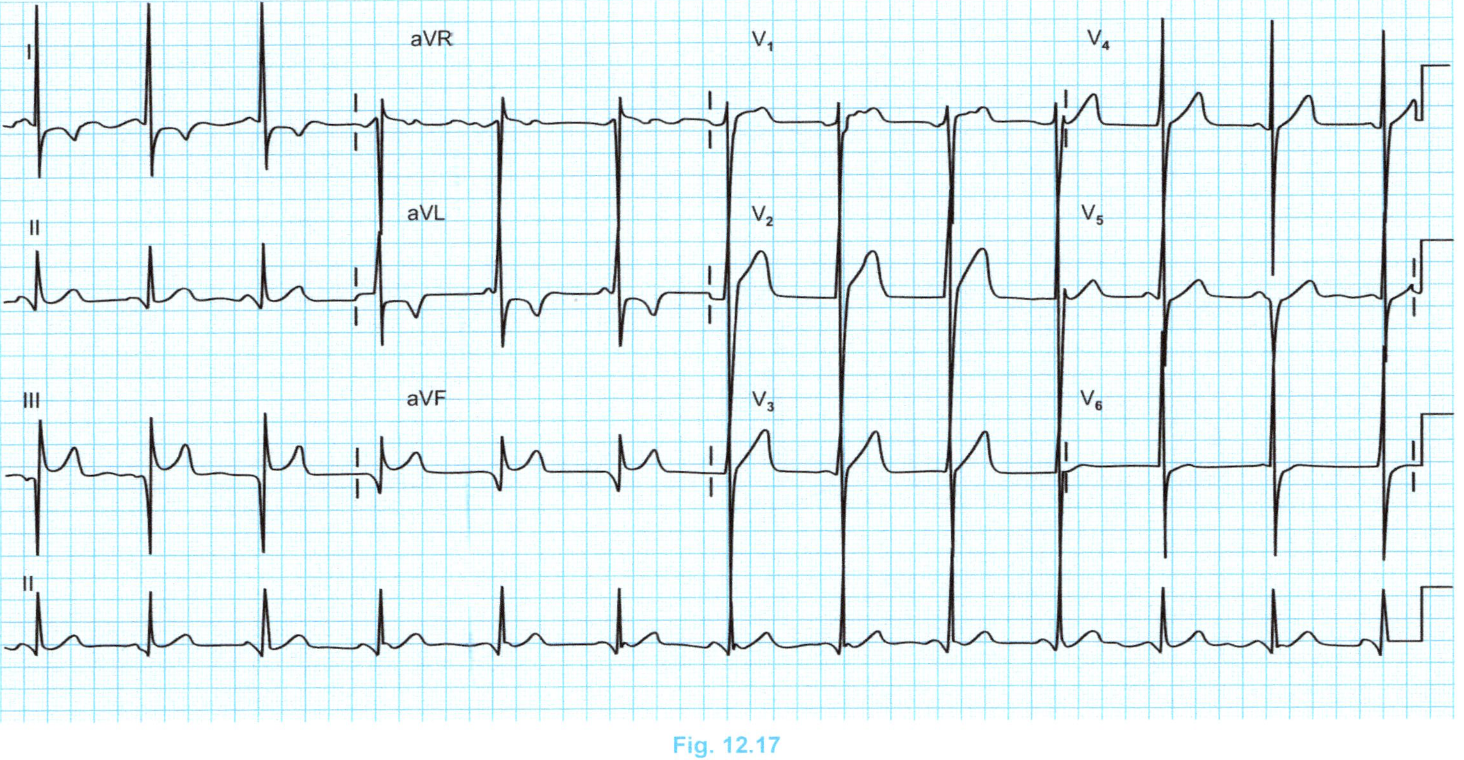

Fig. 12.17

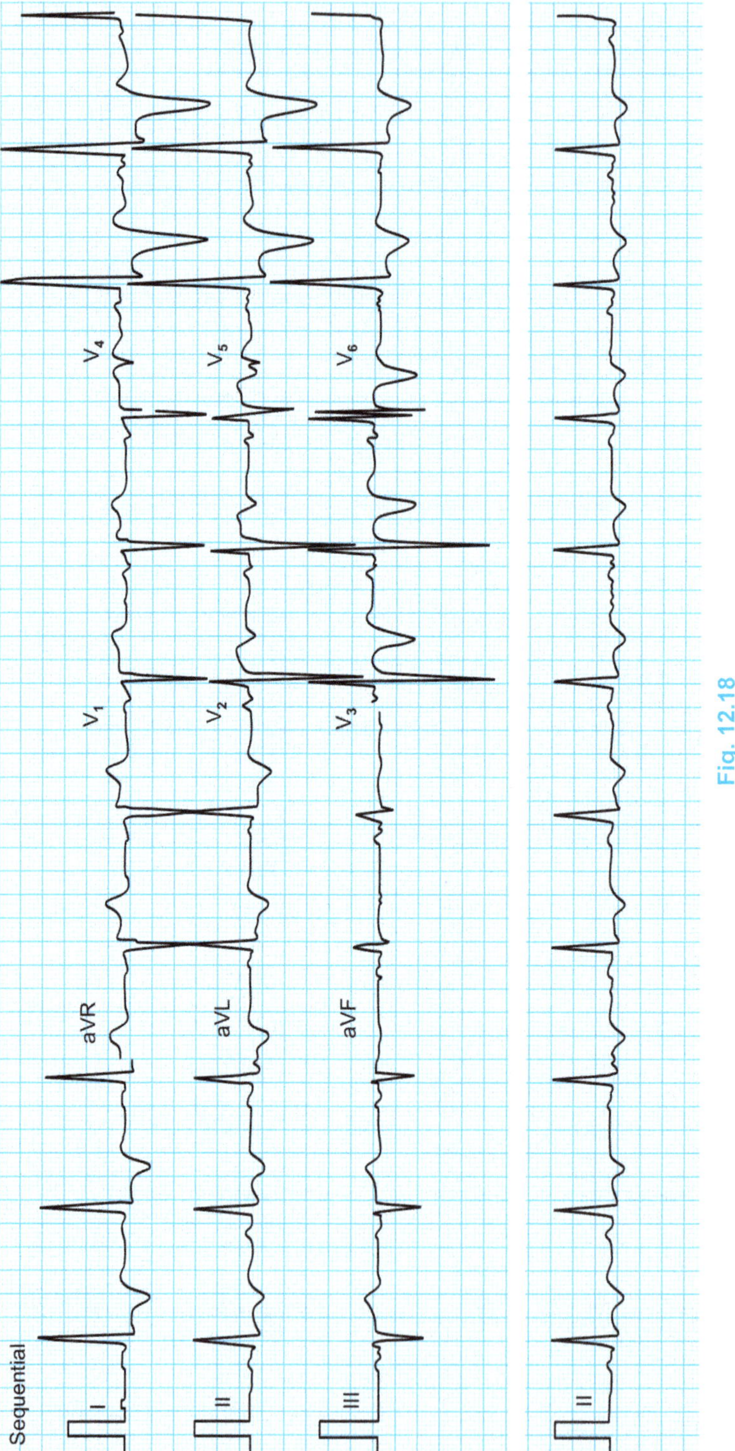

Fig. 12.18

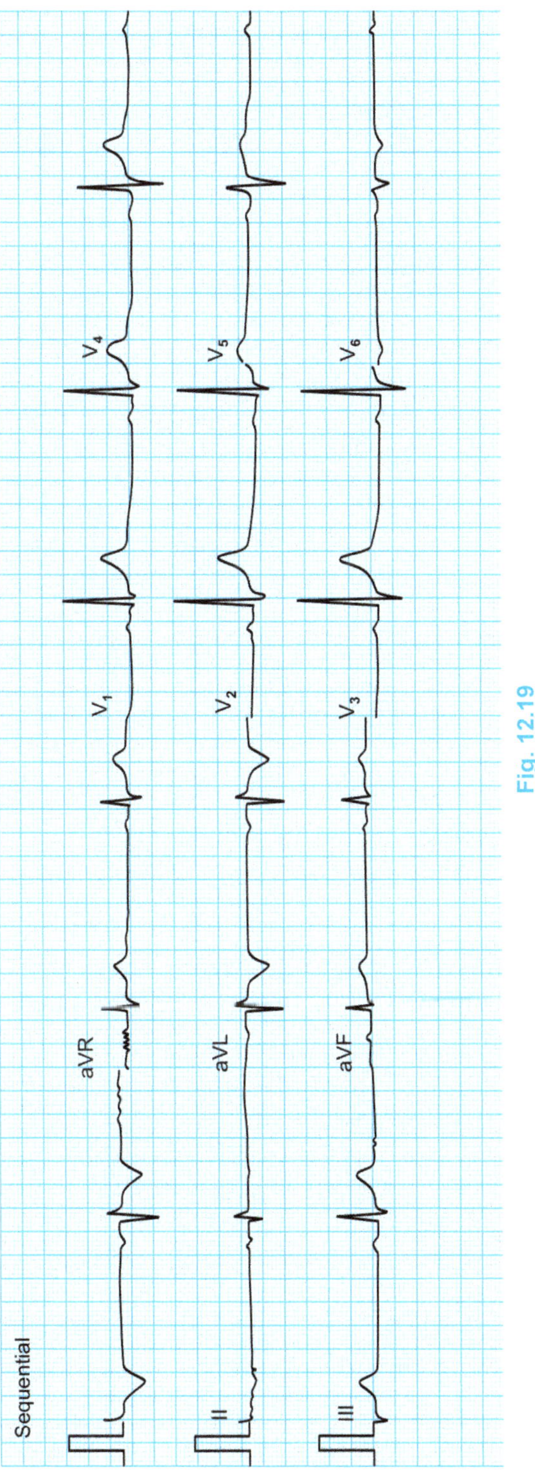

Fig. 12.19

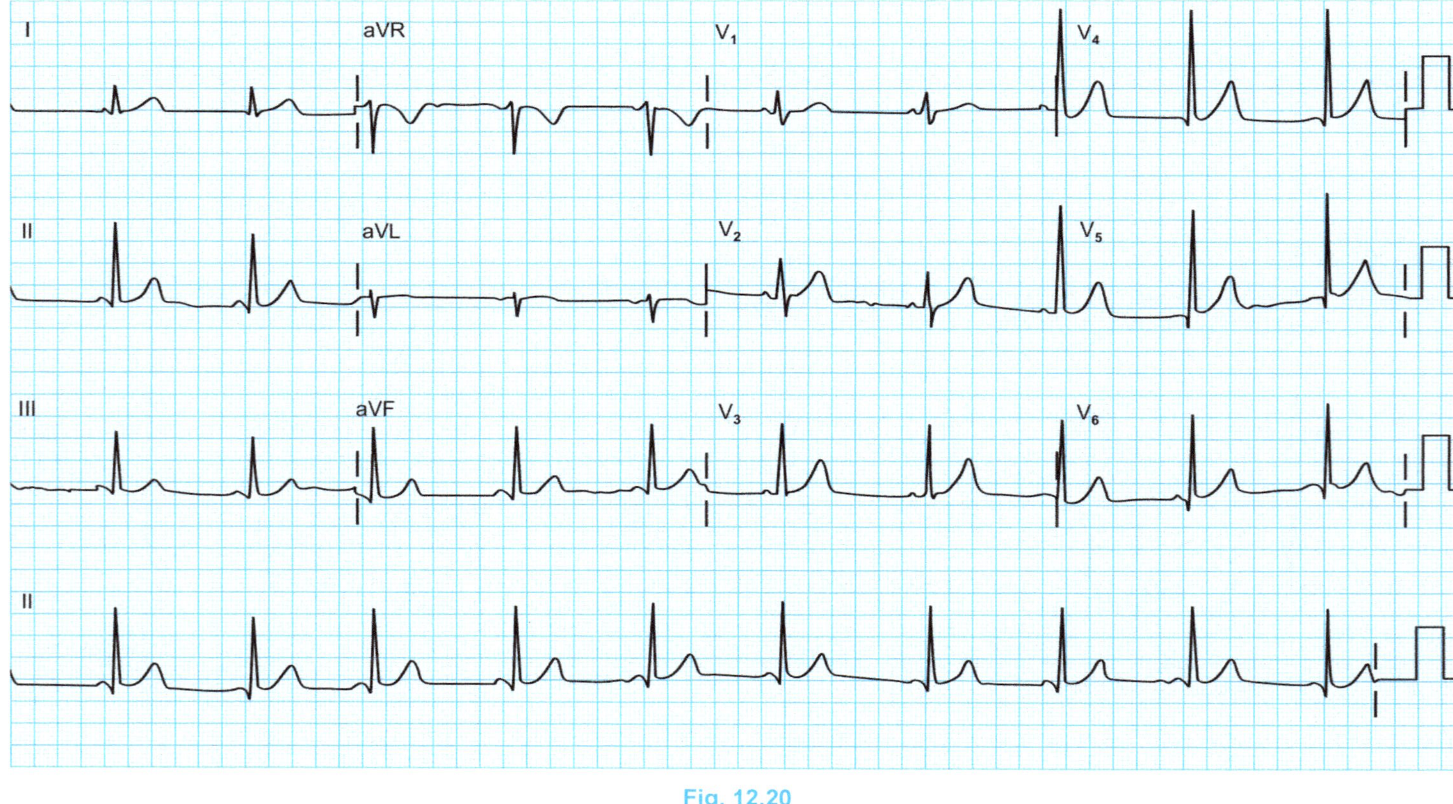

Fig. 12.20

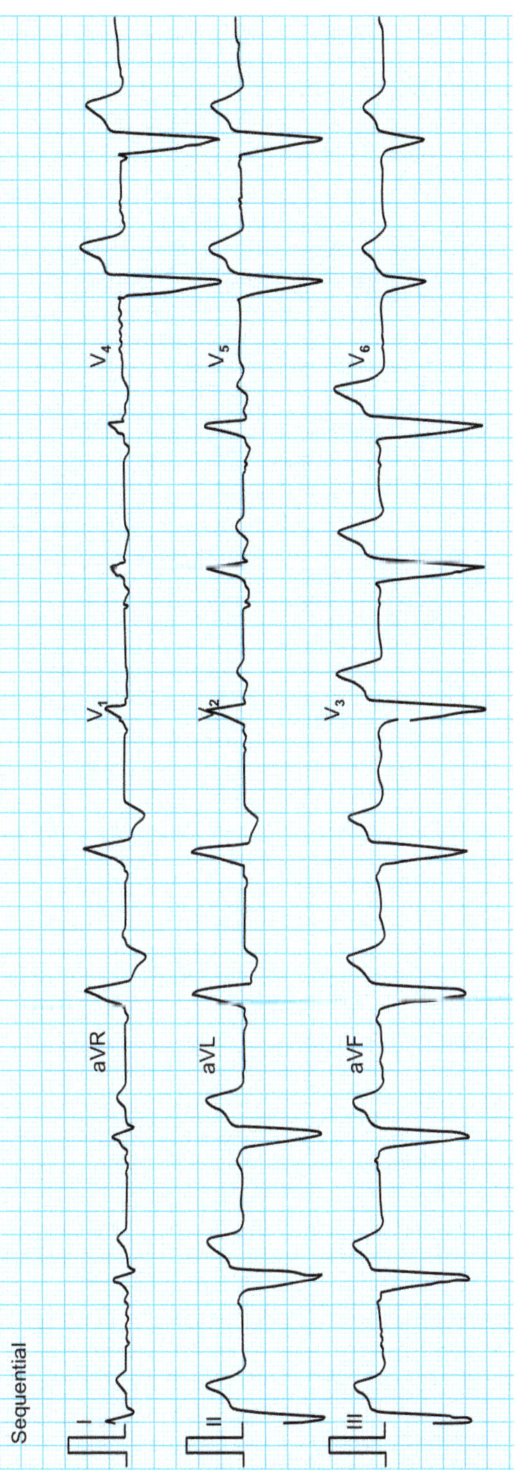

Fig. 12.21

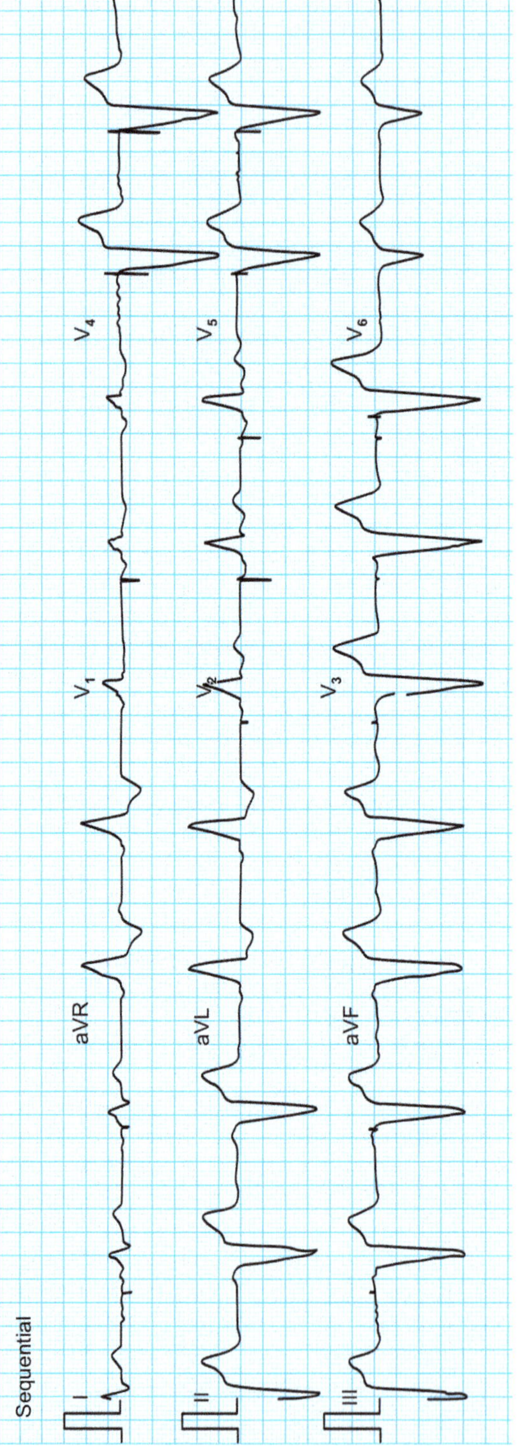

Fig. 12.22

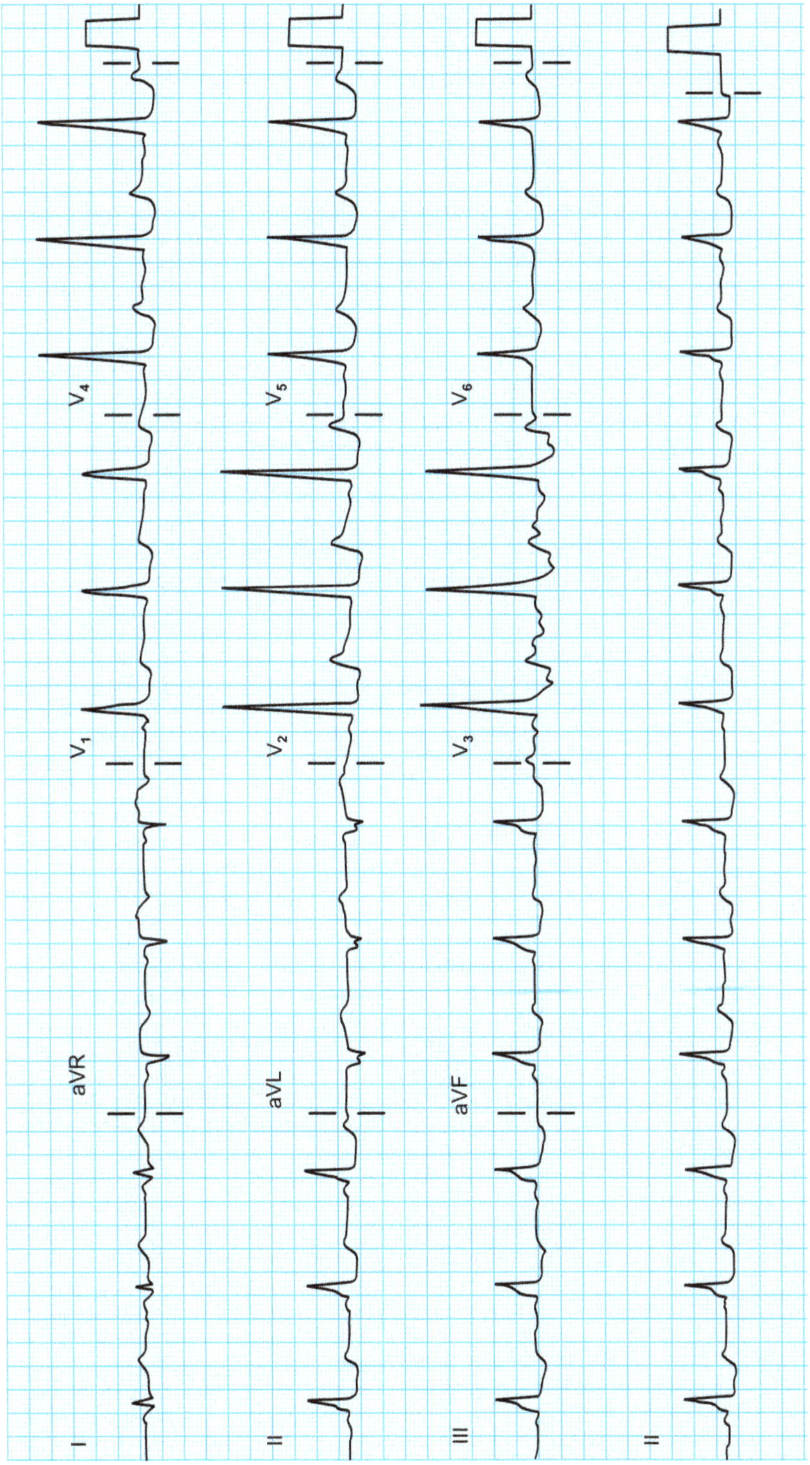

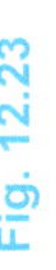

Fig. 12.23

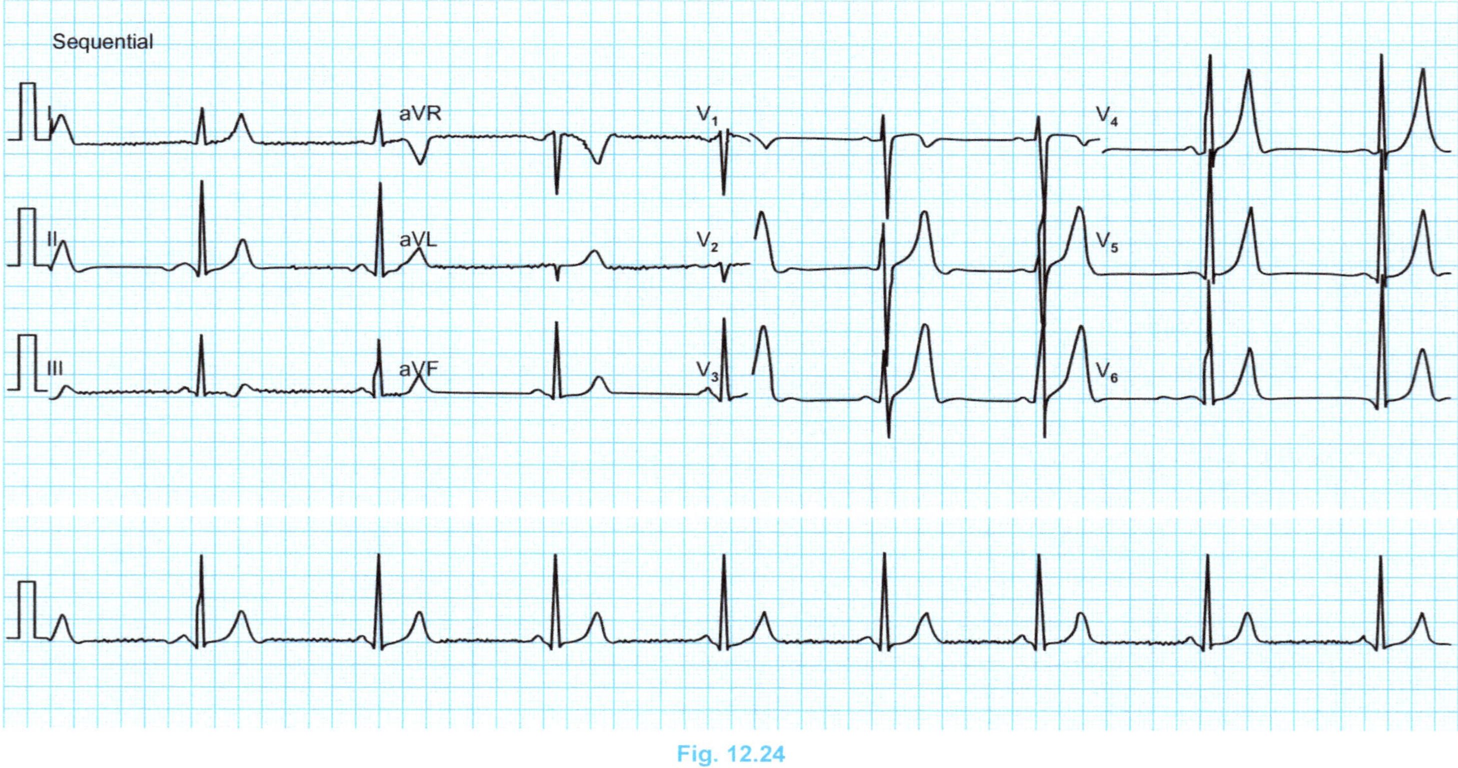

Fig. 12.24

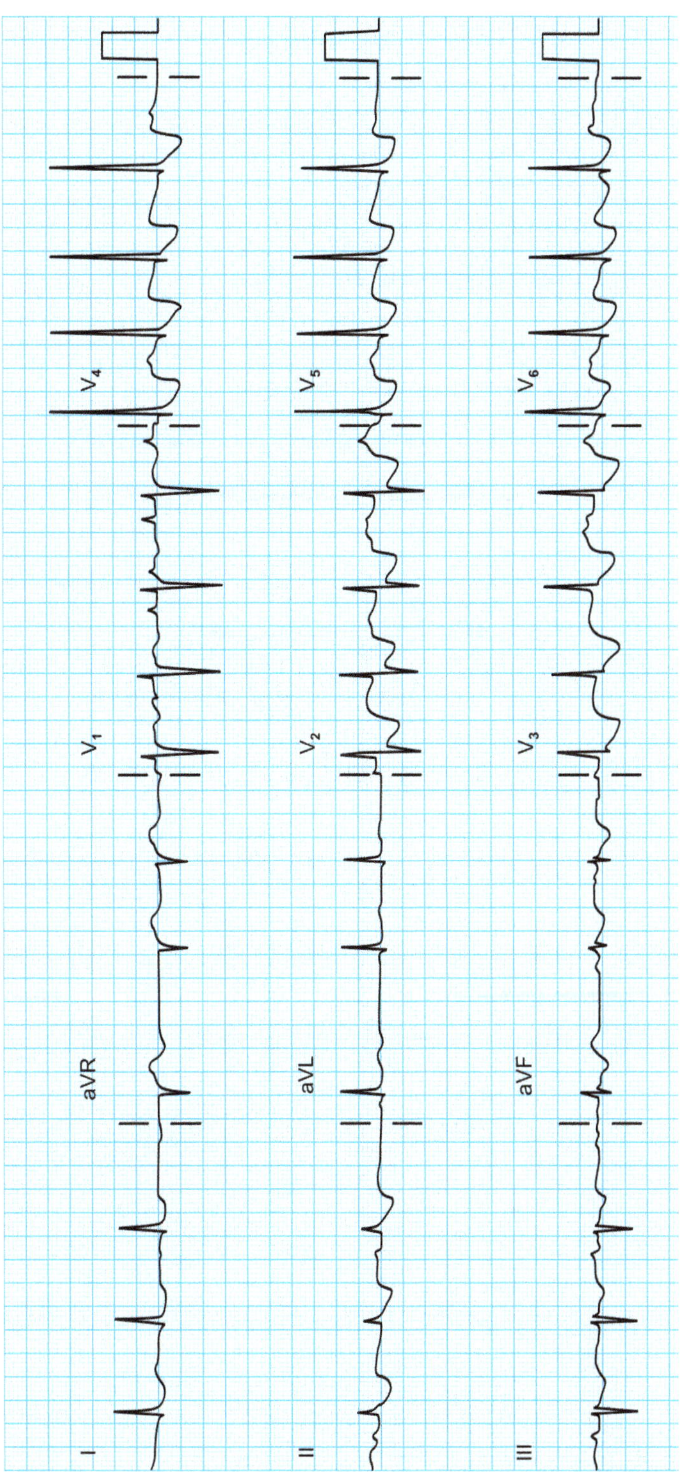

Fig. 12.25

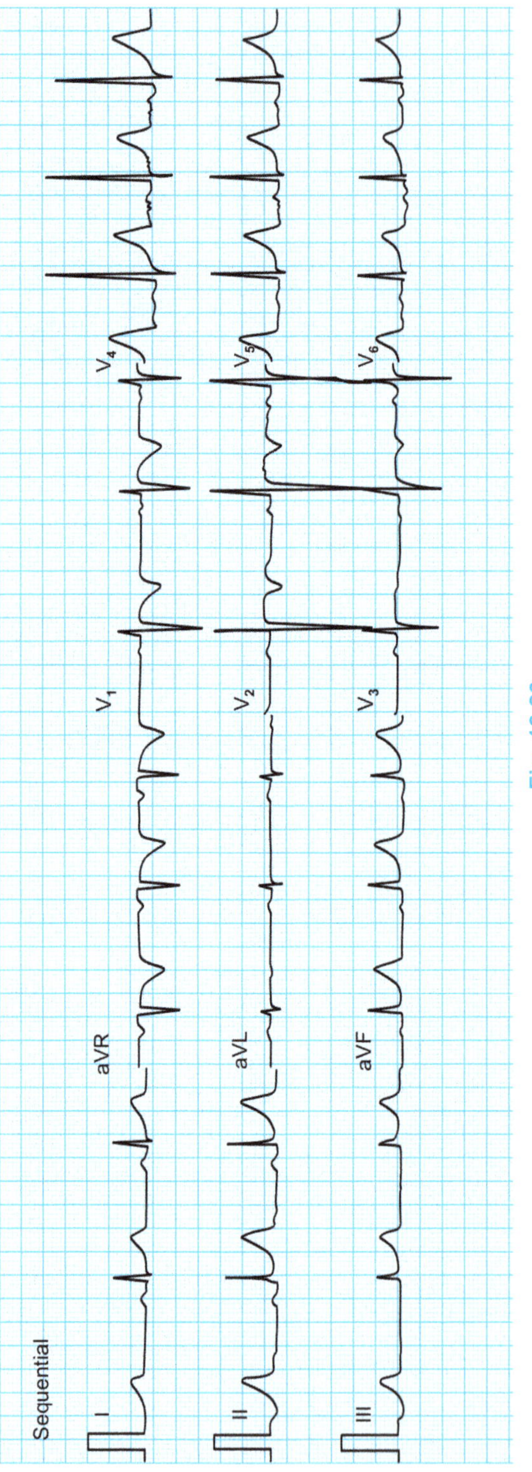

Fig. 12.26

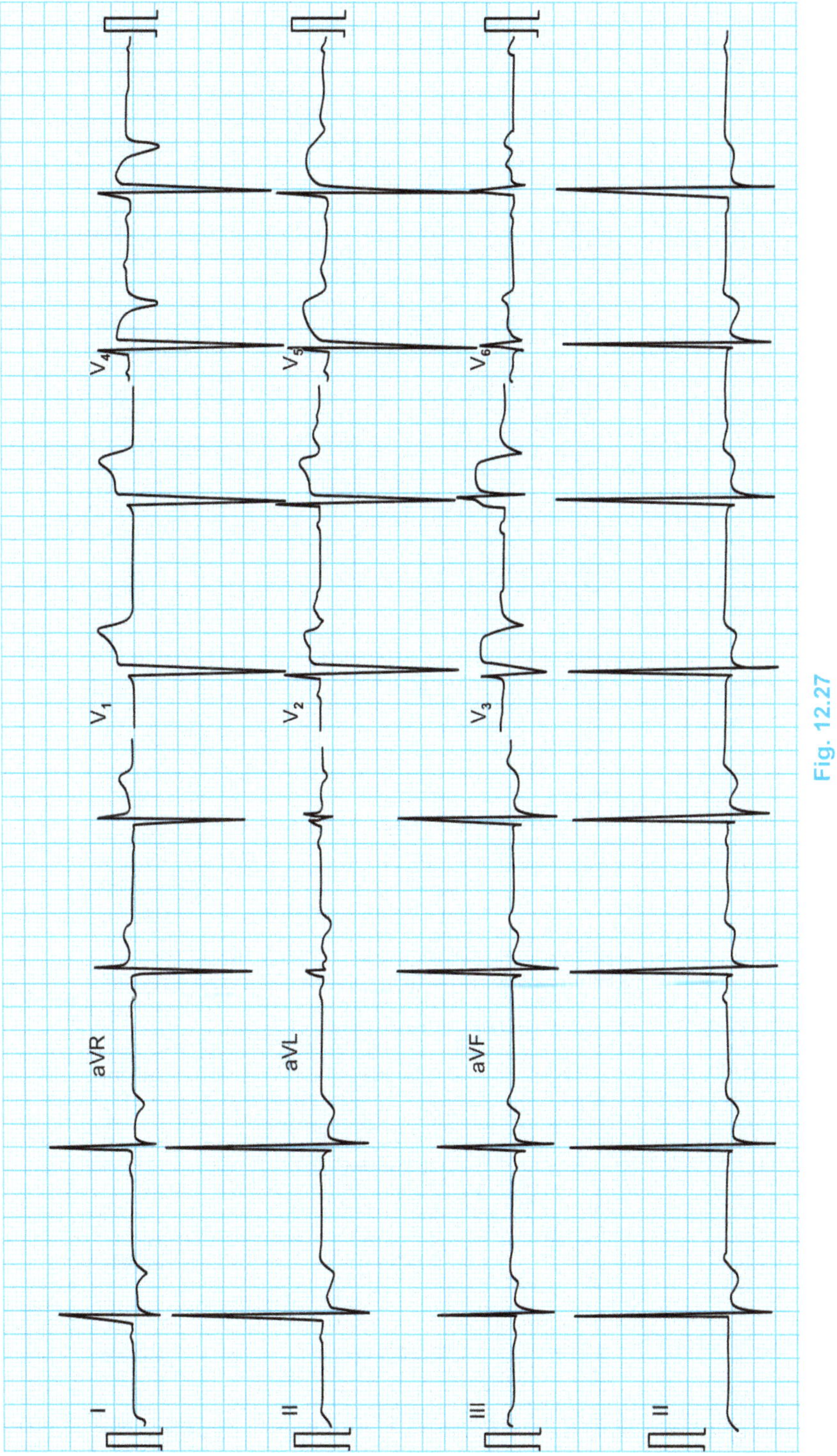

Fig. 12.27

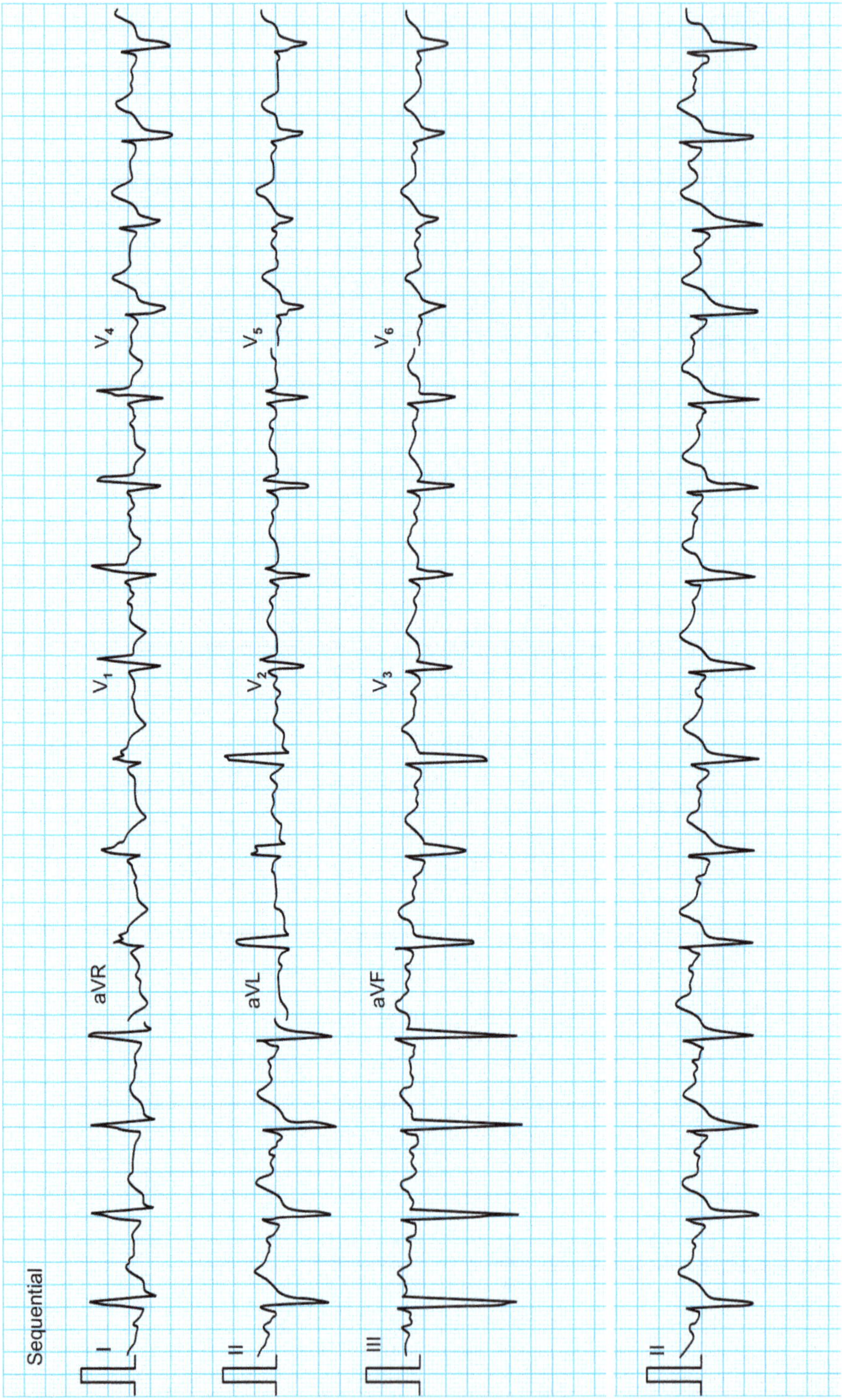

Fig. 12.28

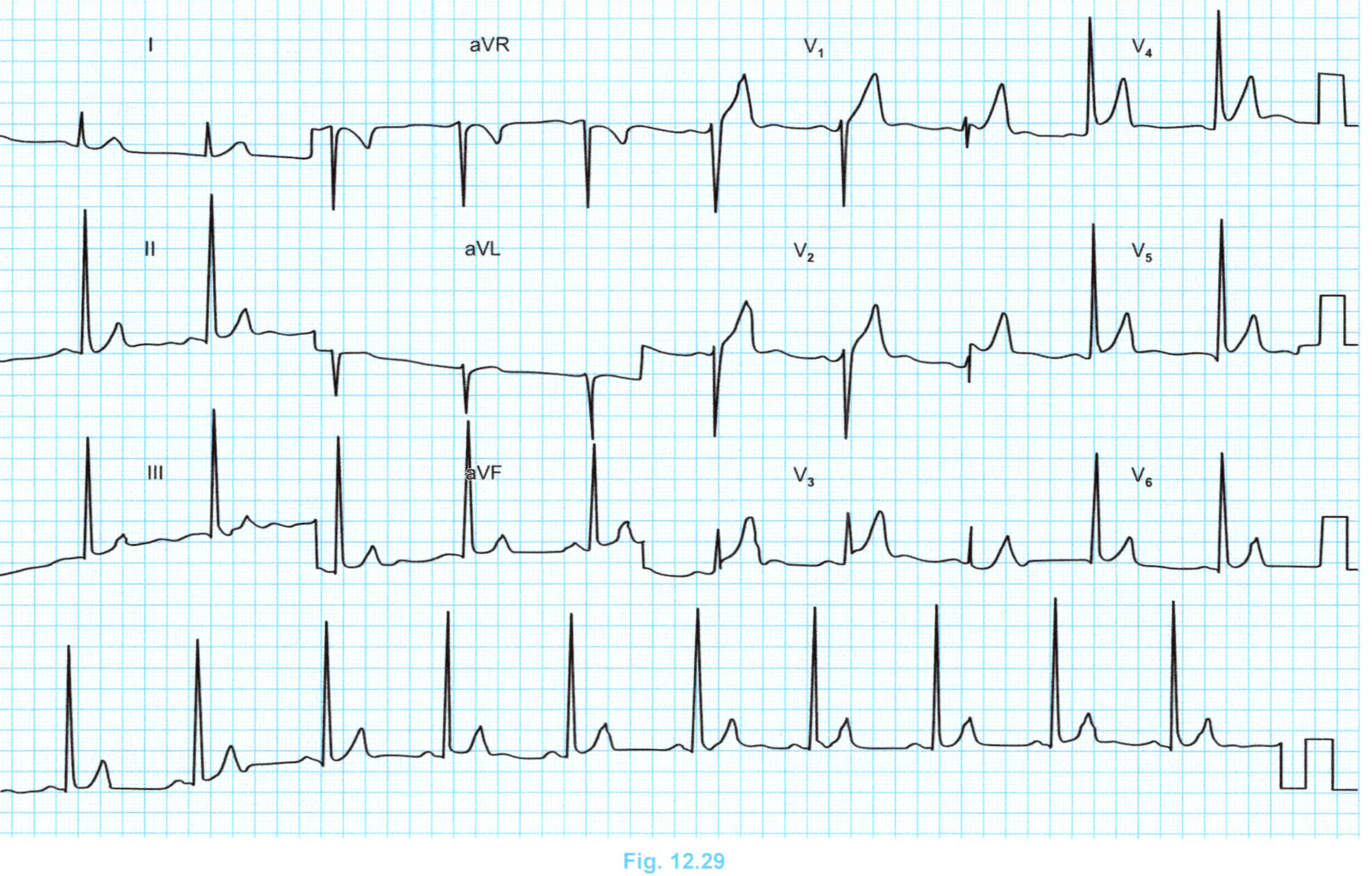

Fig. 12.29

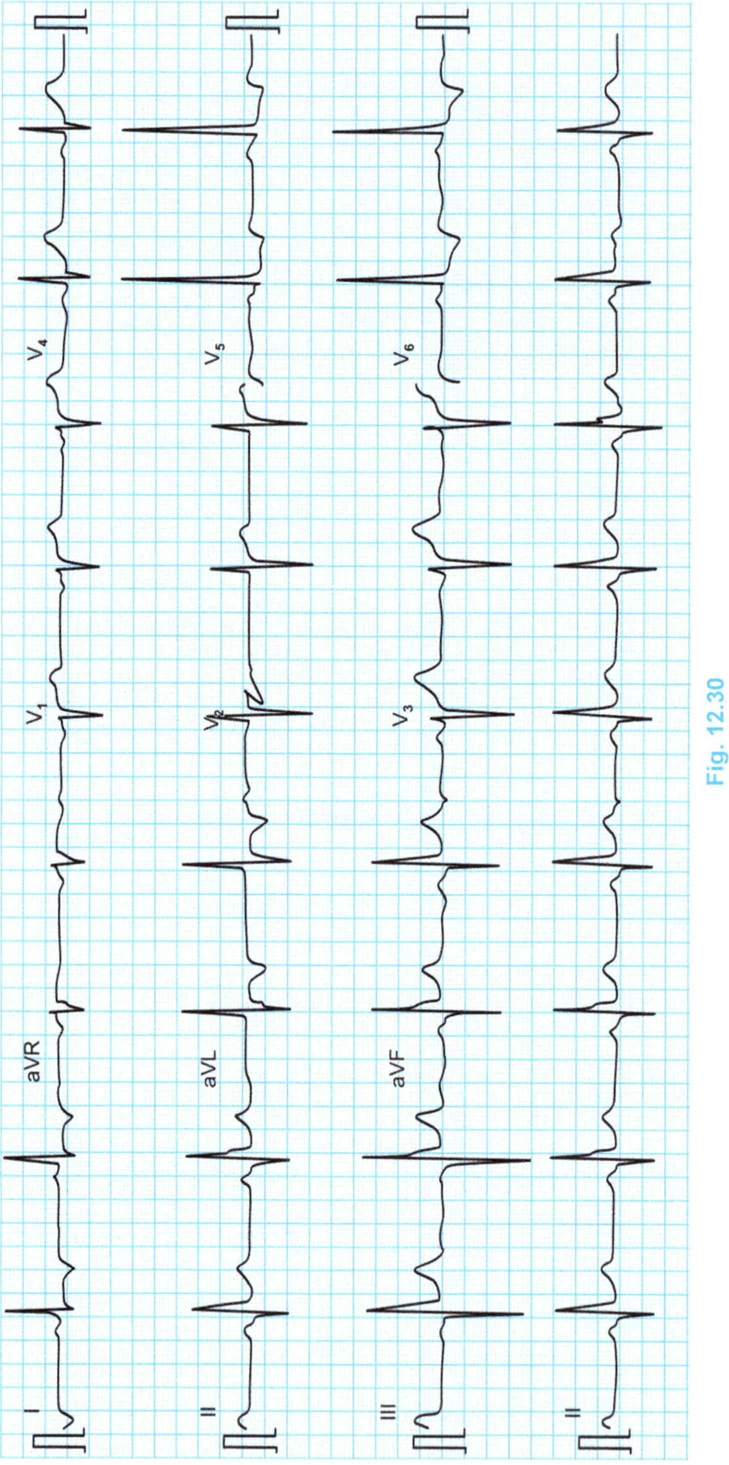

Fig. 12.30

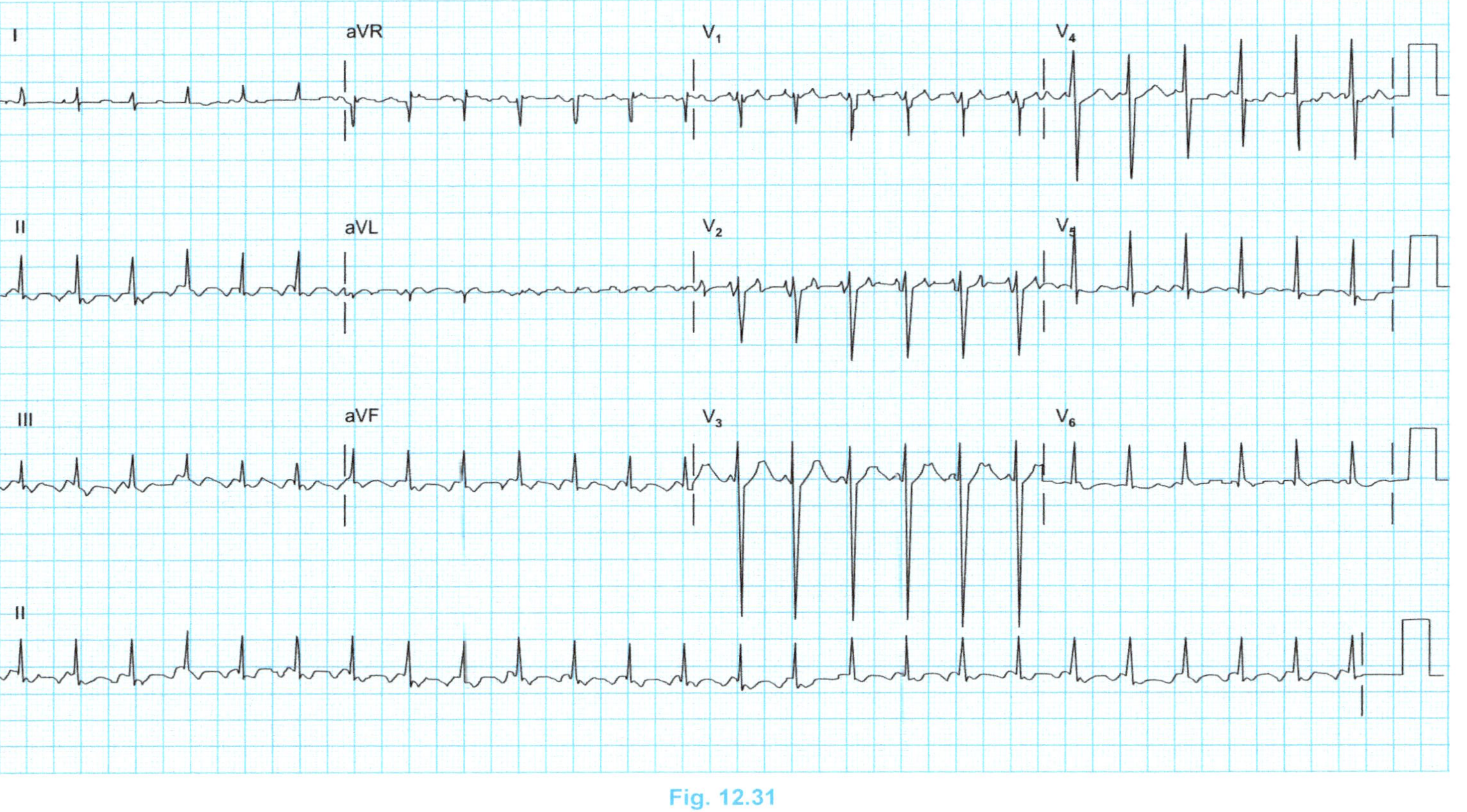

Fig. 12.31

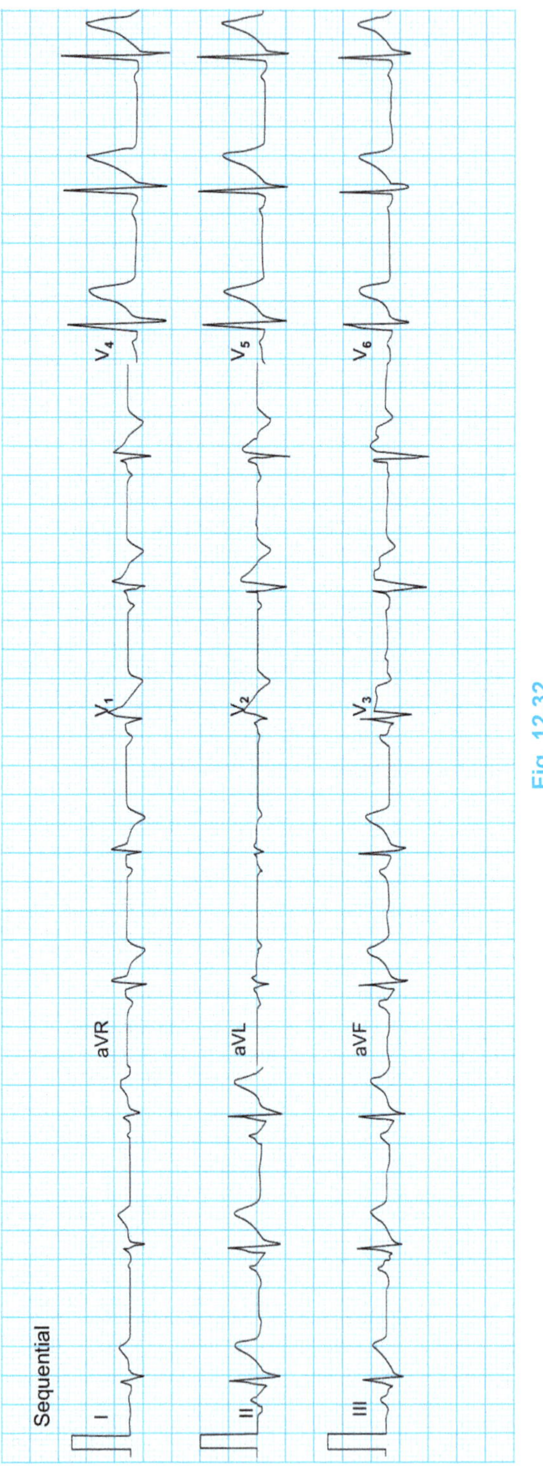

Fig. 12.32

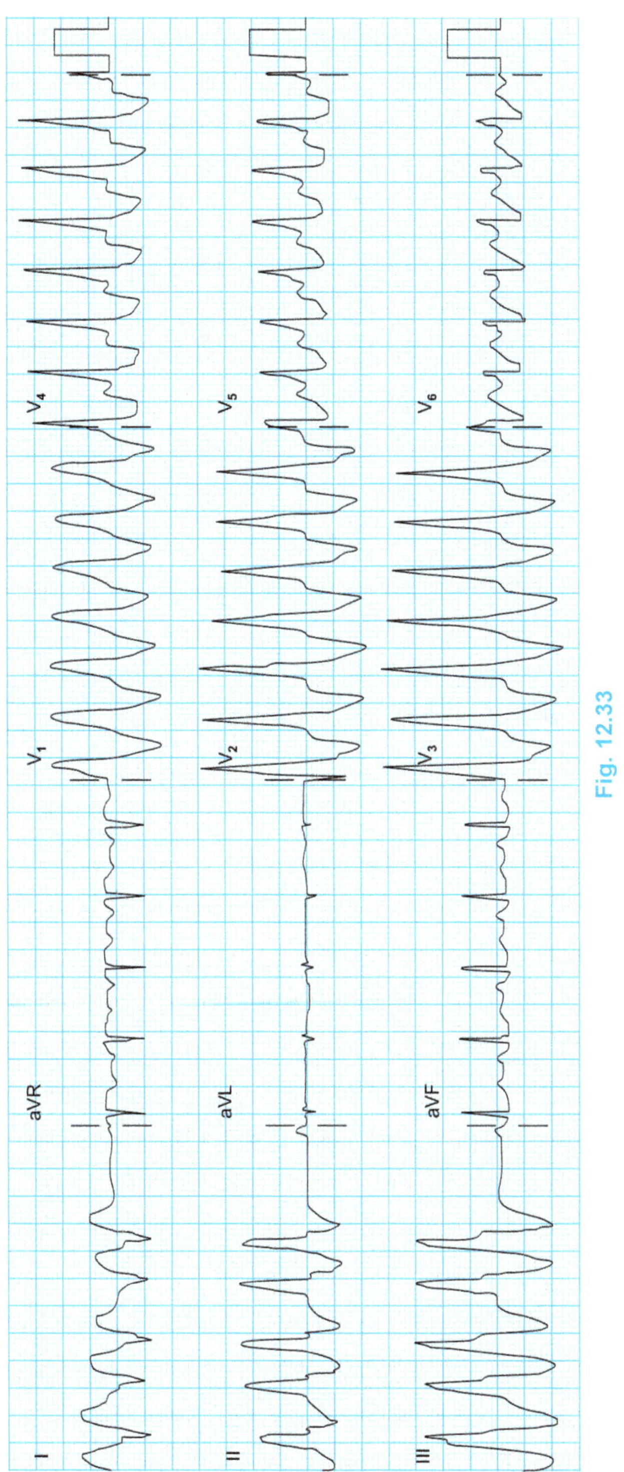

Fig. 12.33

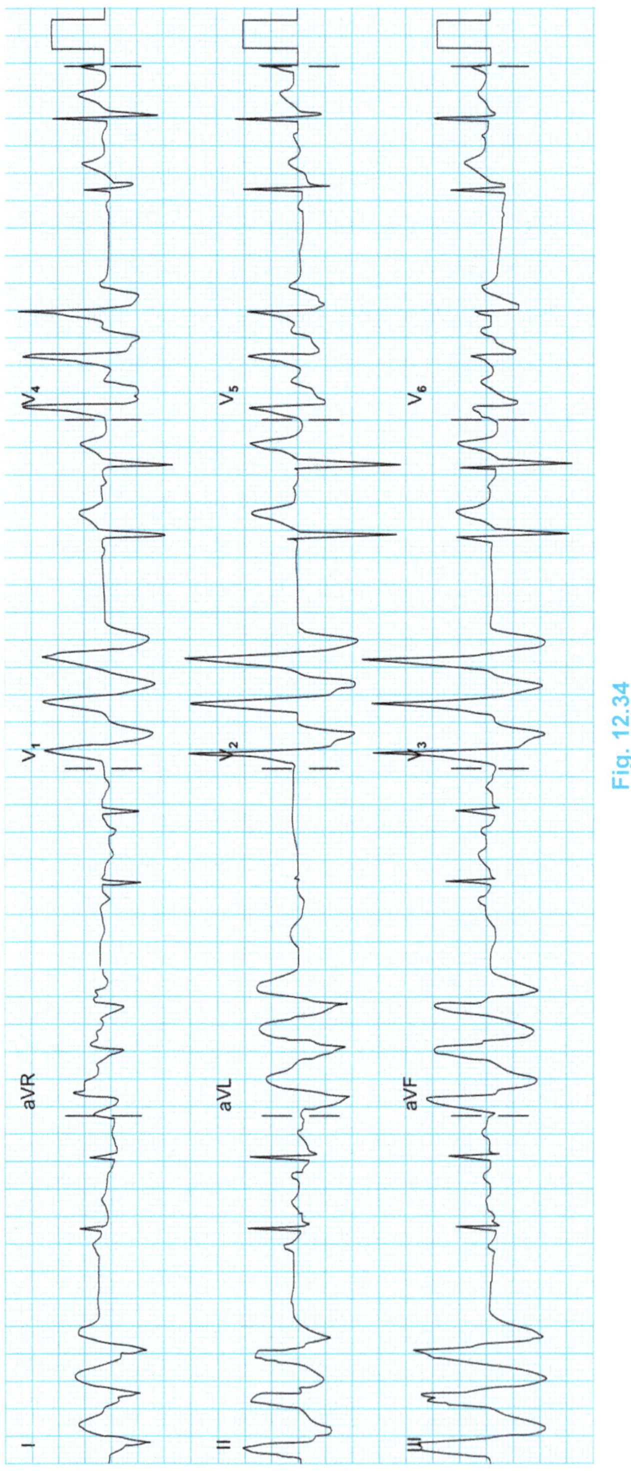

Fig. 12.34

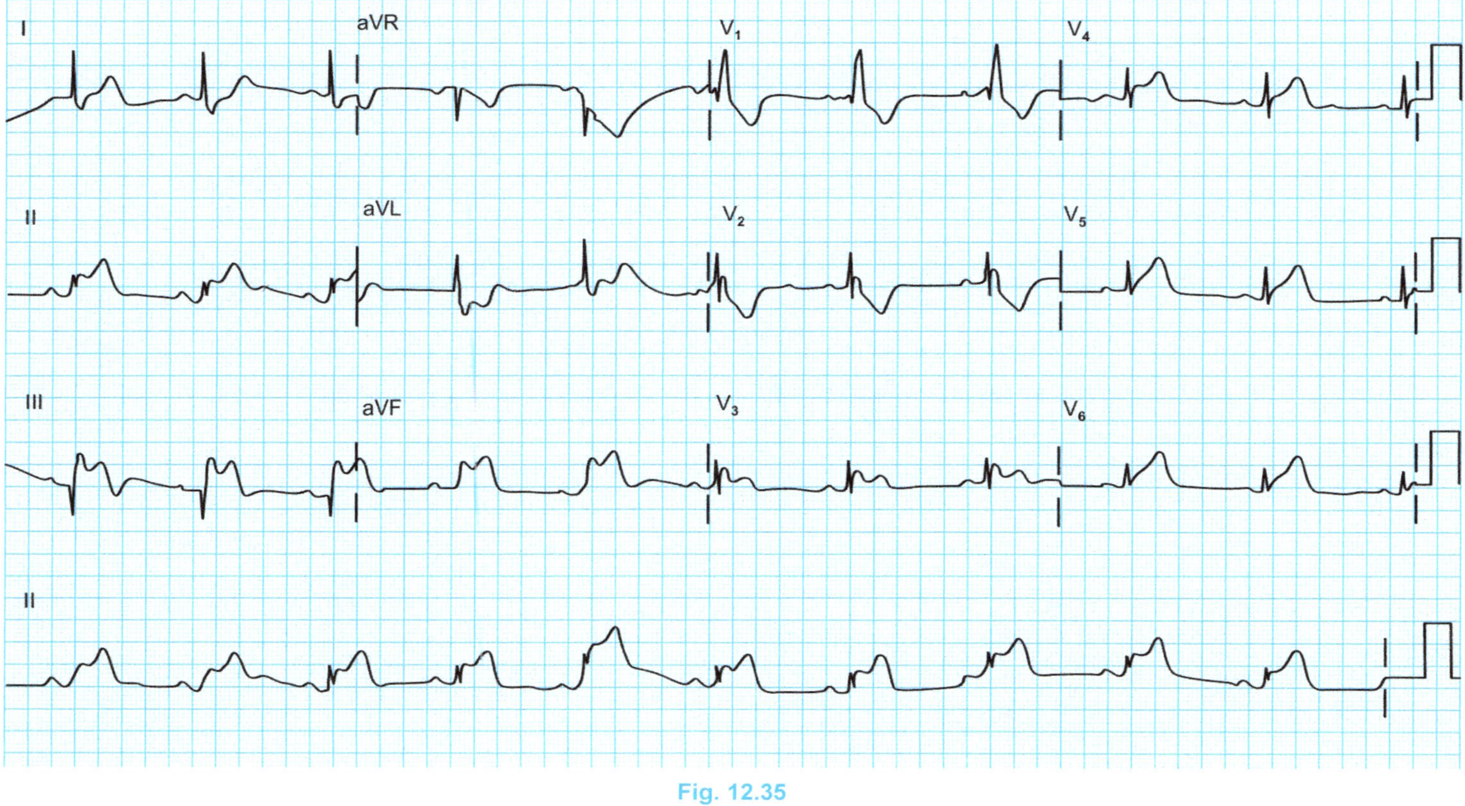

Fig. 12.35

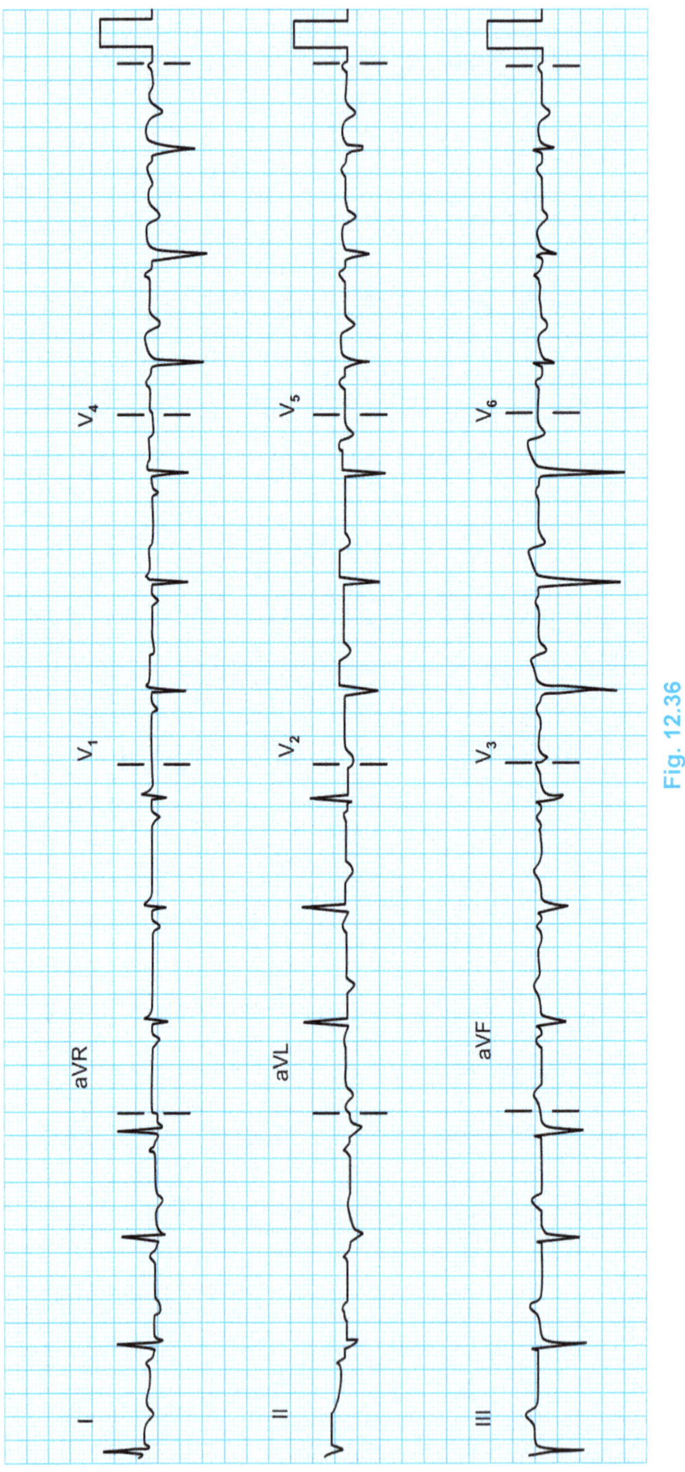

Fig. 12.36

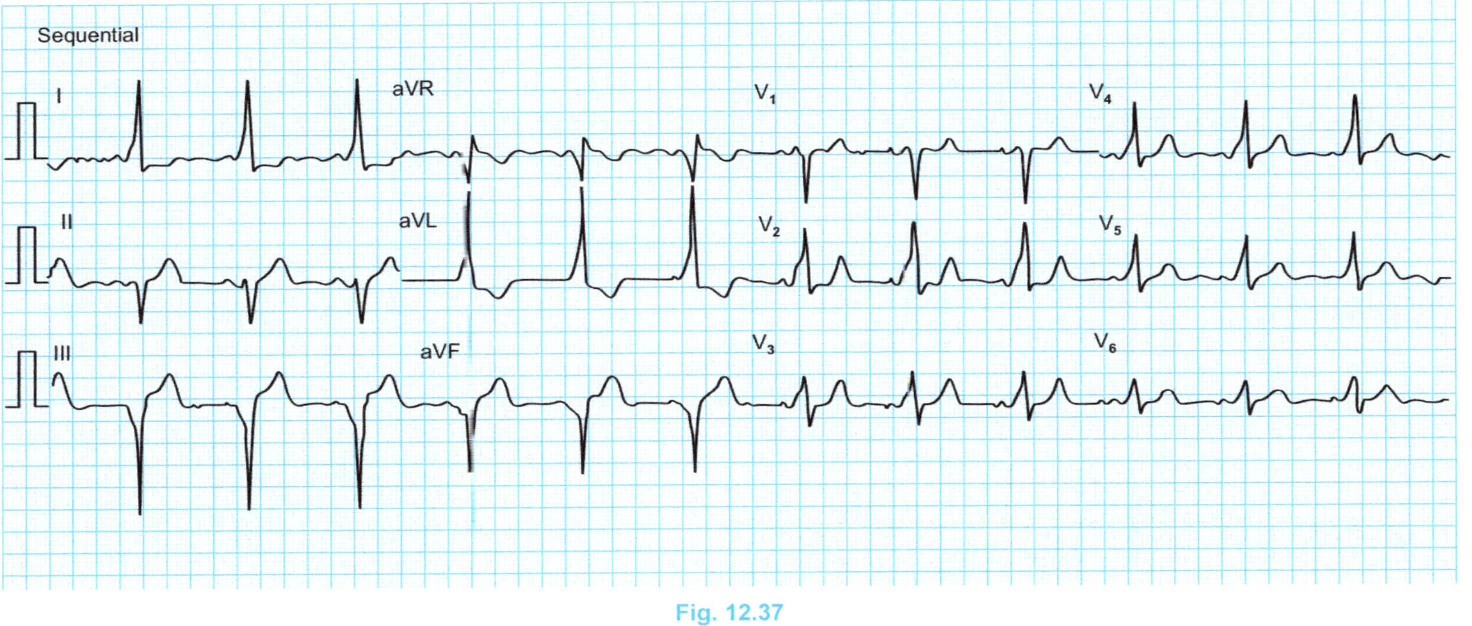

Fig. 12.37

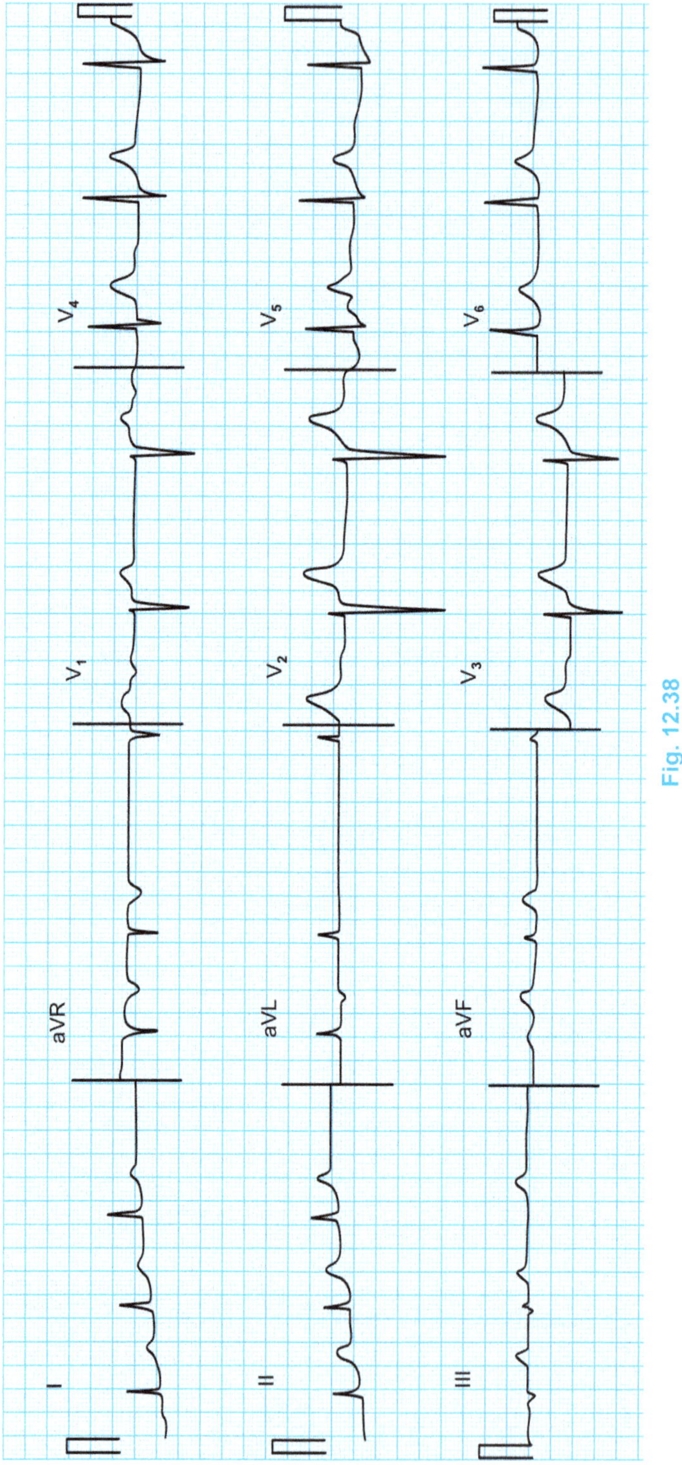

Fig. 12.38

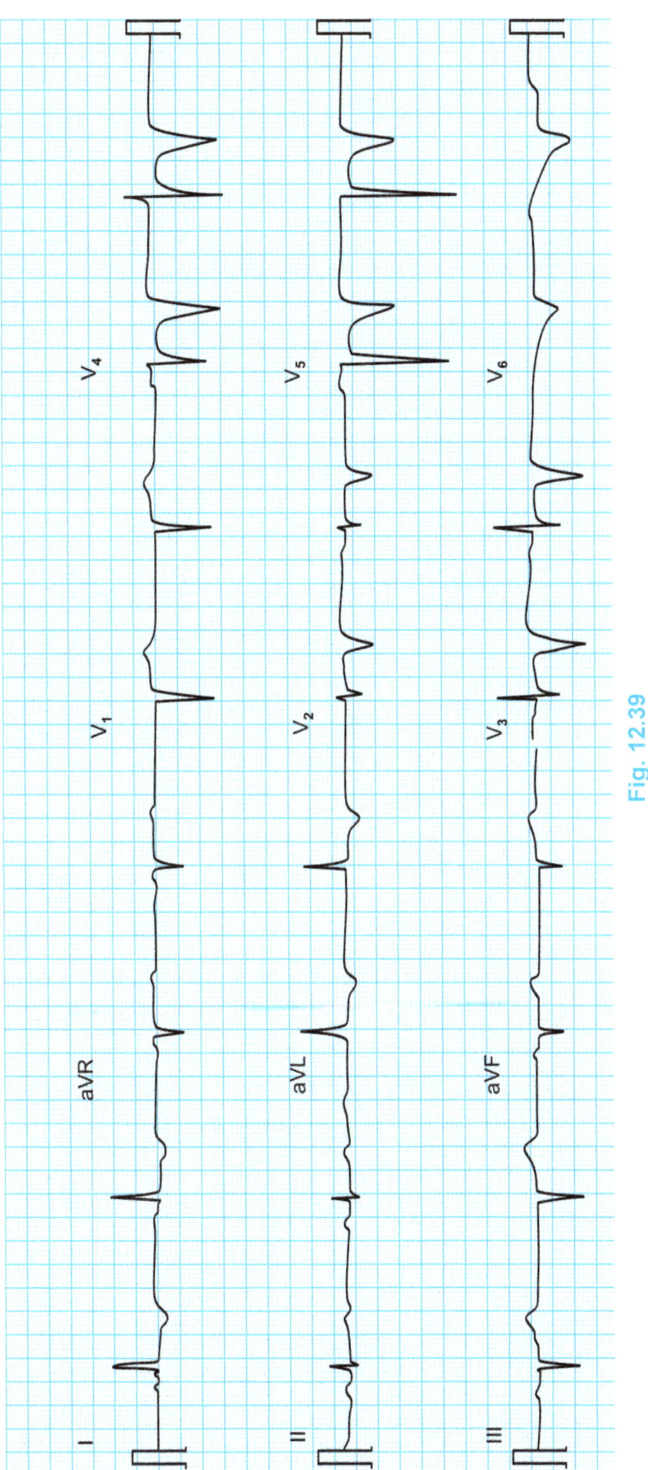

Fig. 12.39

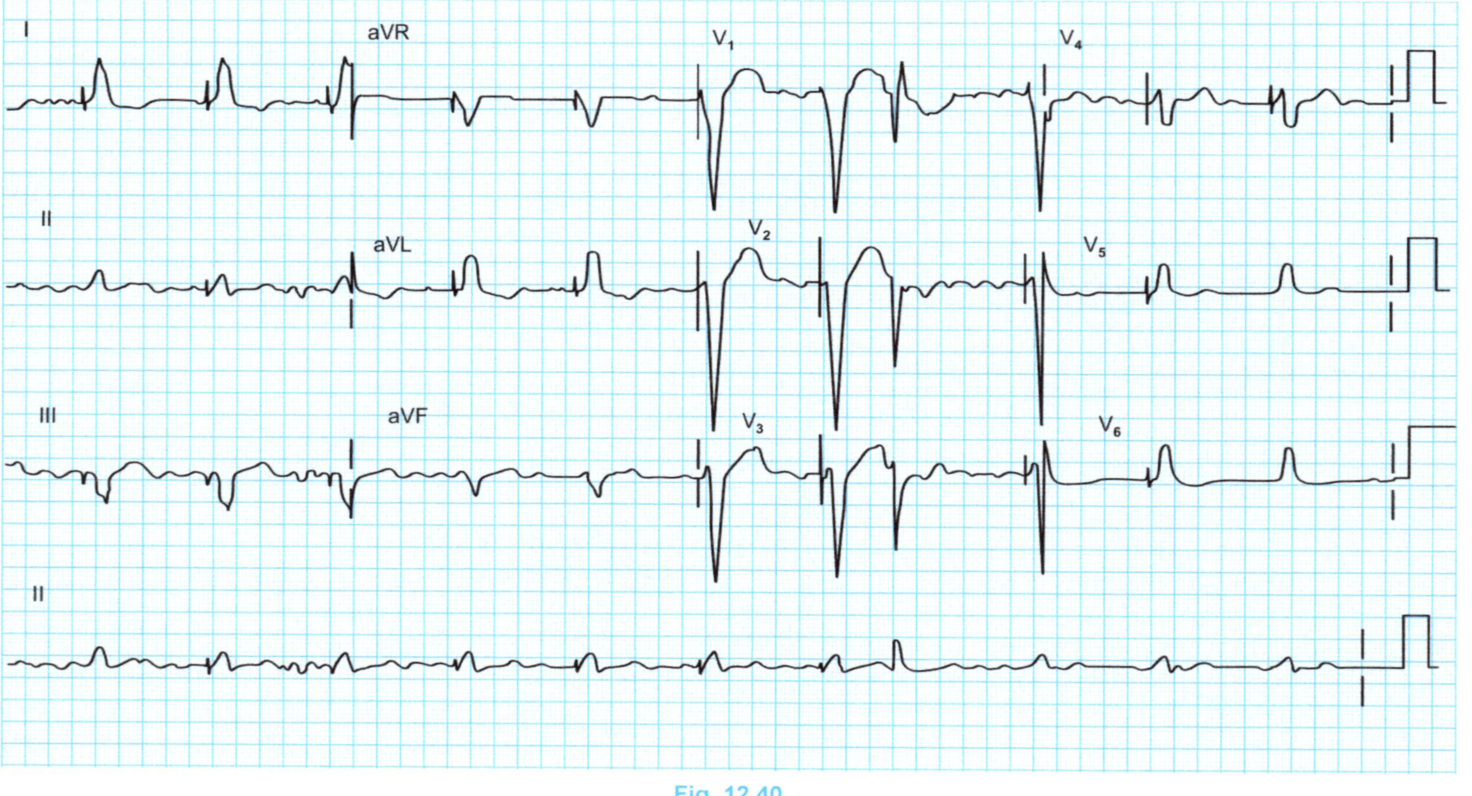

Fig. 12.40

Findings of different pathological significance

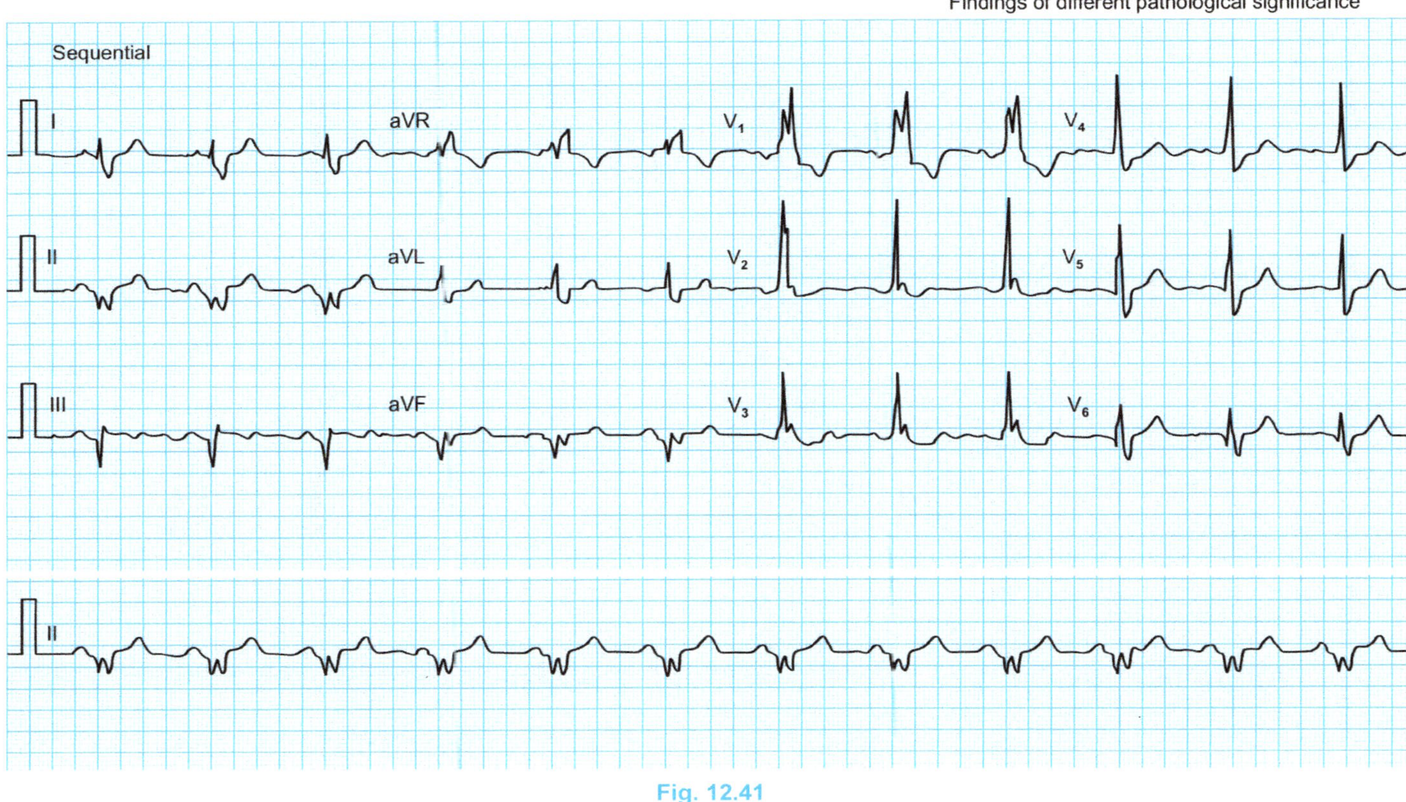

Fig. 12.41

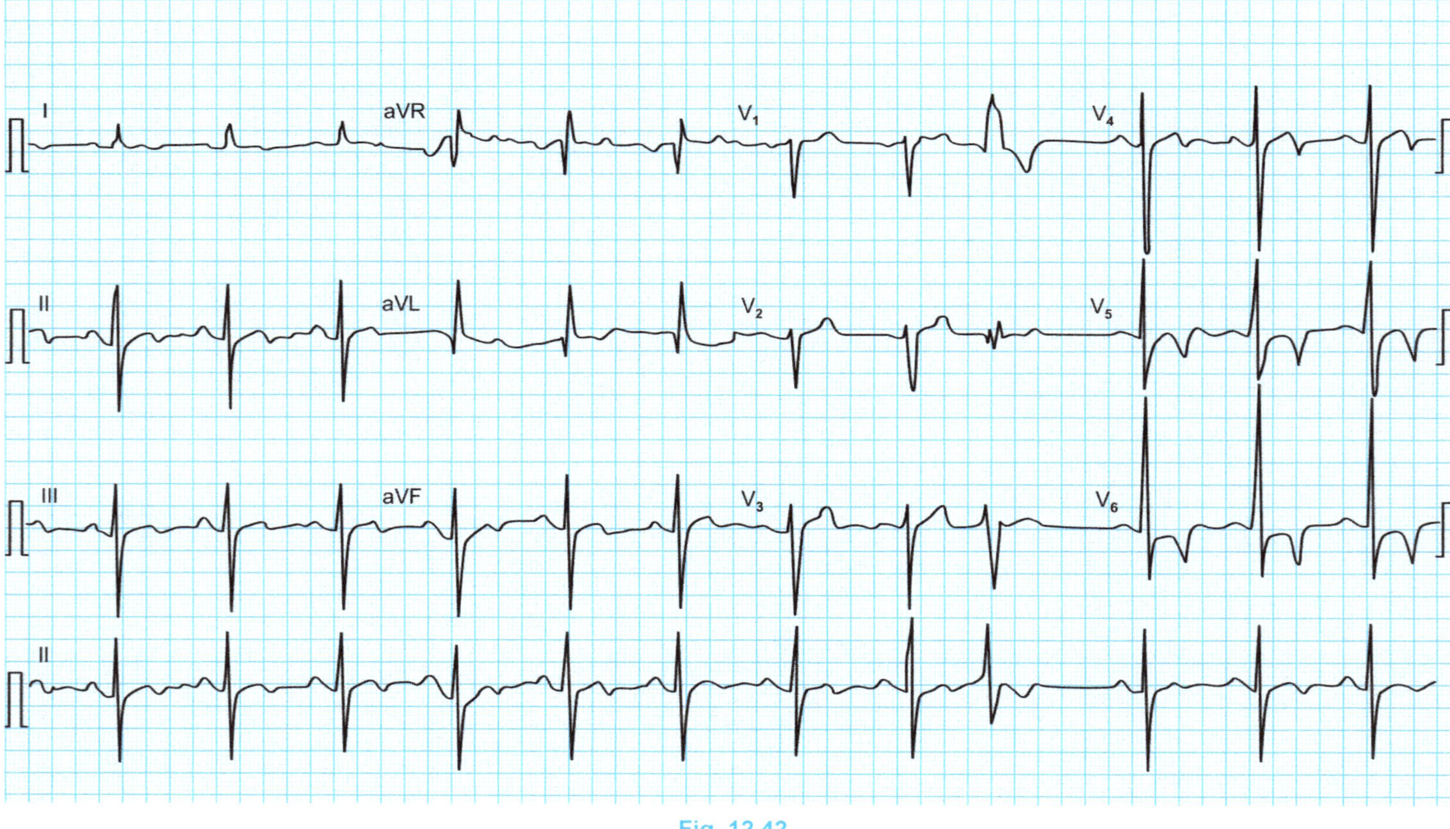

Fig. 12.42

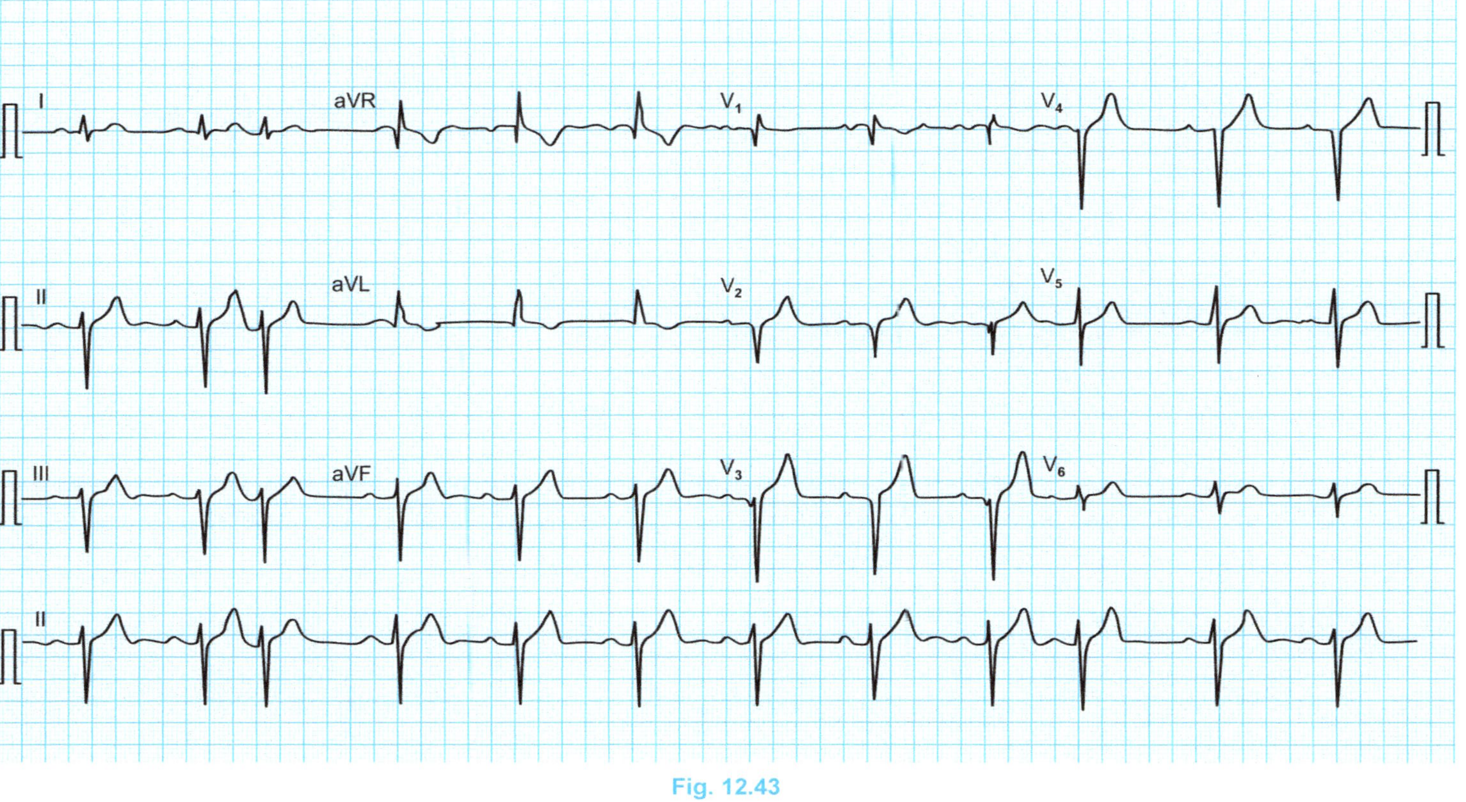

Fig. 12.43

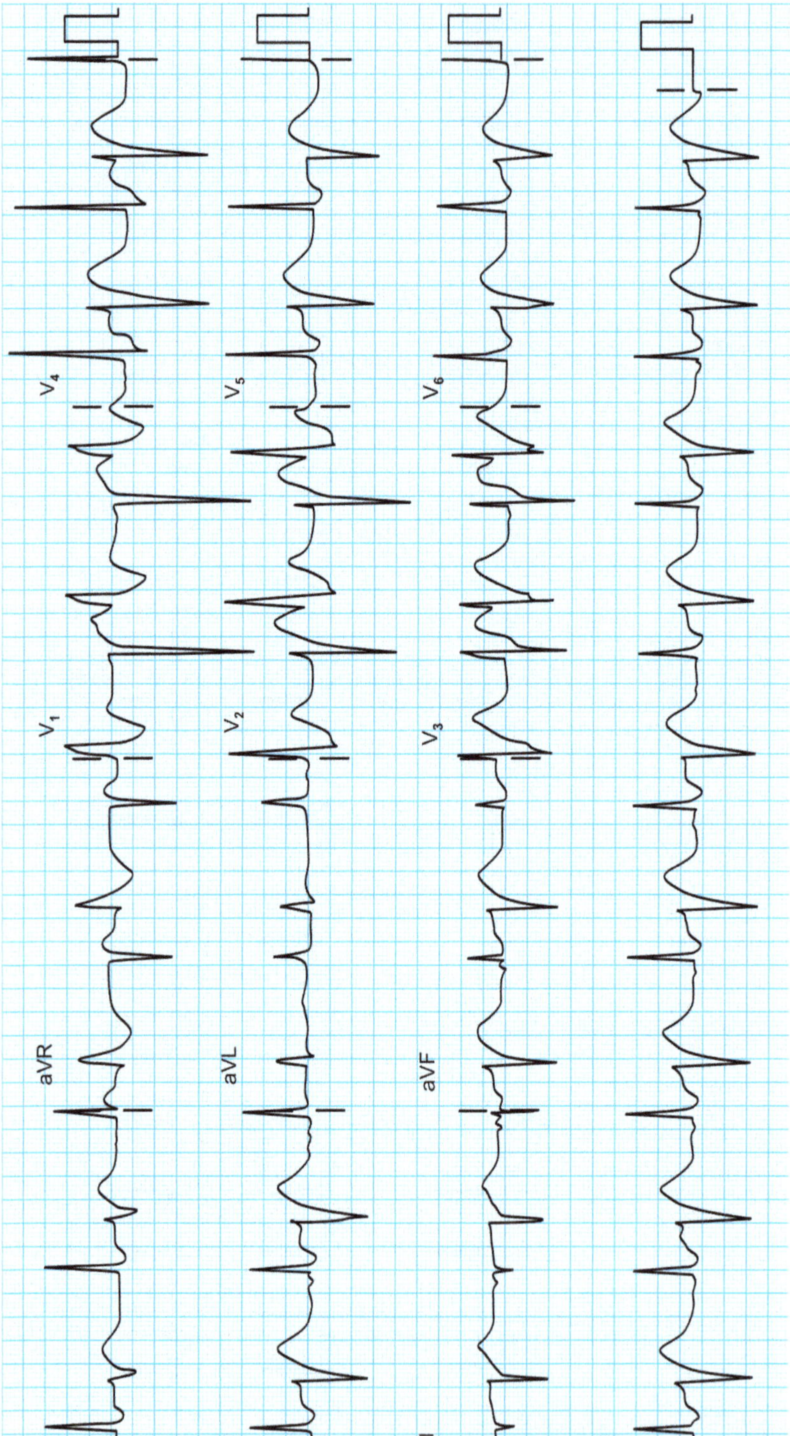

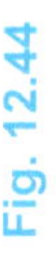

Fig. 12.44

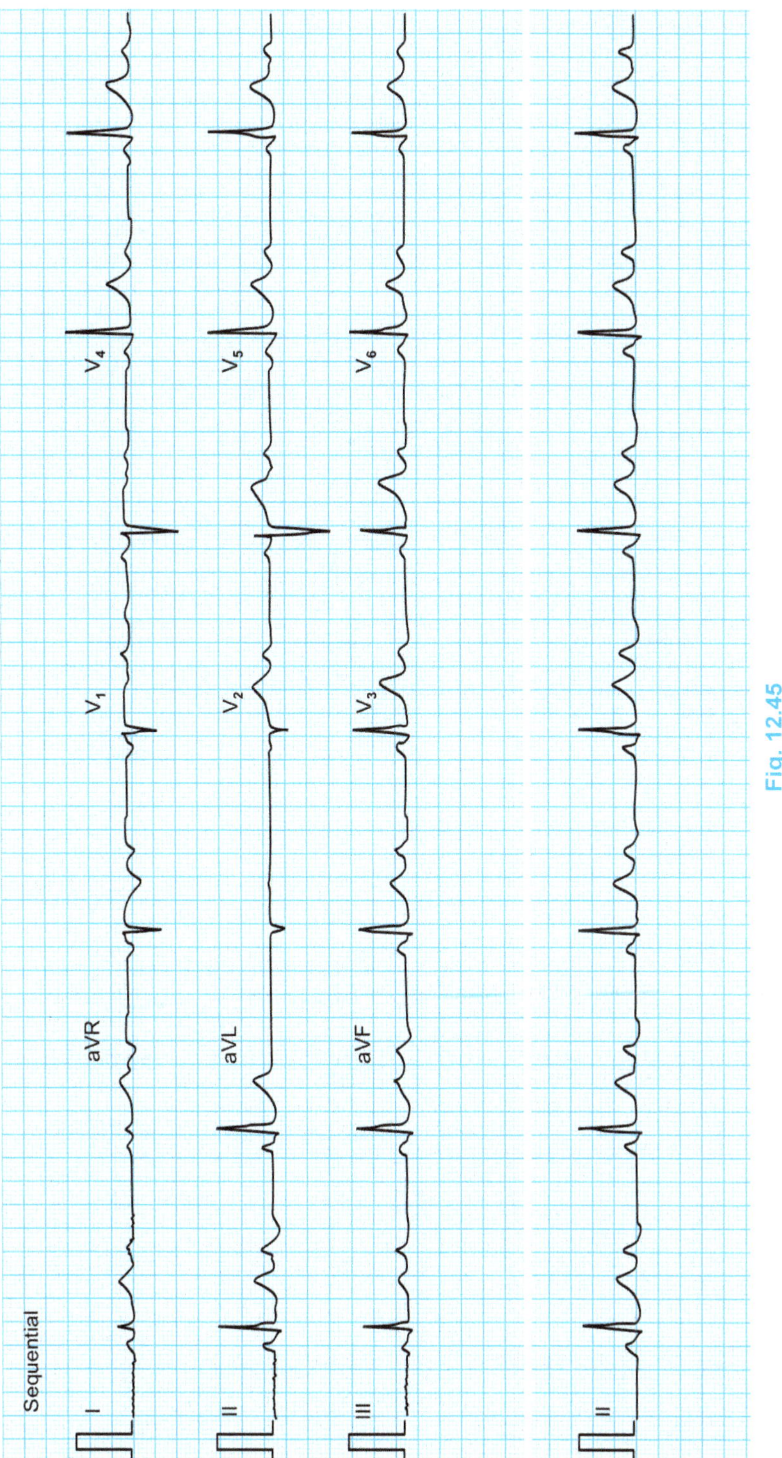

Fig. 12.45

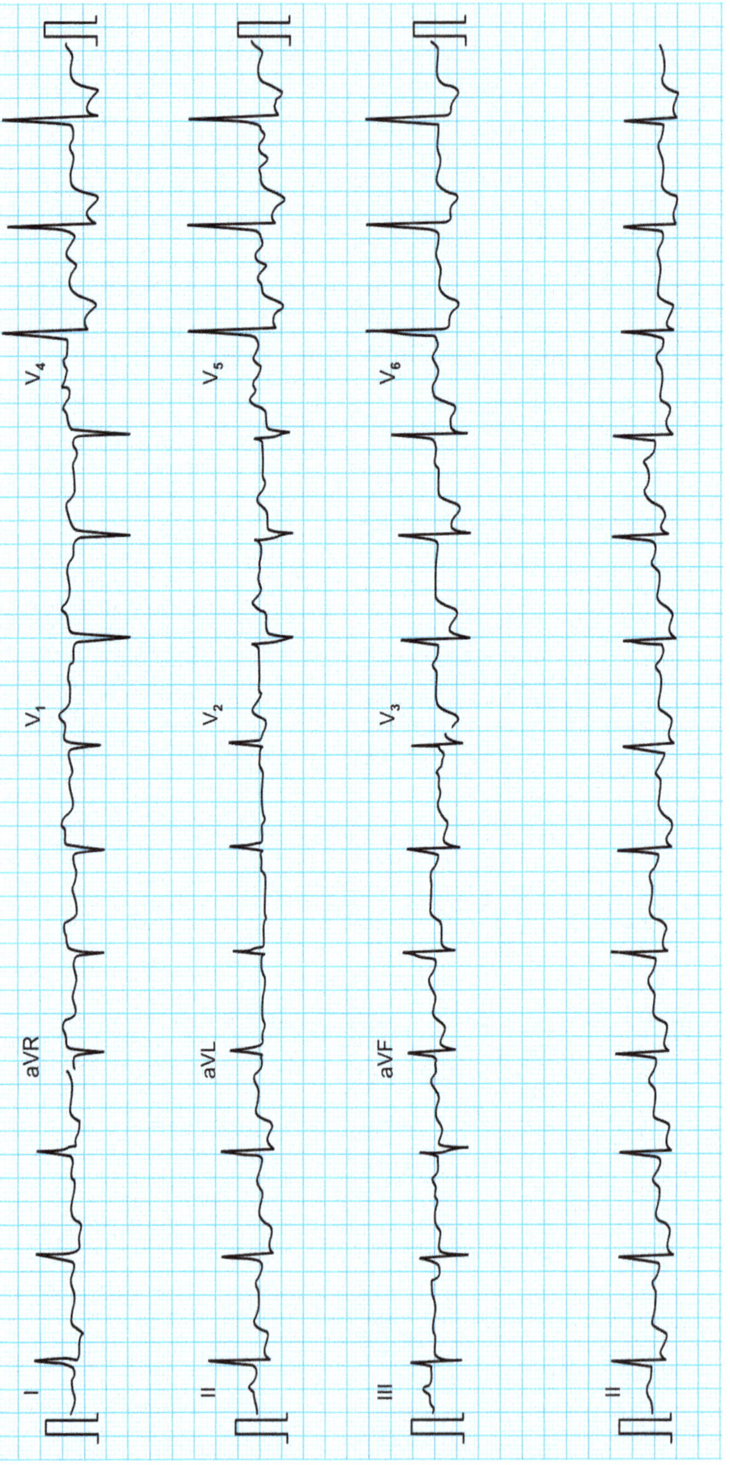

Fig. 12.46

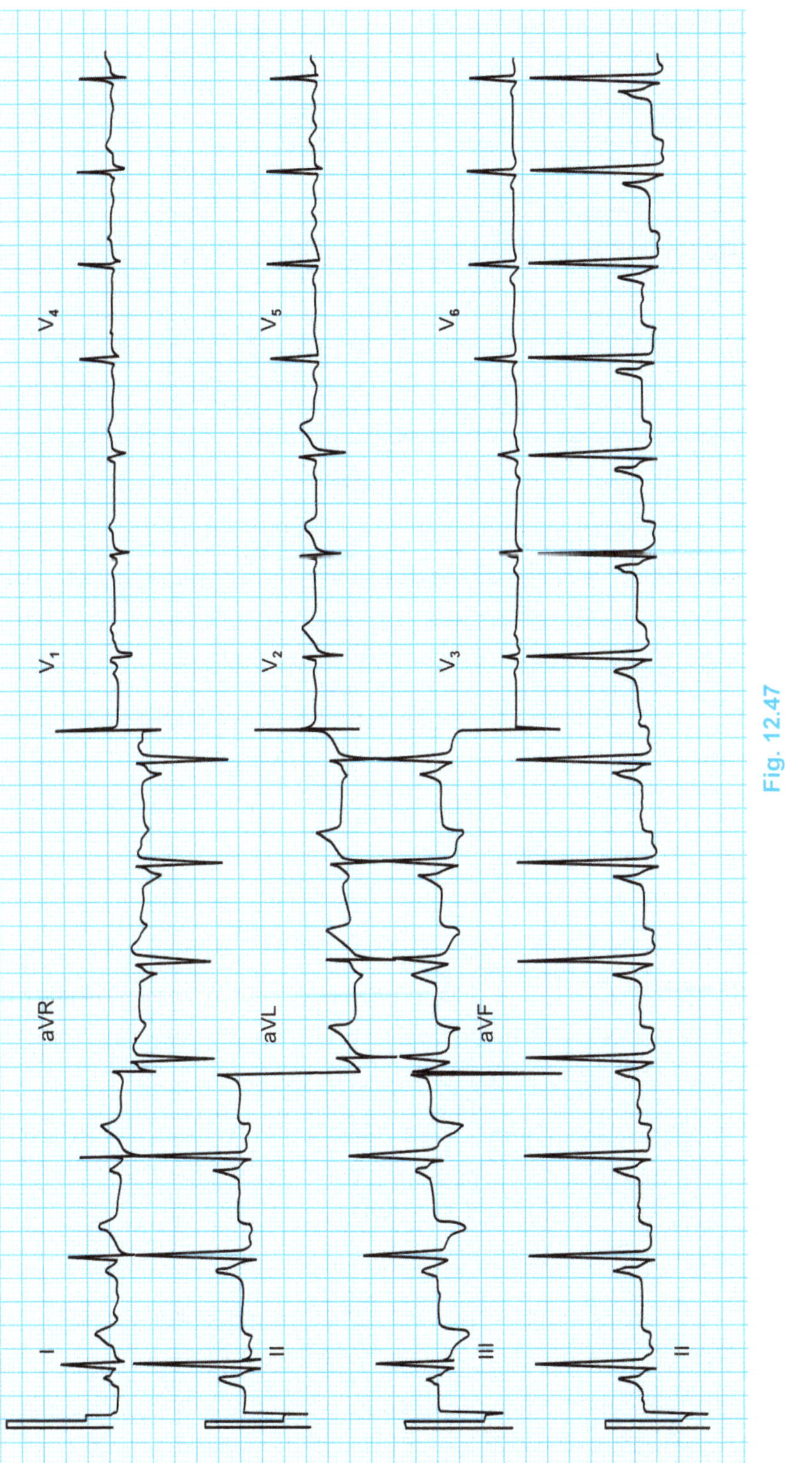

Fig. 12.47

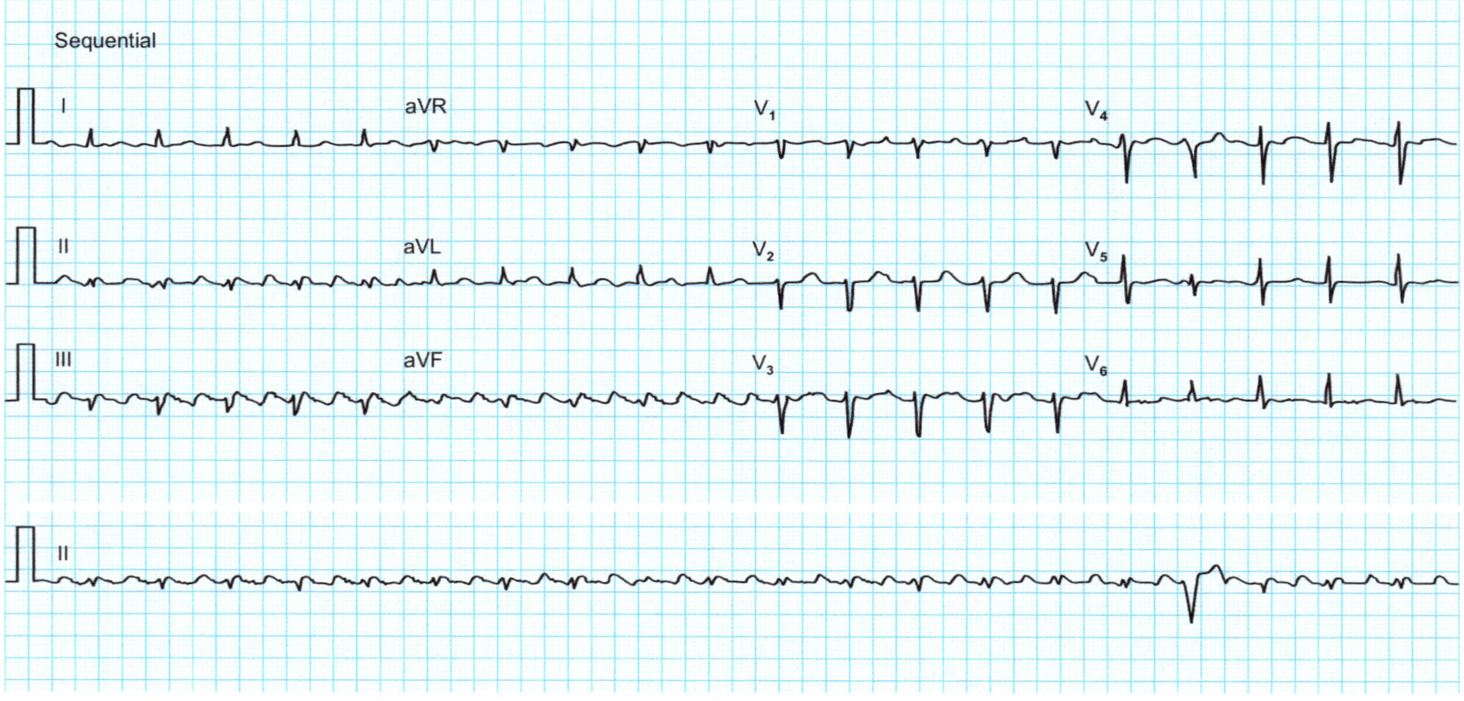

Fig. 12.48

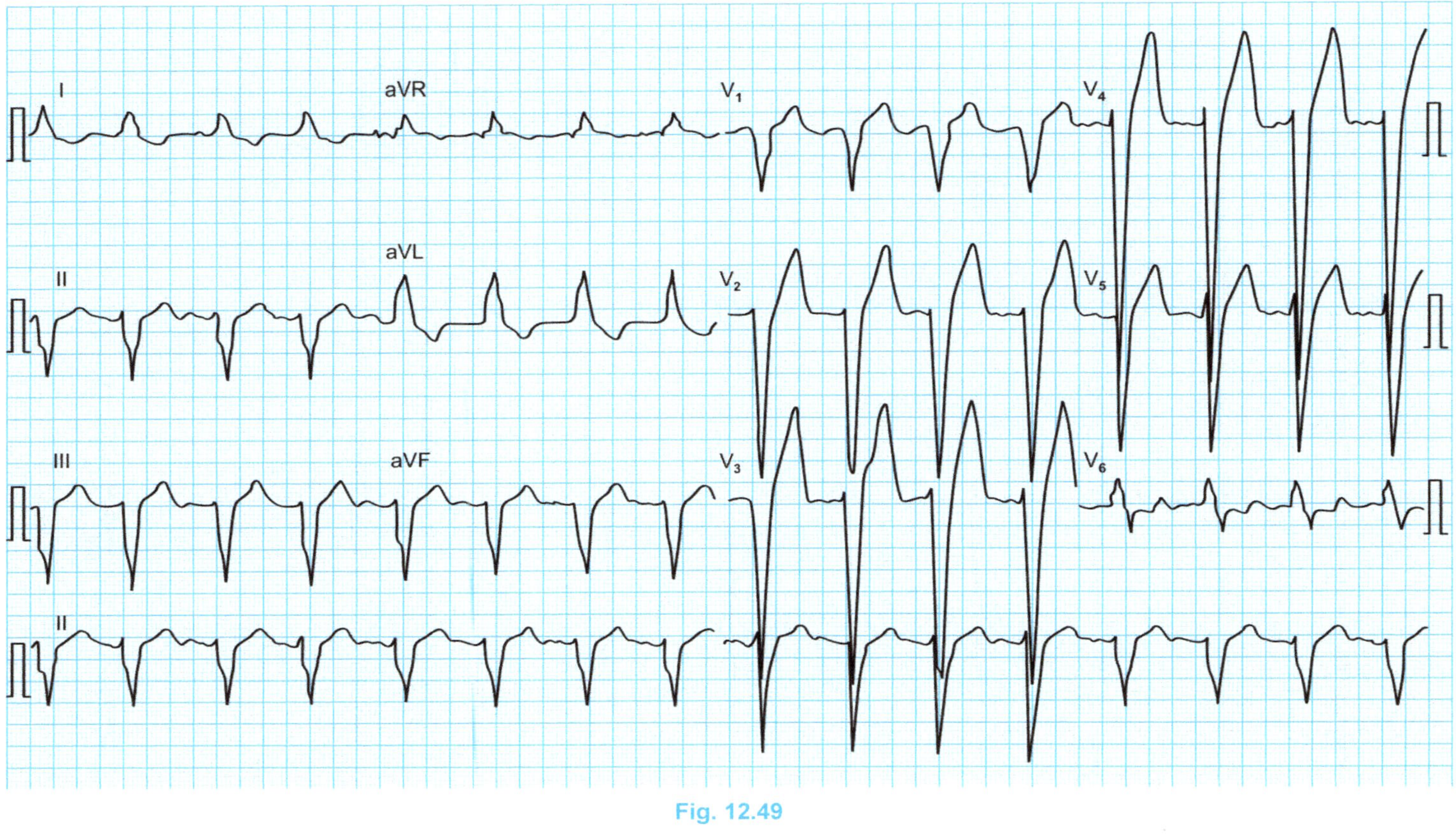

Fig. 12.49

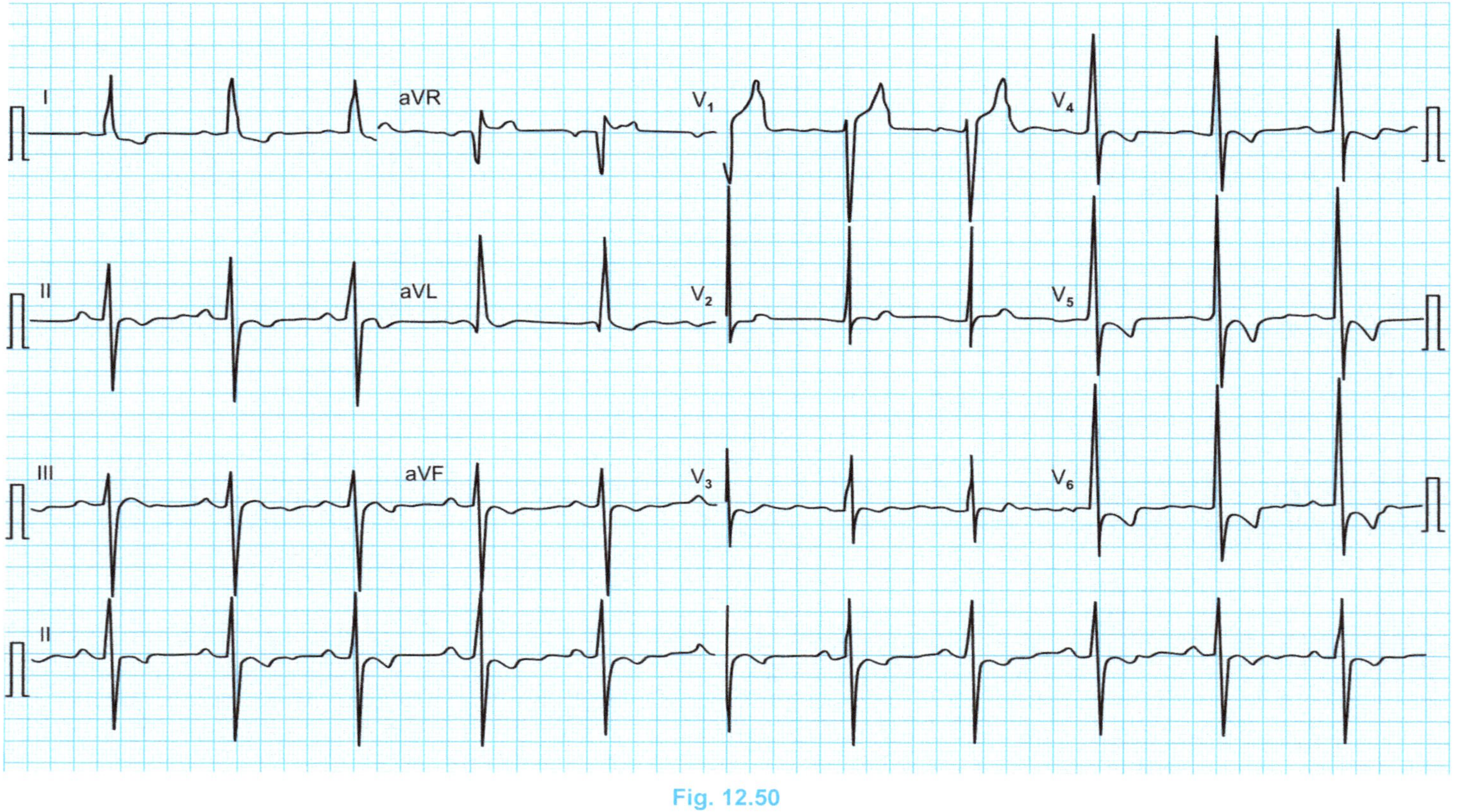

Fig. 12.50

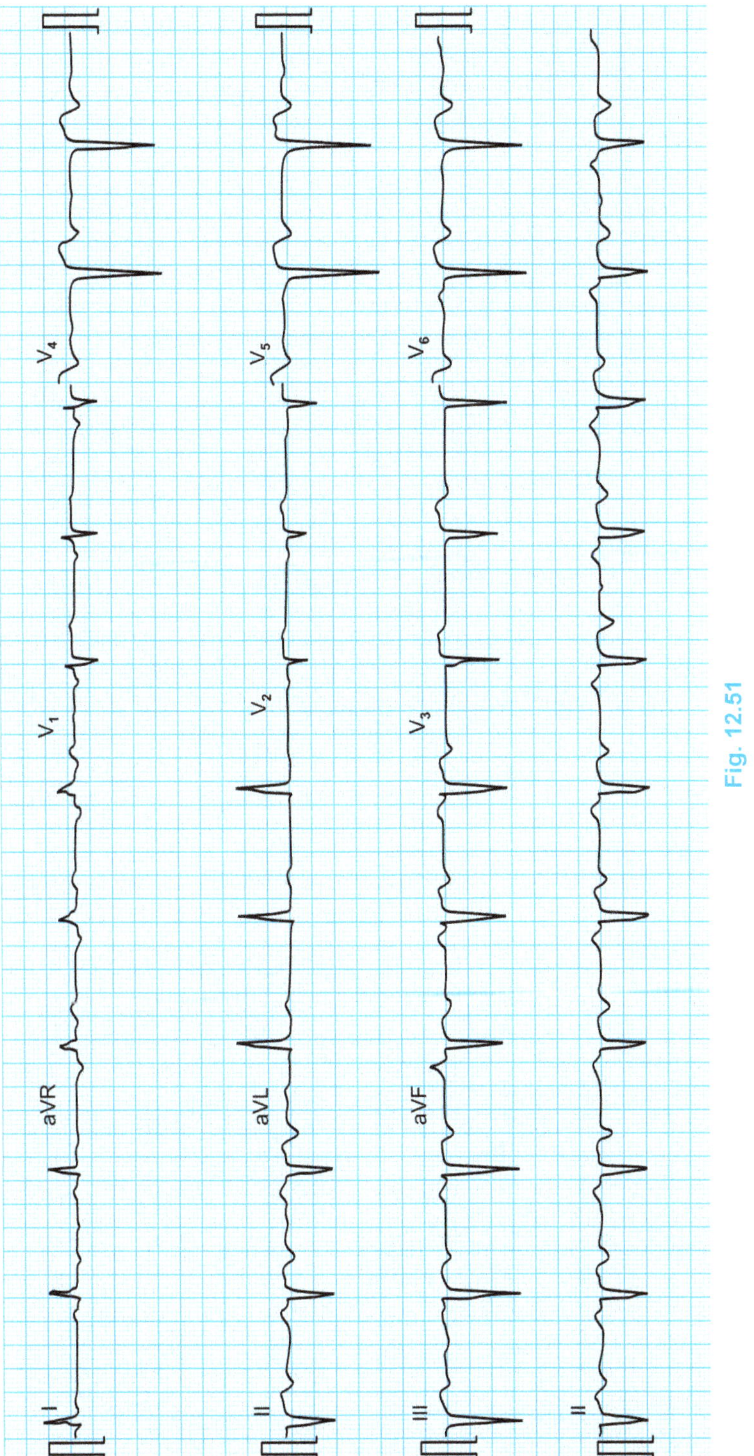

Fig. 12.51

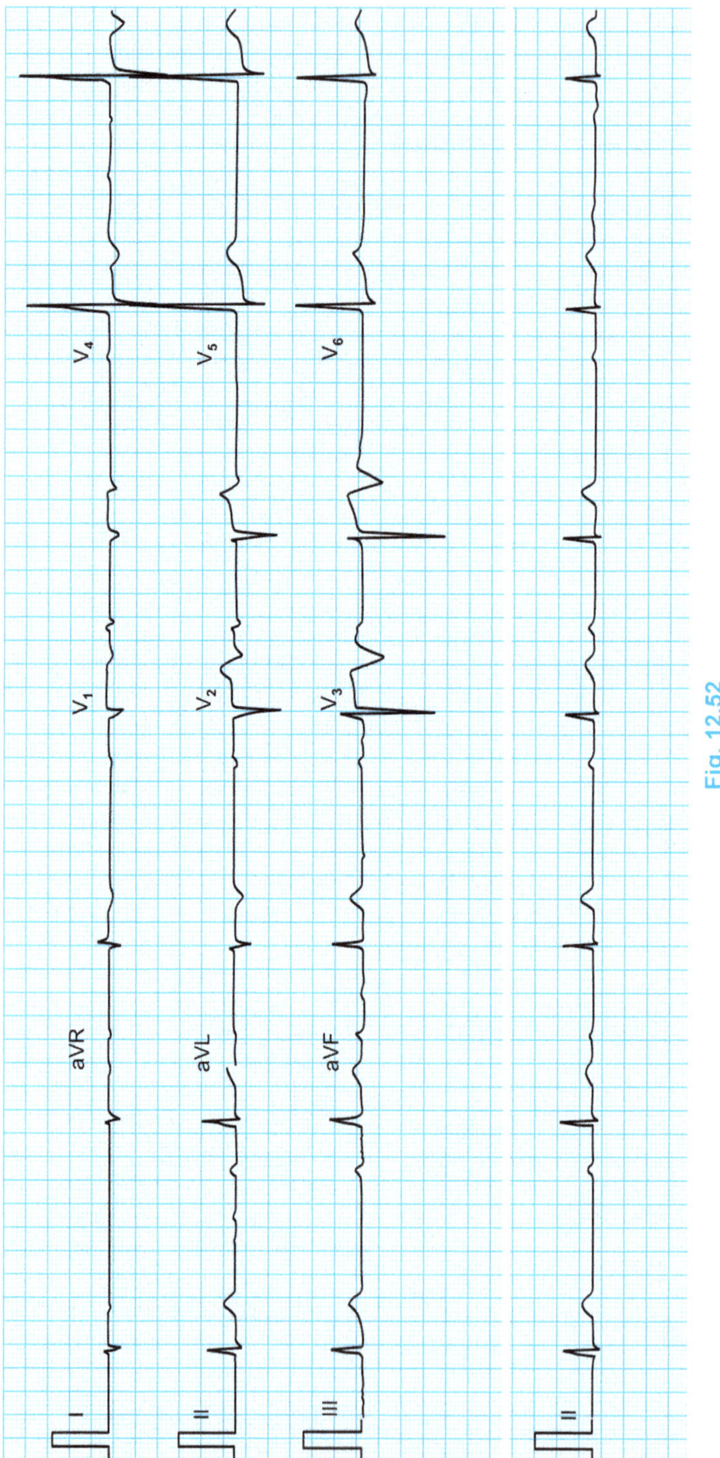

Fig. 12.52

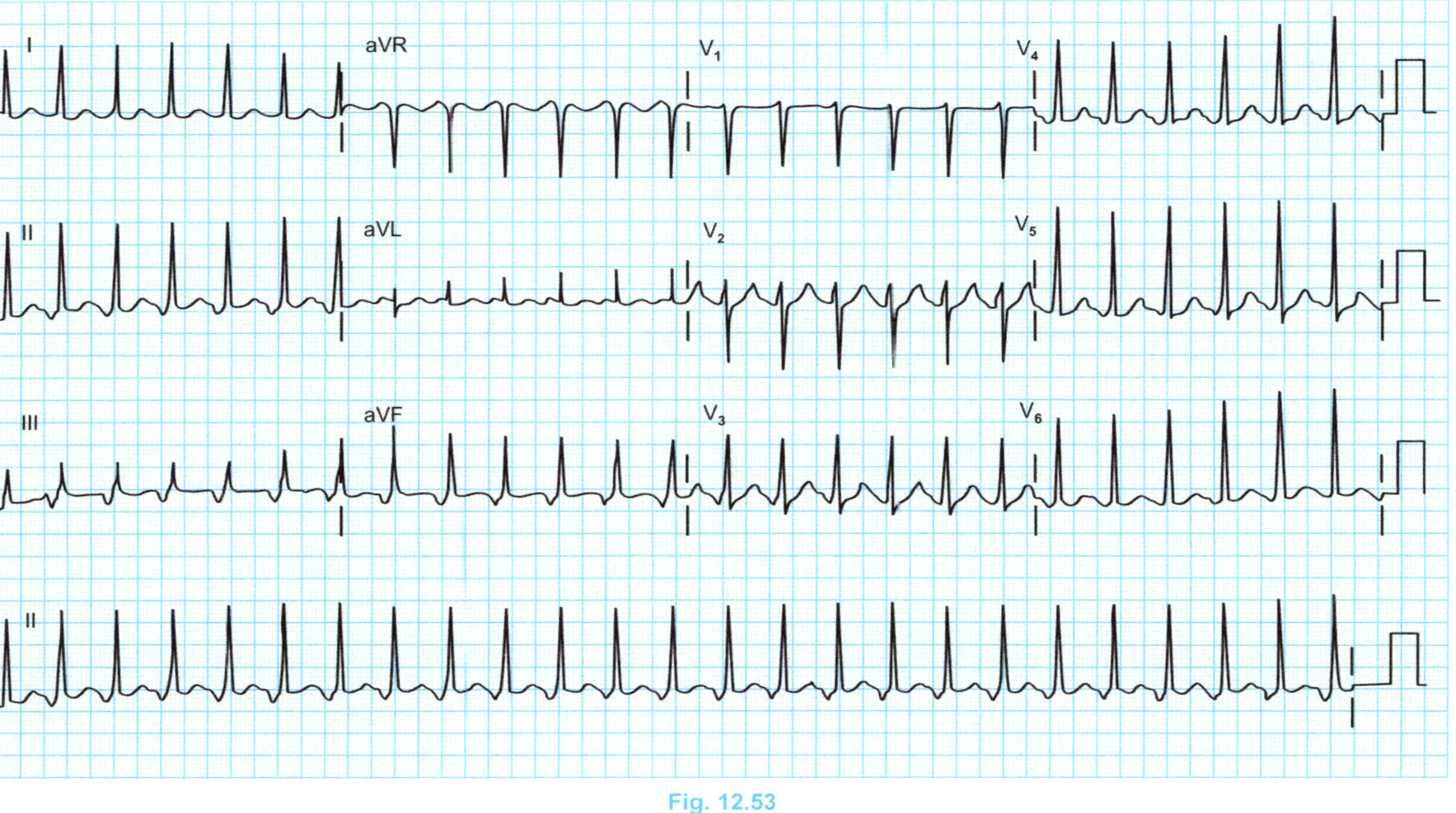

Fig. 12.53

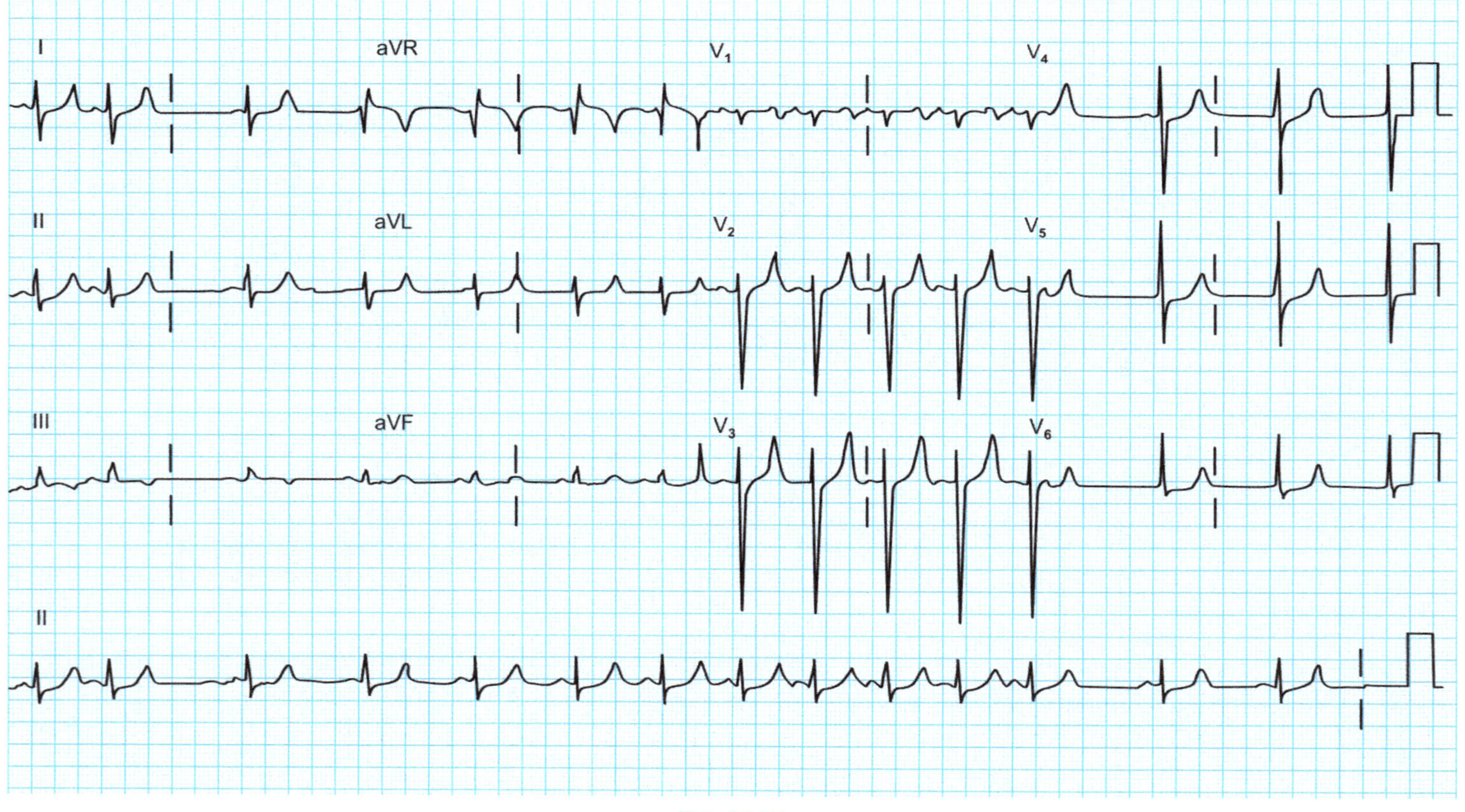

Fig. 12.54

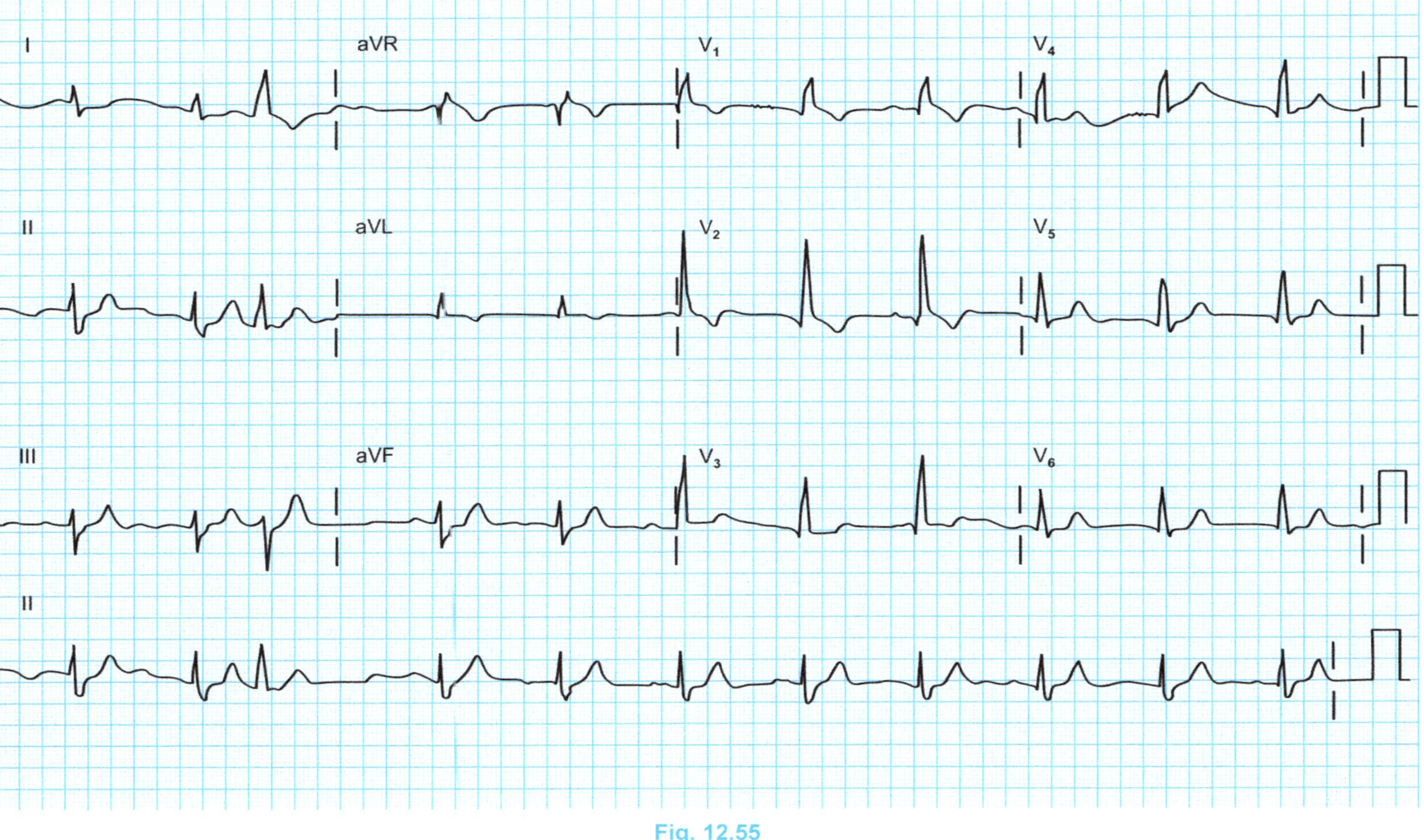

Fig. 12.55

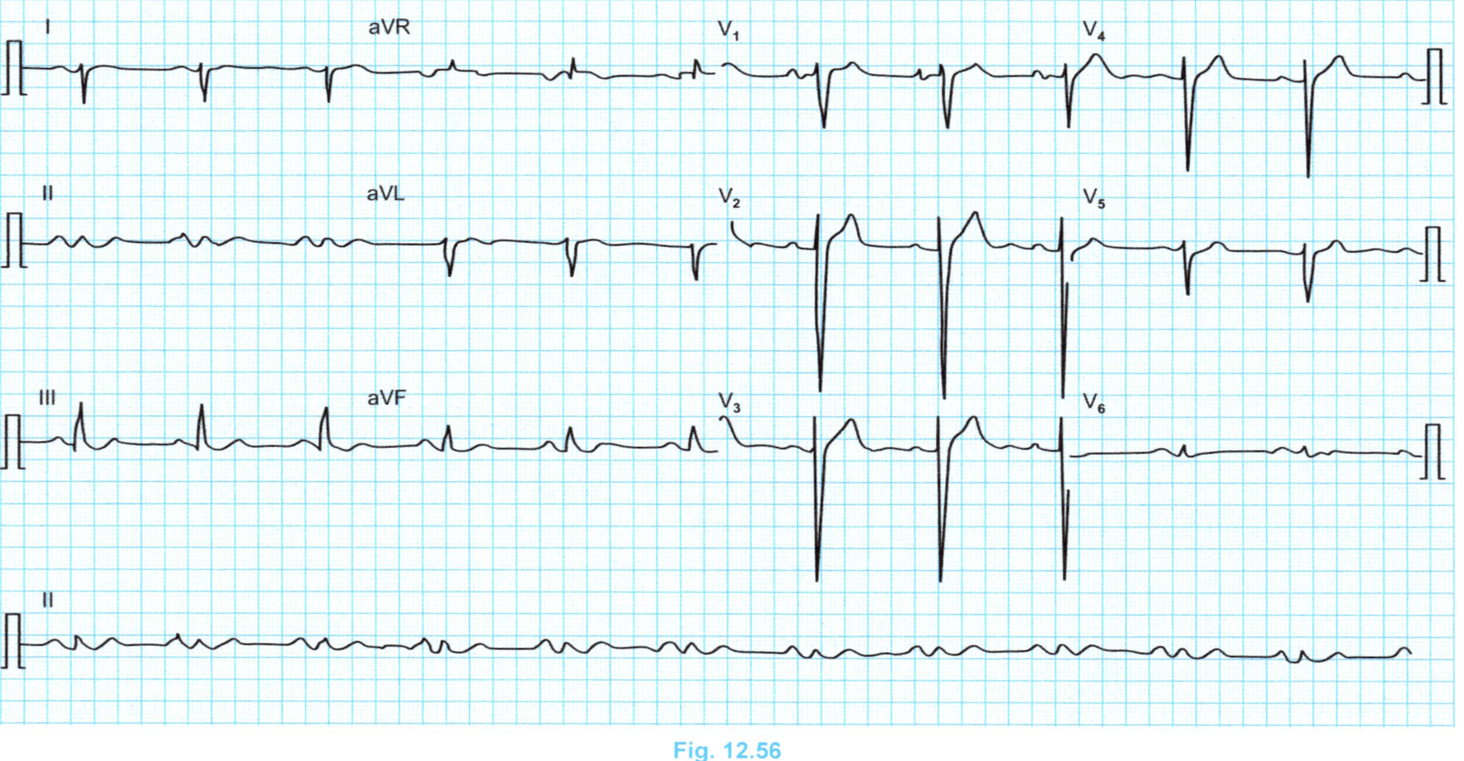

Fig. 12.56

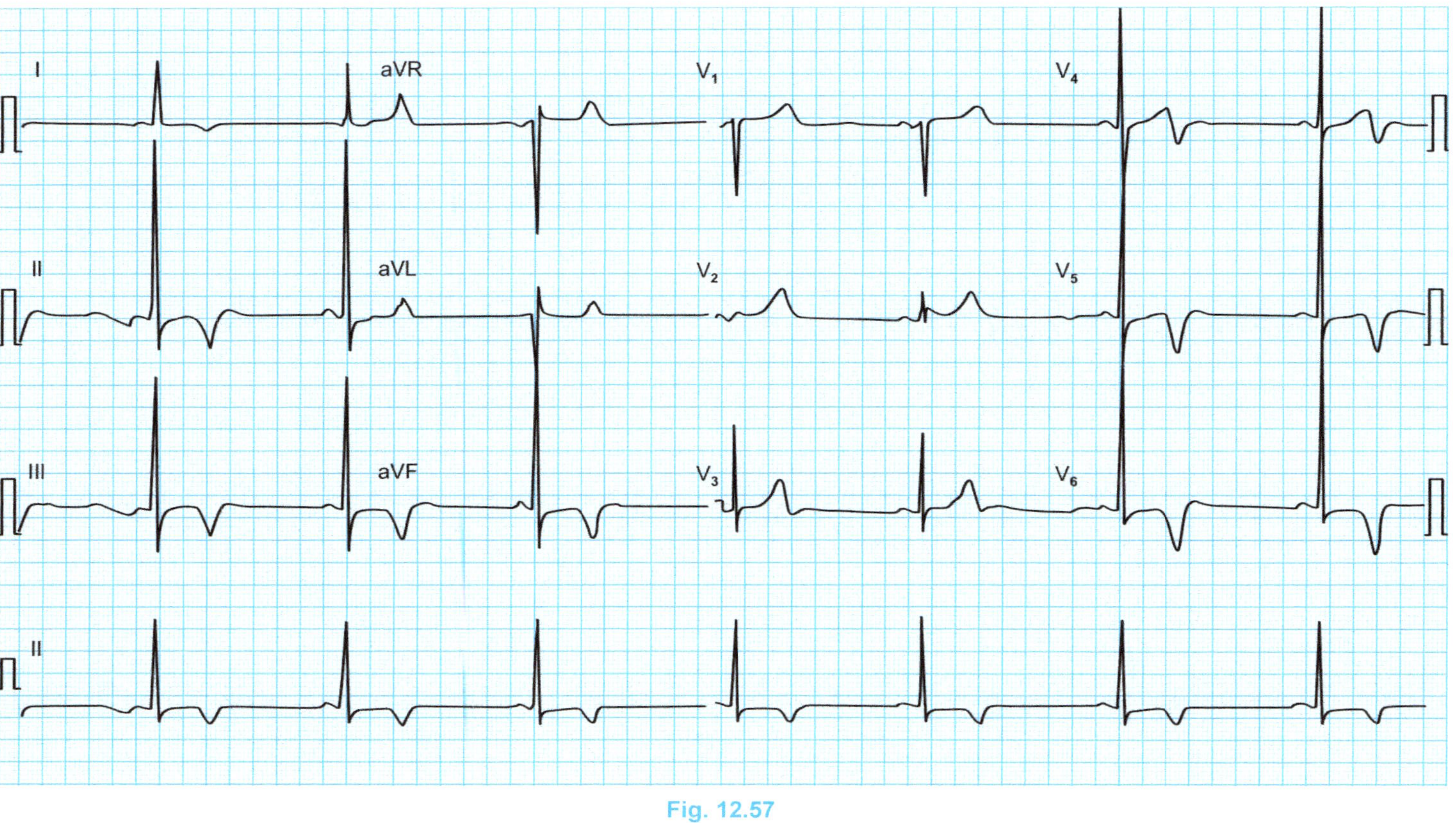

Fig. 12.57

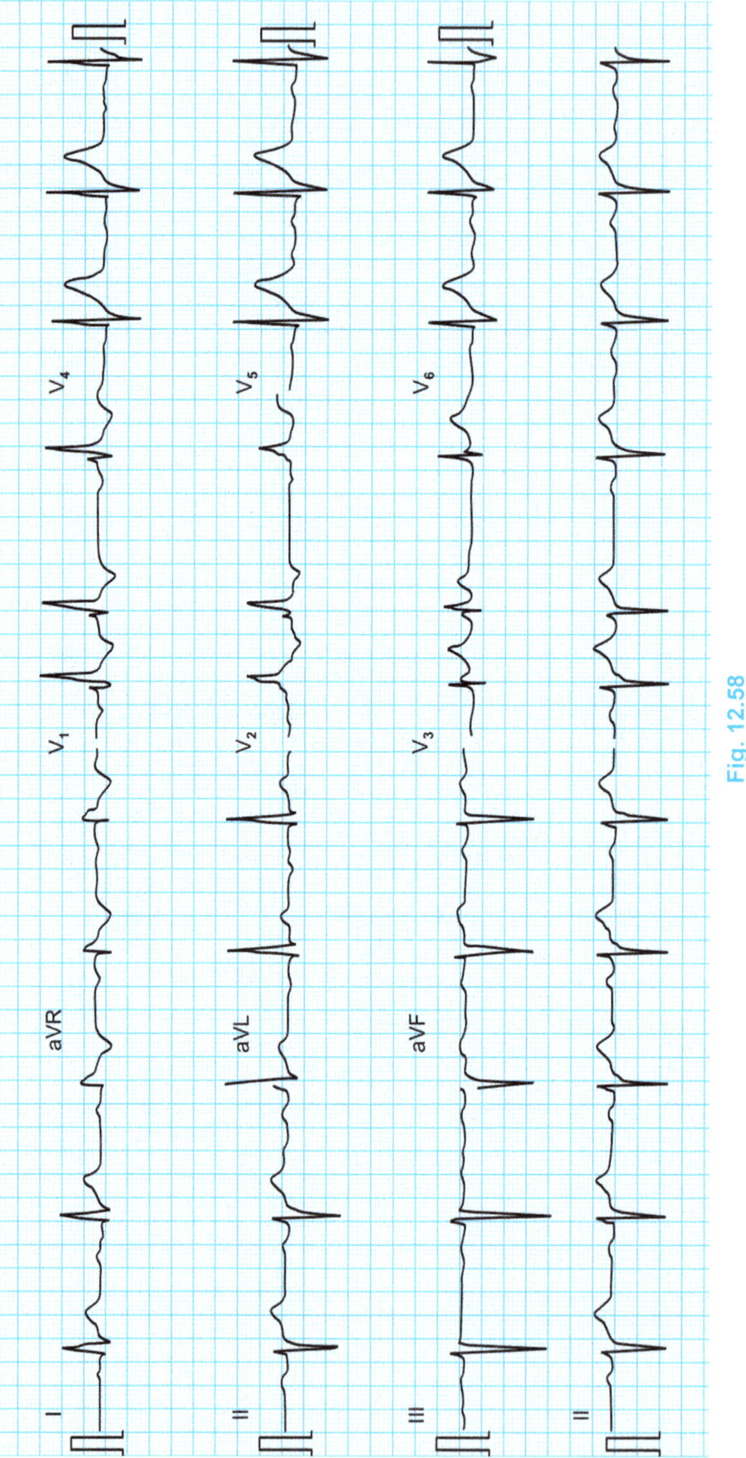

Fig. 12.58

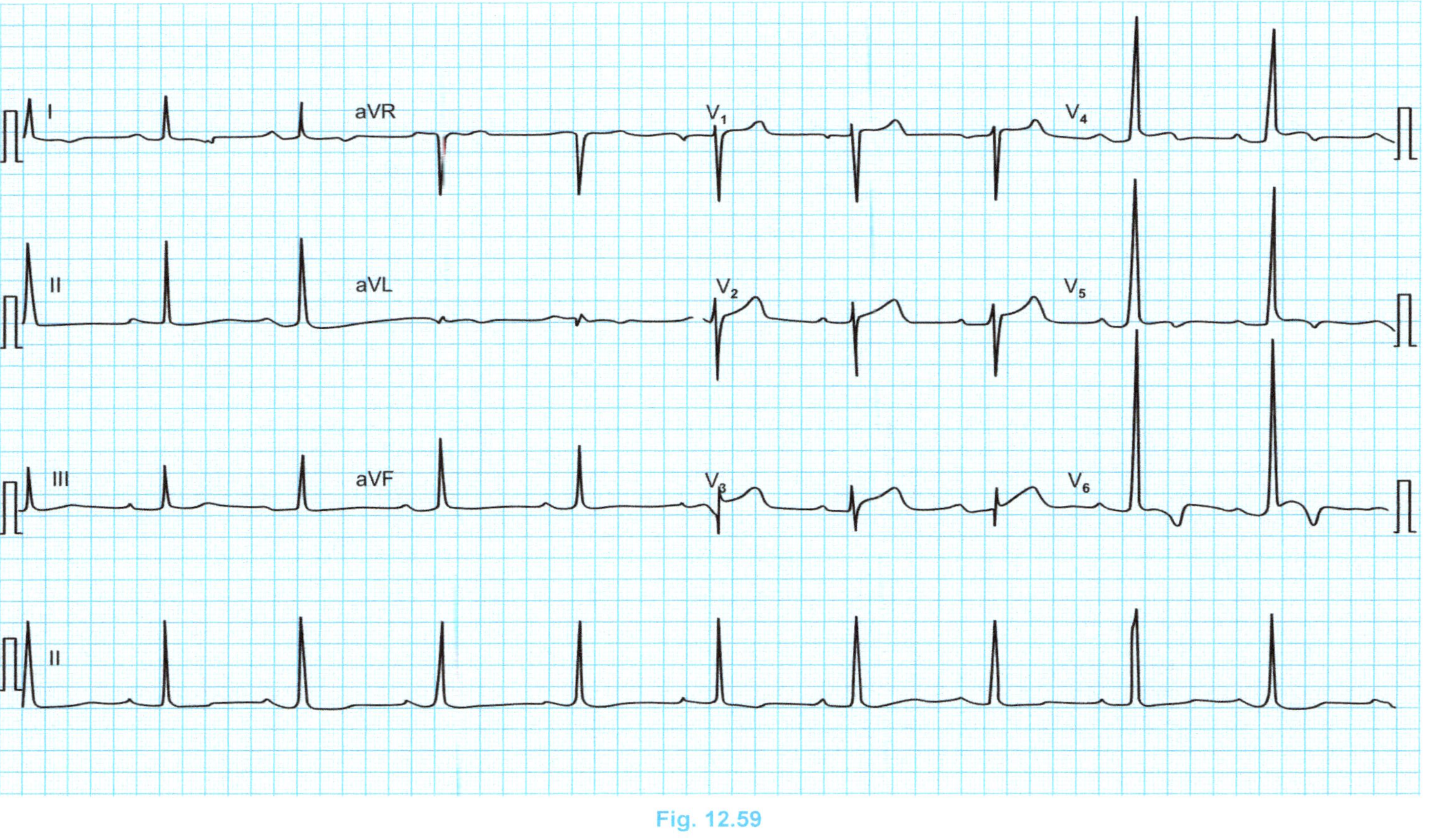

Fig. 12.59

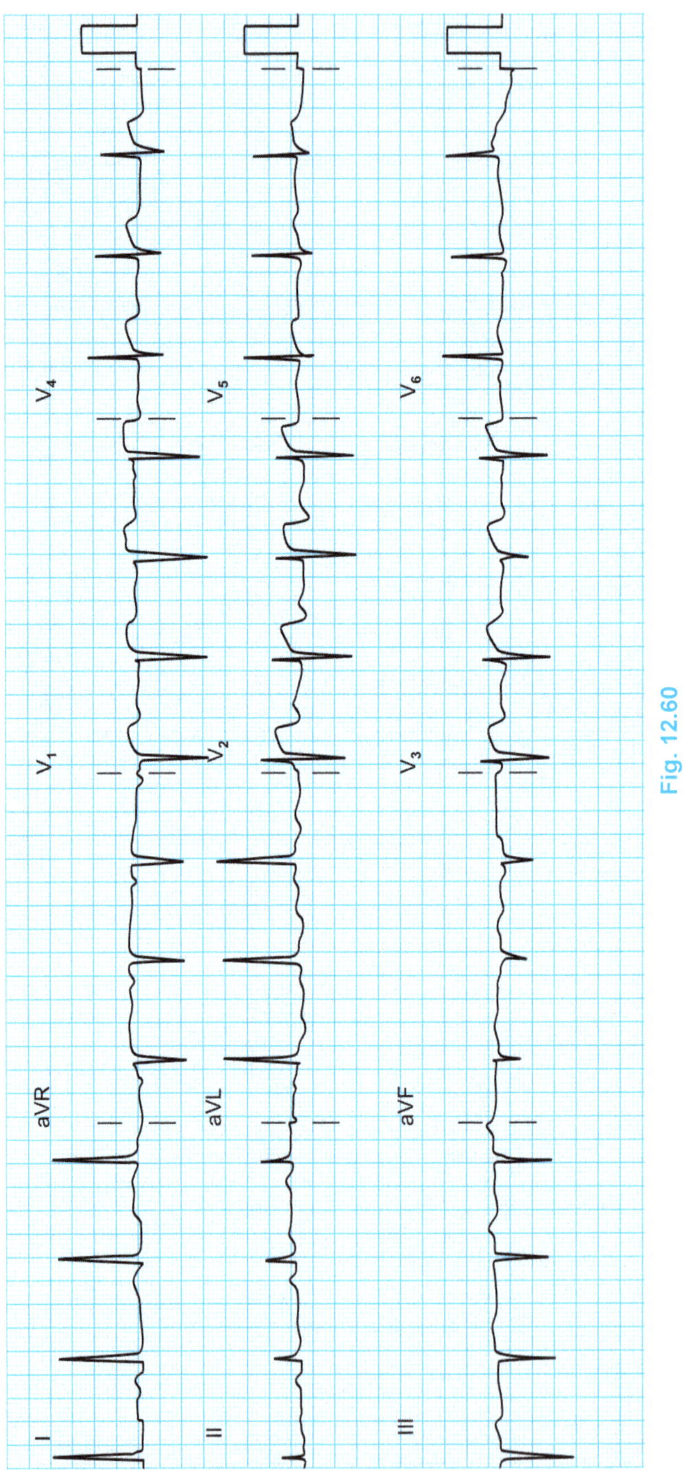

Fig. 12.60

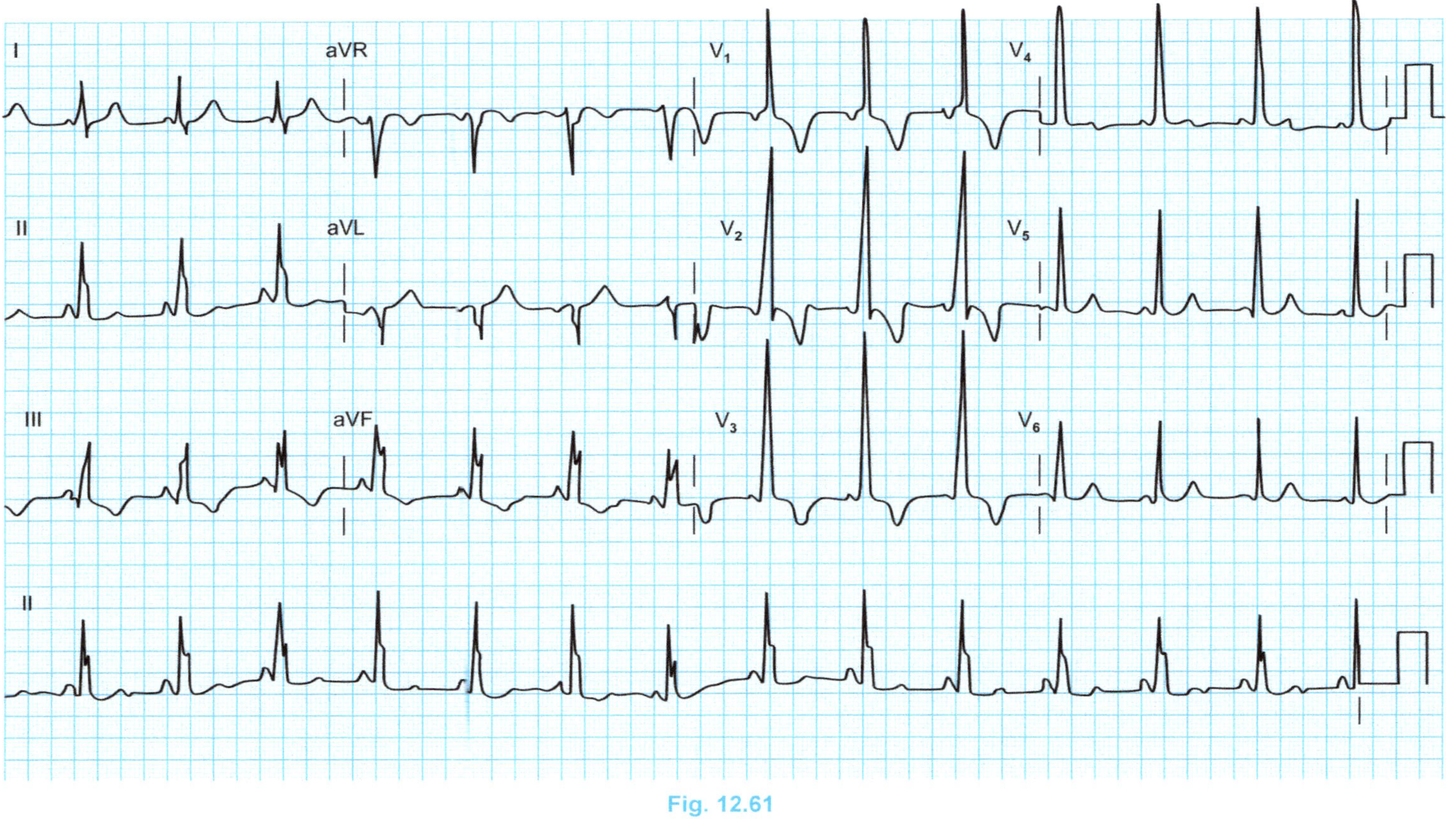

Fig. 12.61

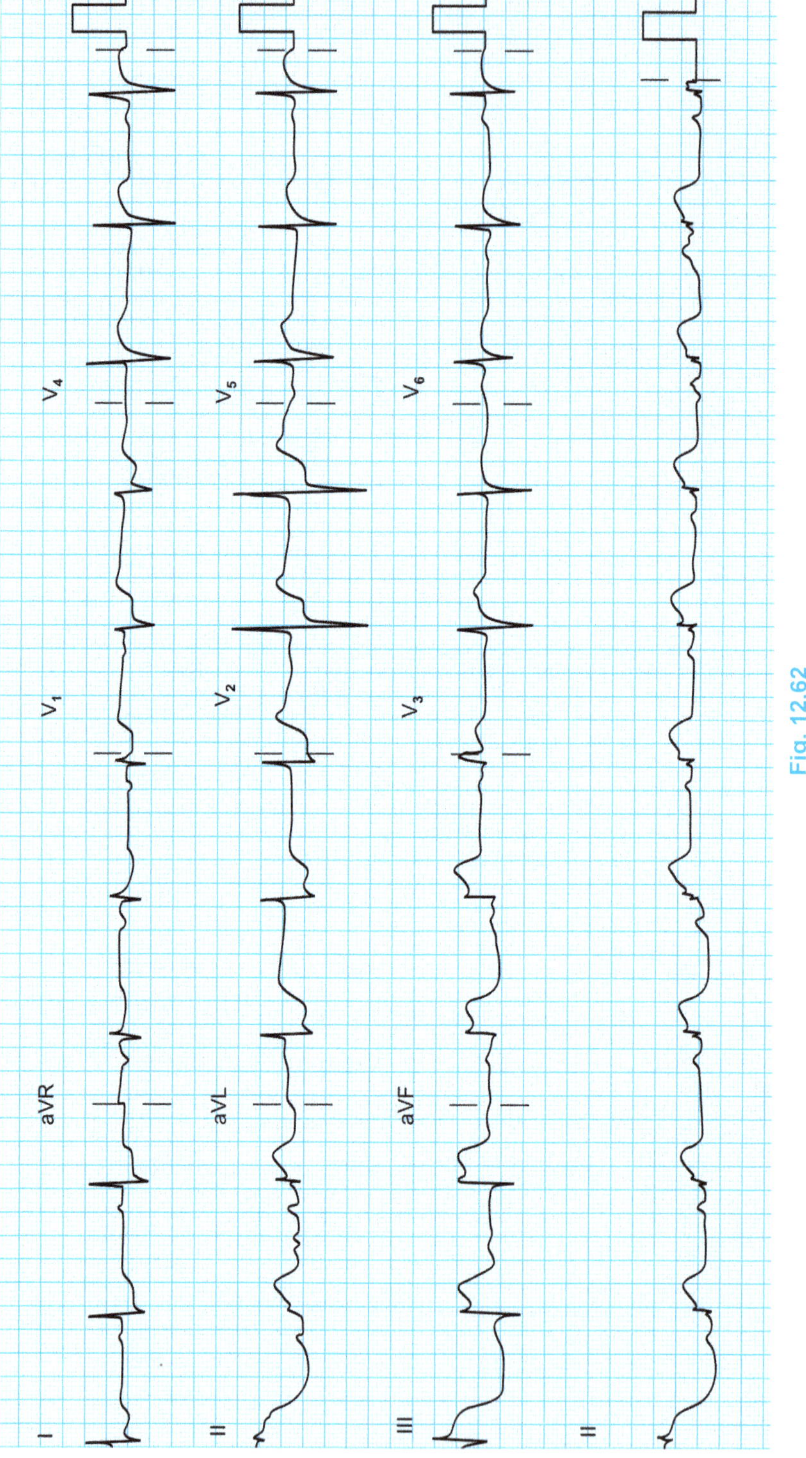

Fig. 12.62

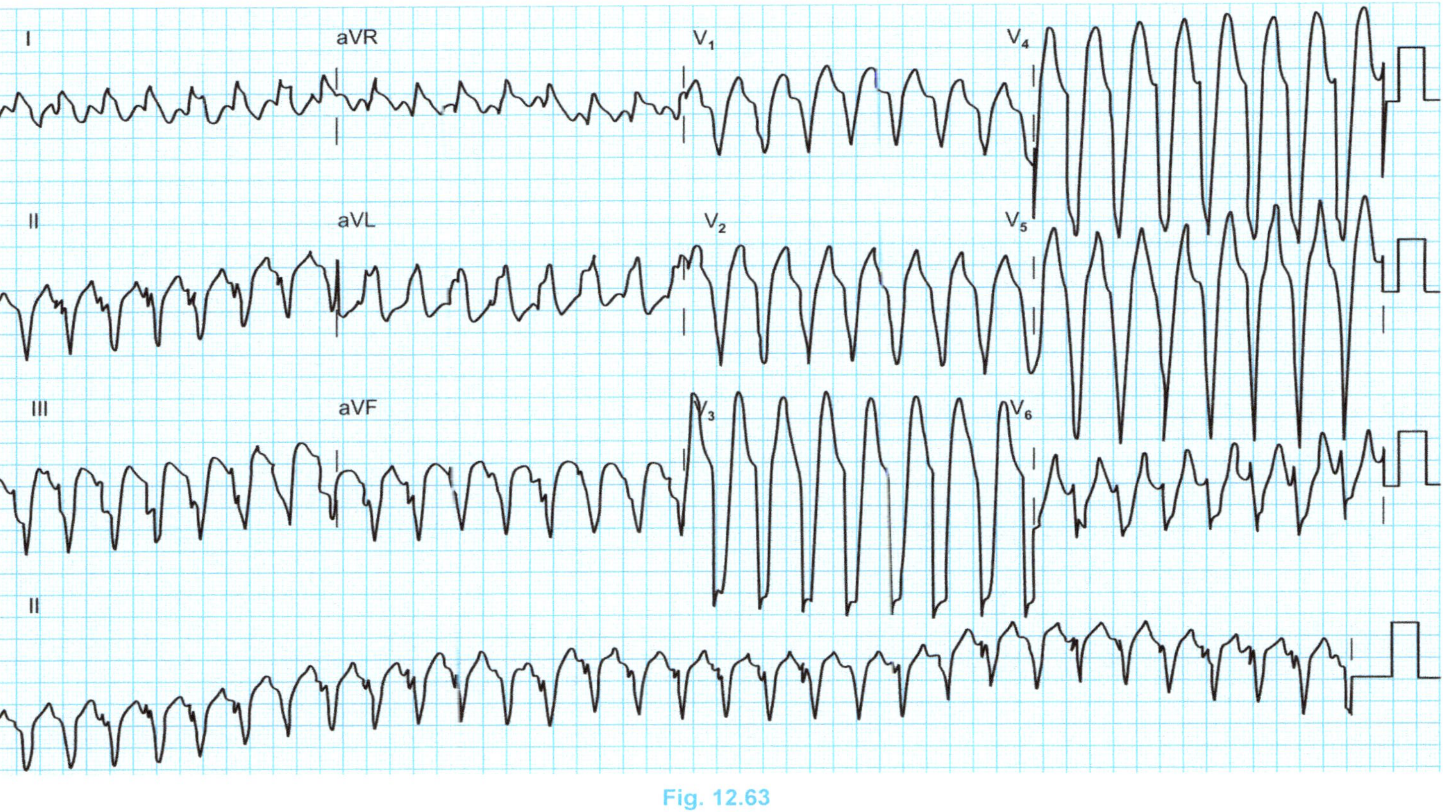

Fig. 12.63

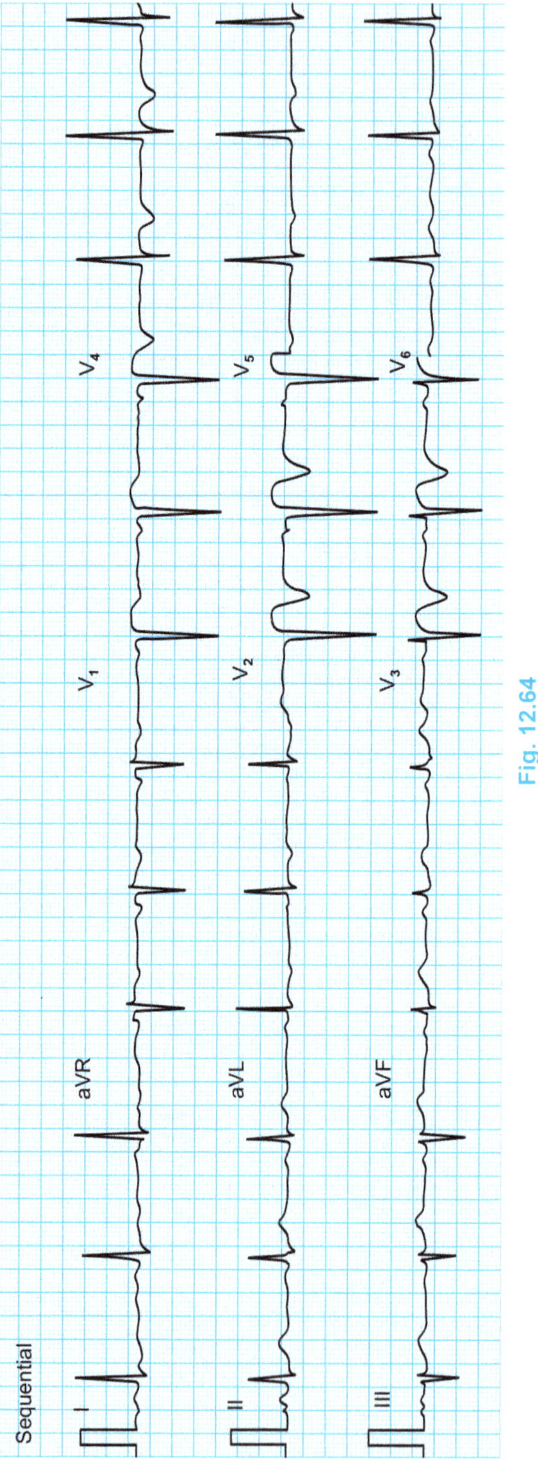

Fig. 12.64

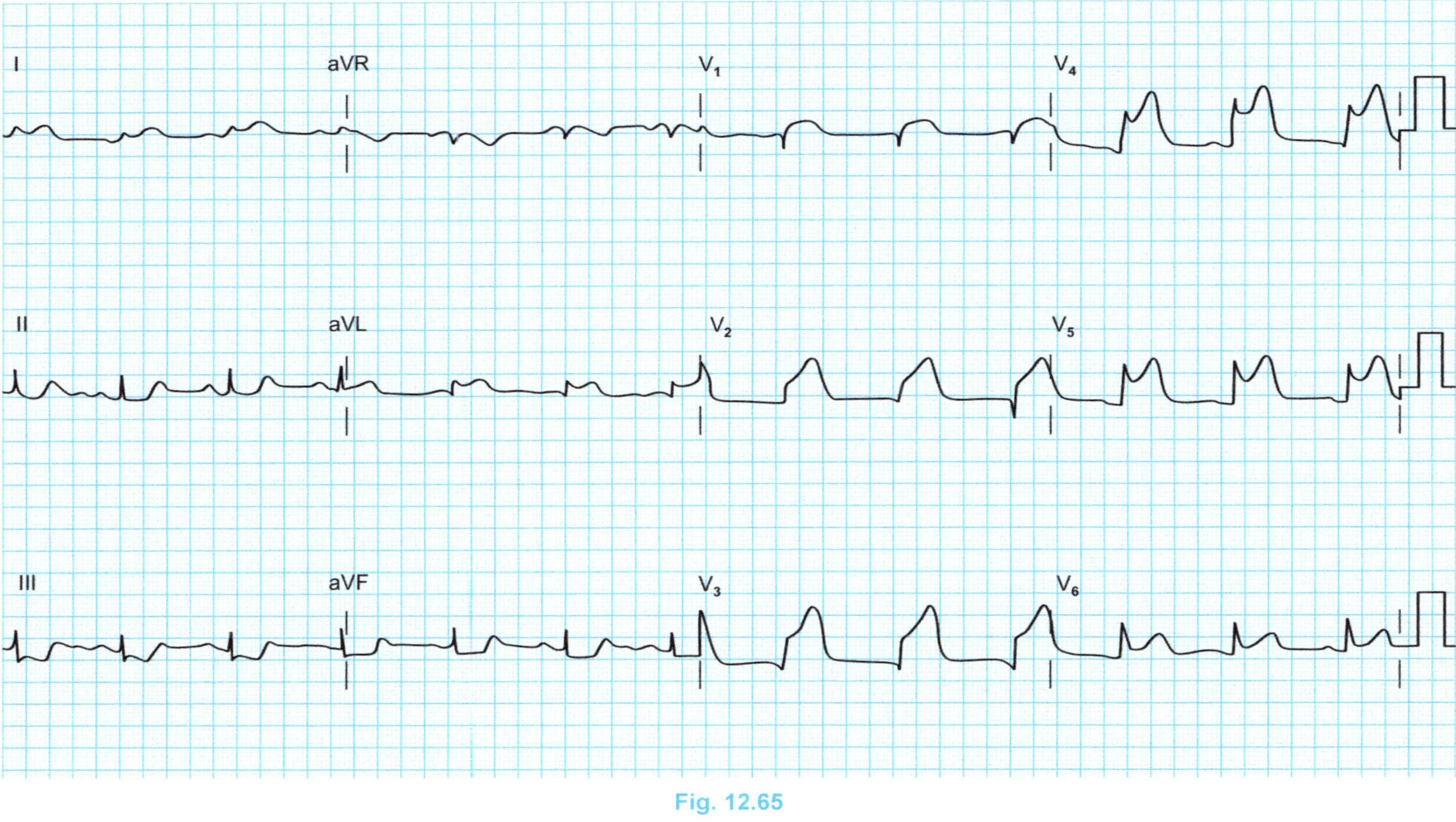

Fig. 12.65

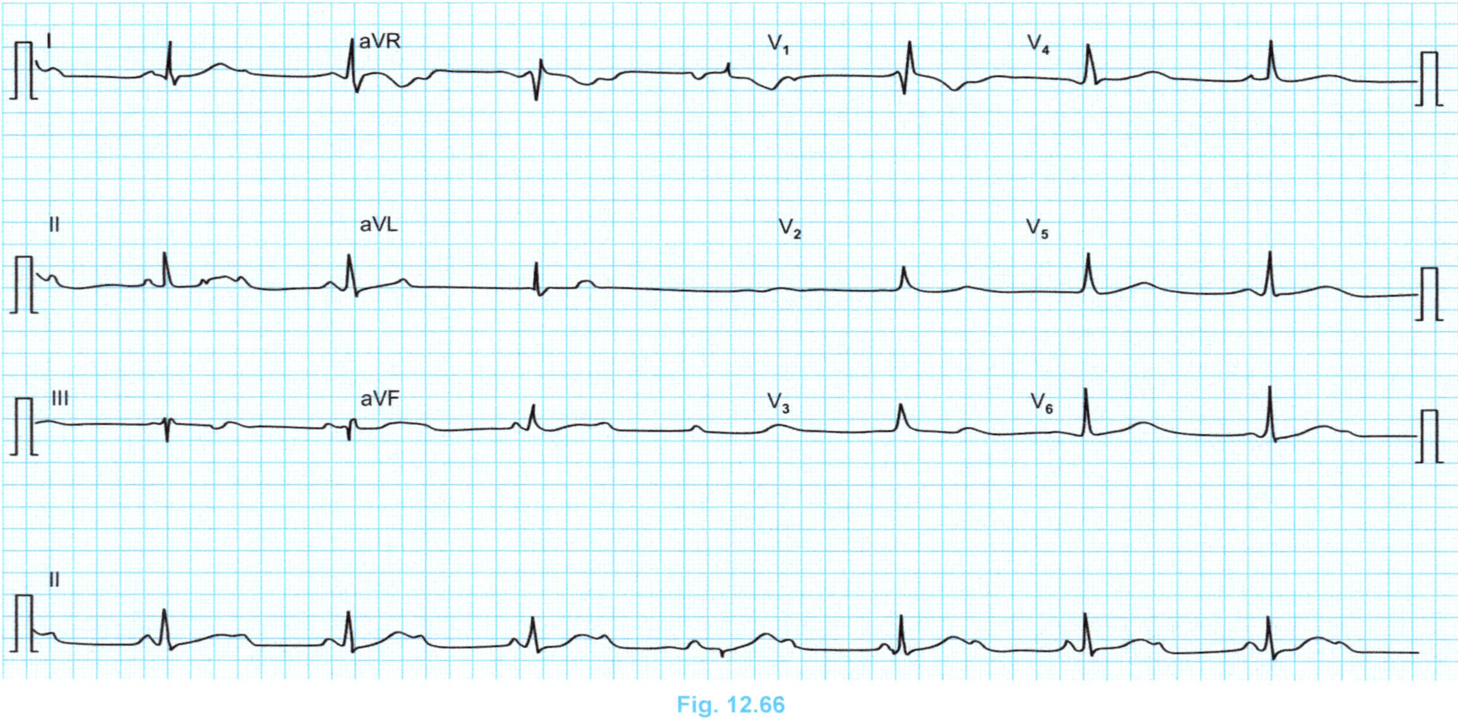

Fig. 12.66

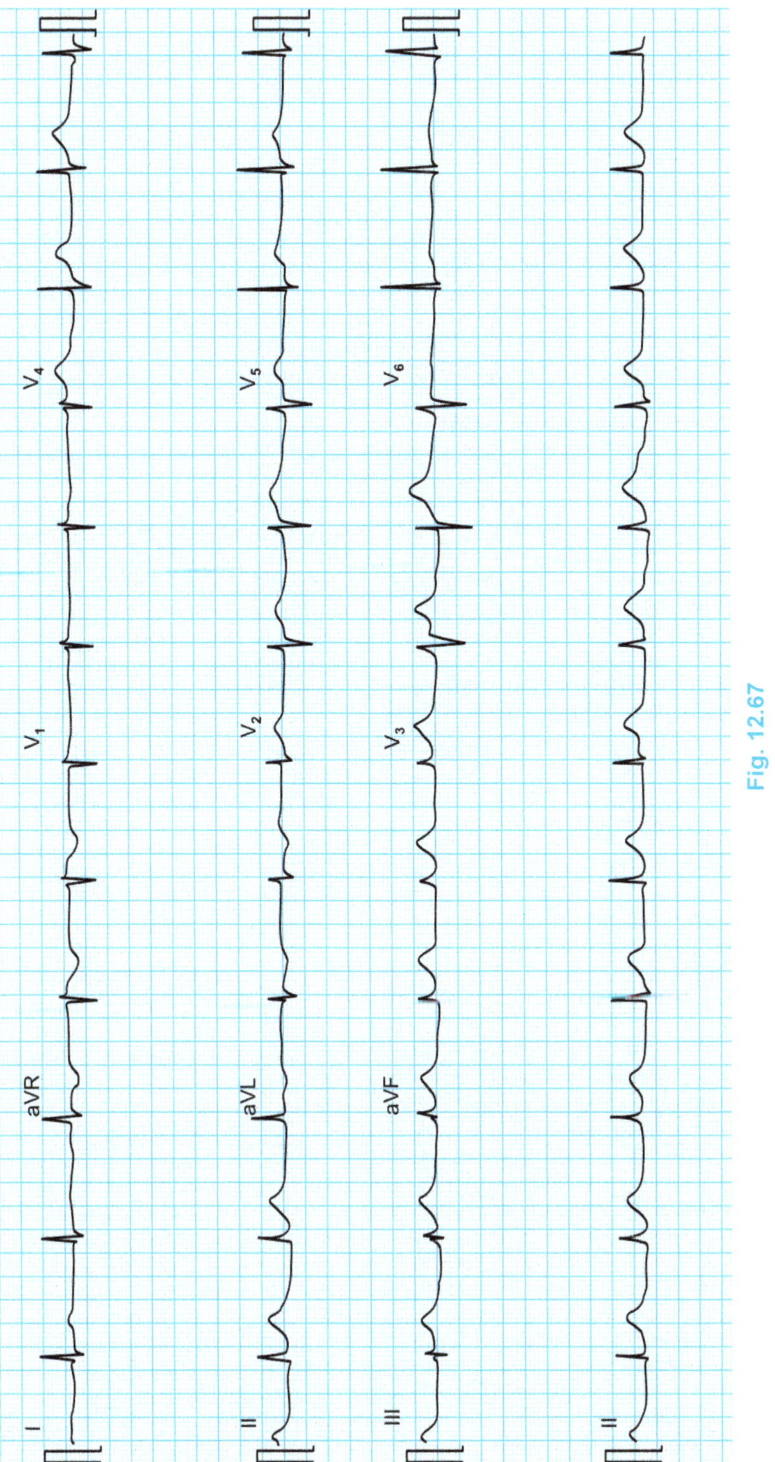

Fig. 12.67

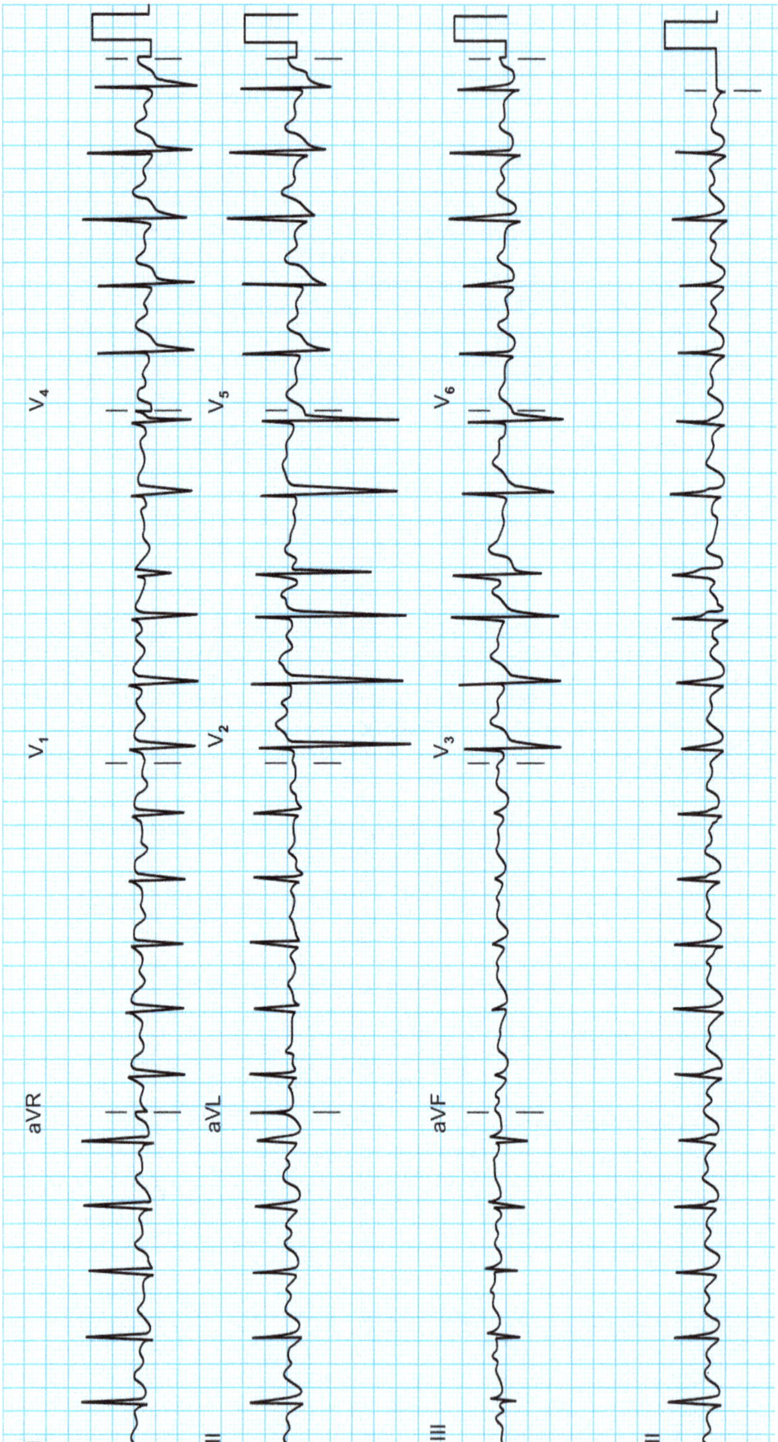

Fig. 12.68

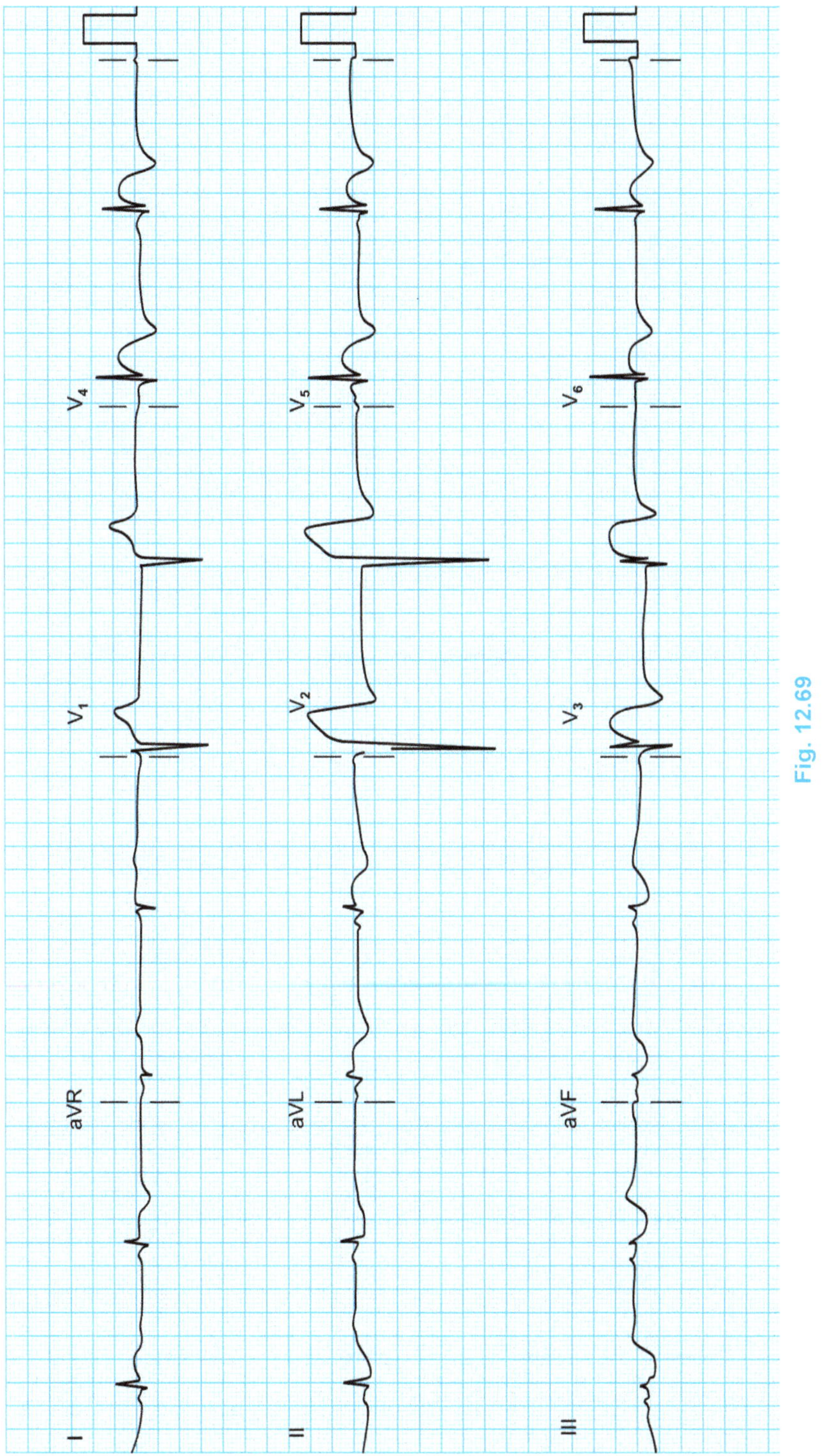

Fig. 12.69

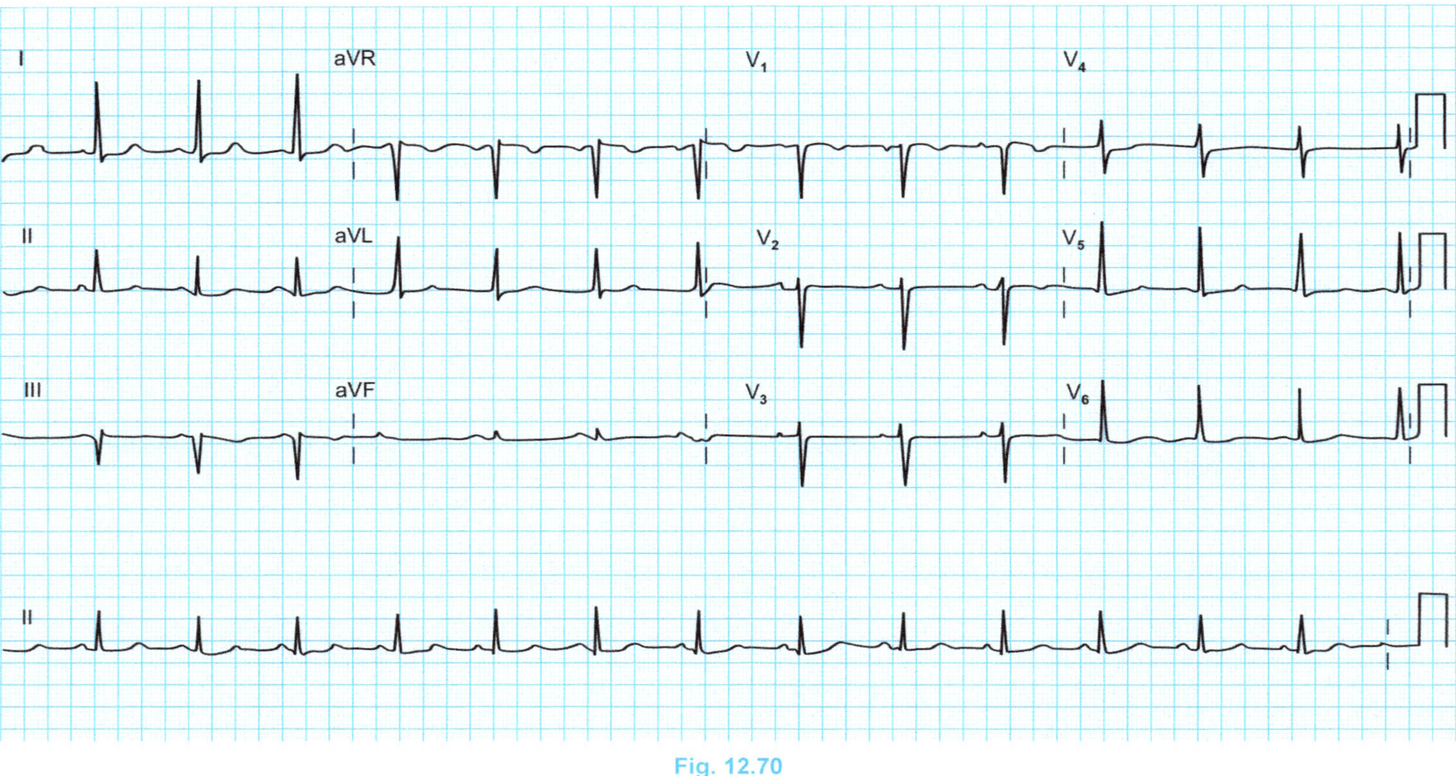

Fig. 12.70

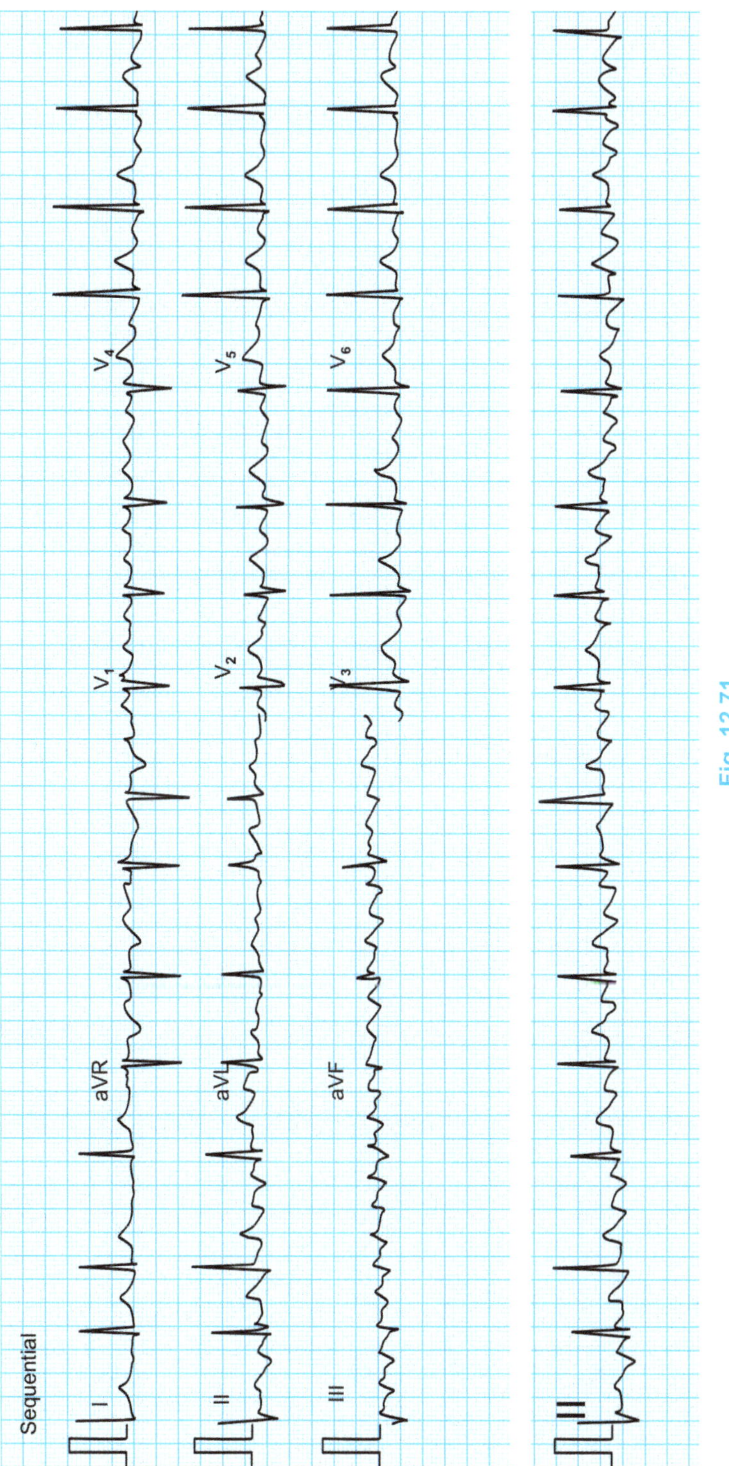

Fig. 12.71

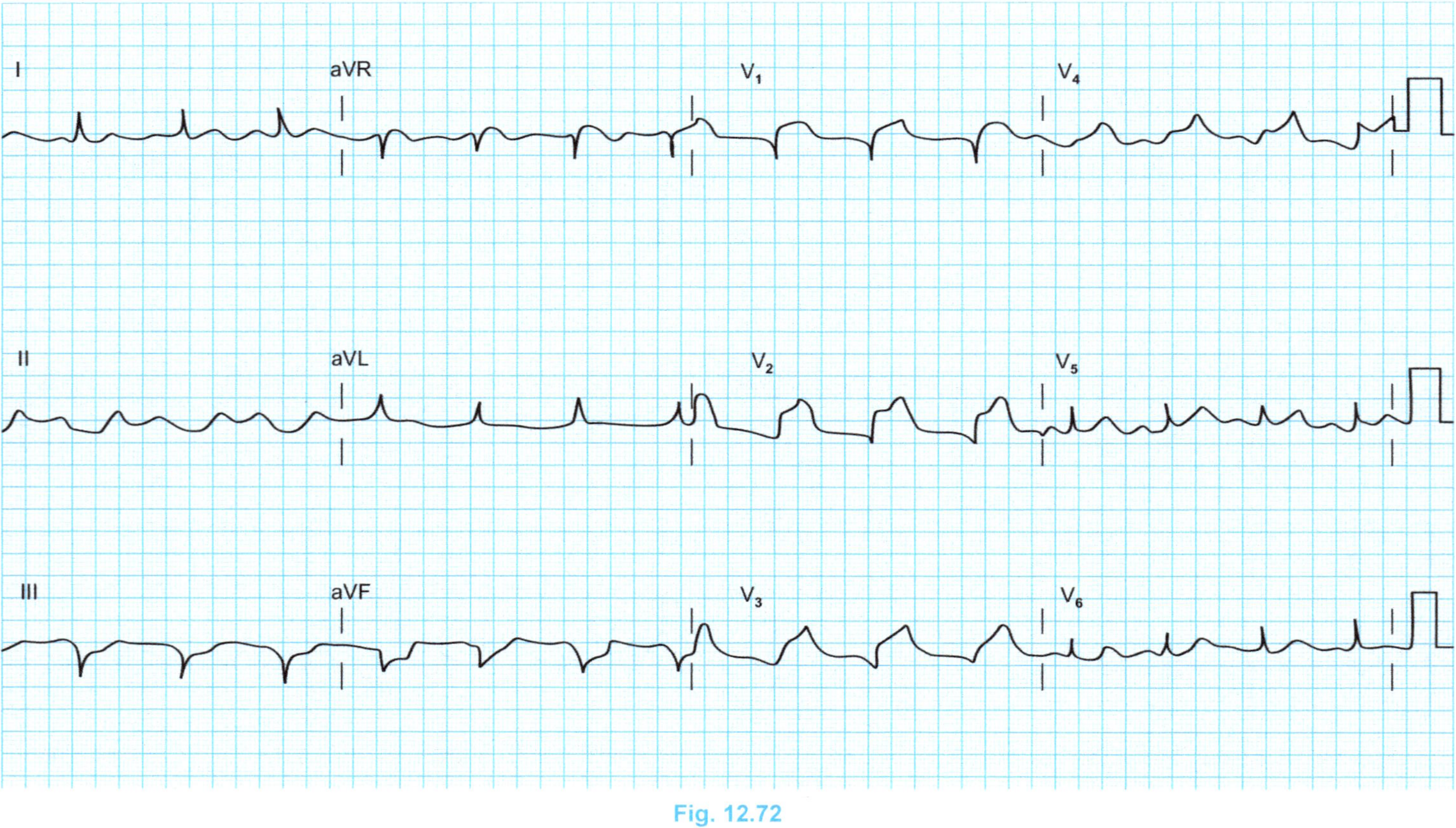

Fig. 12.72

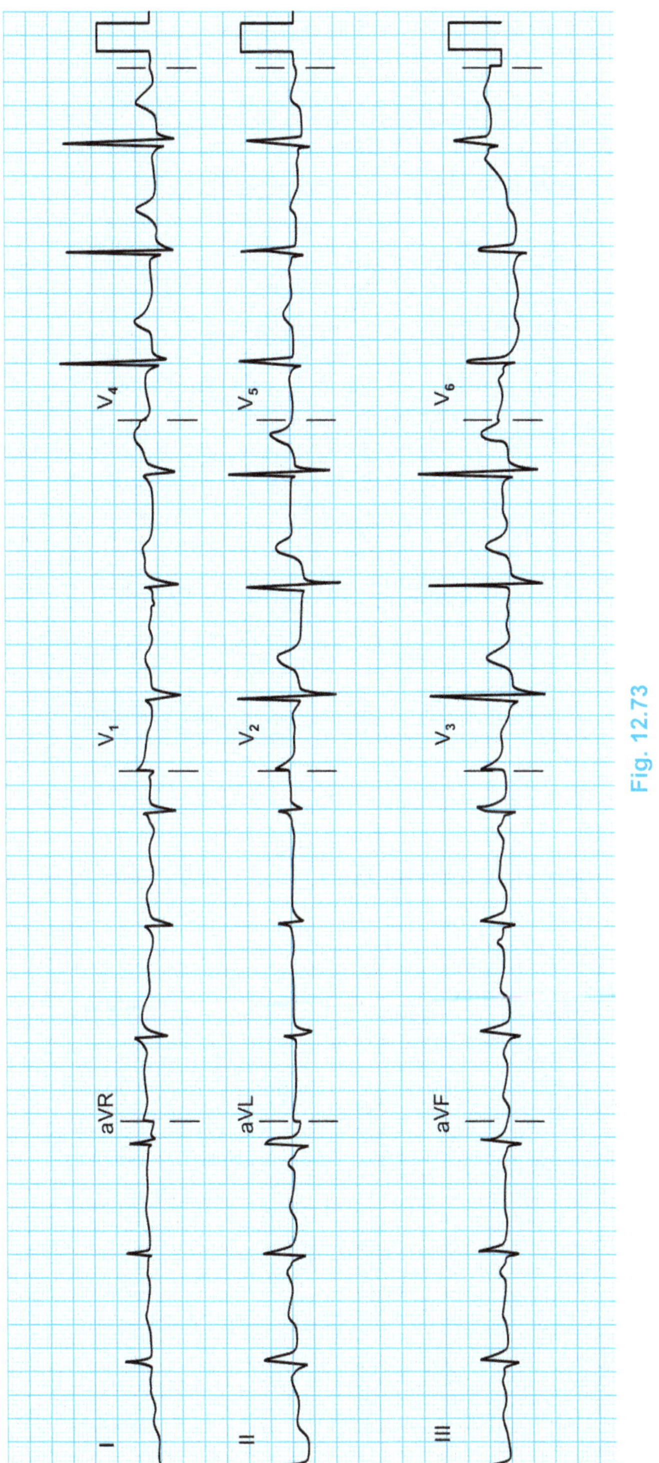

Fig. 12.73

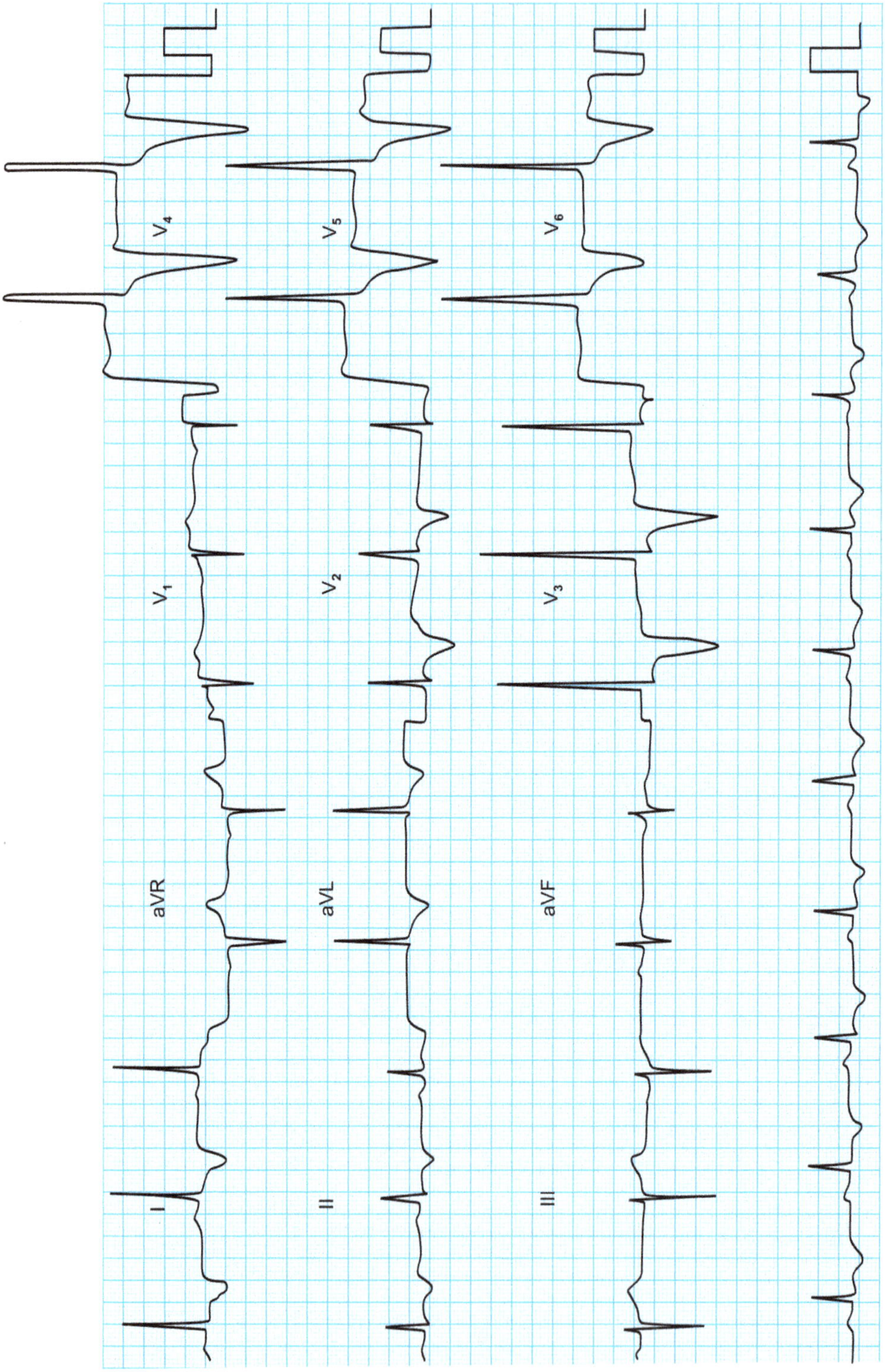

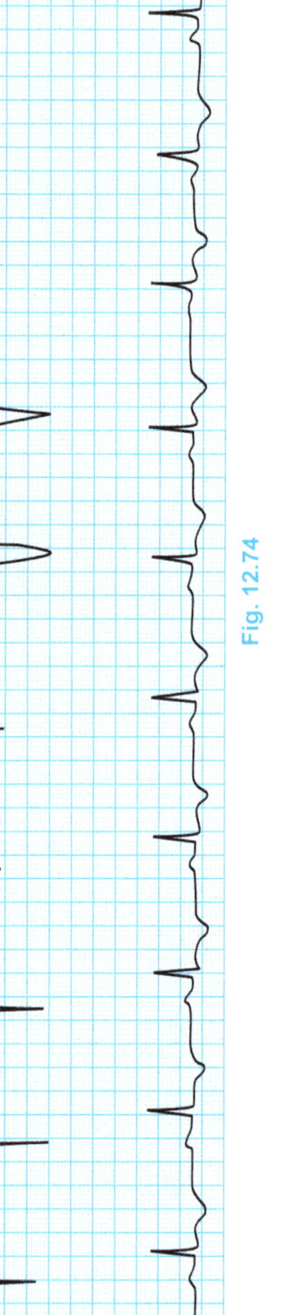

Fig. 12.74

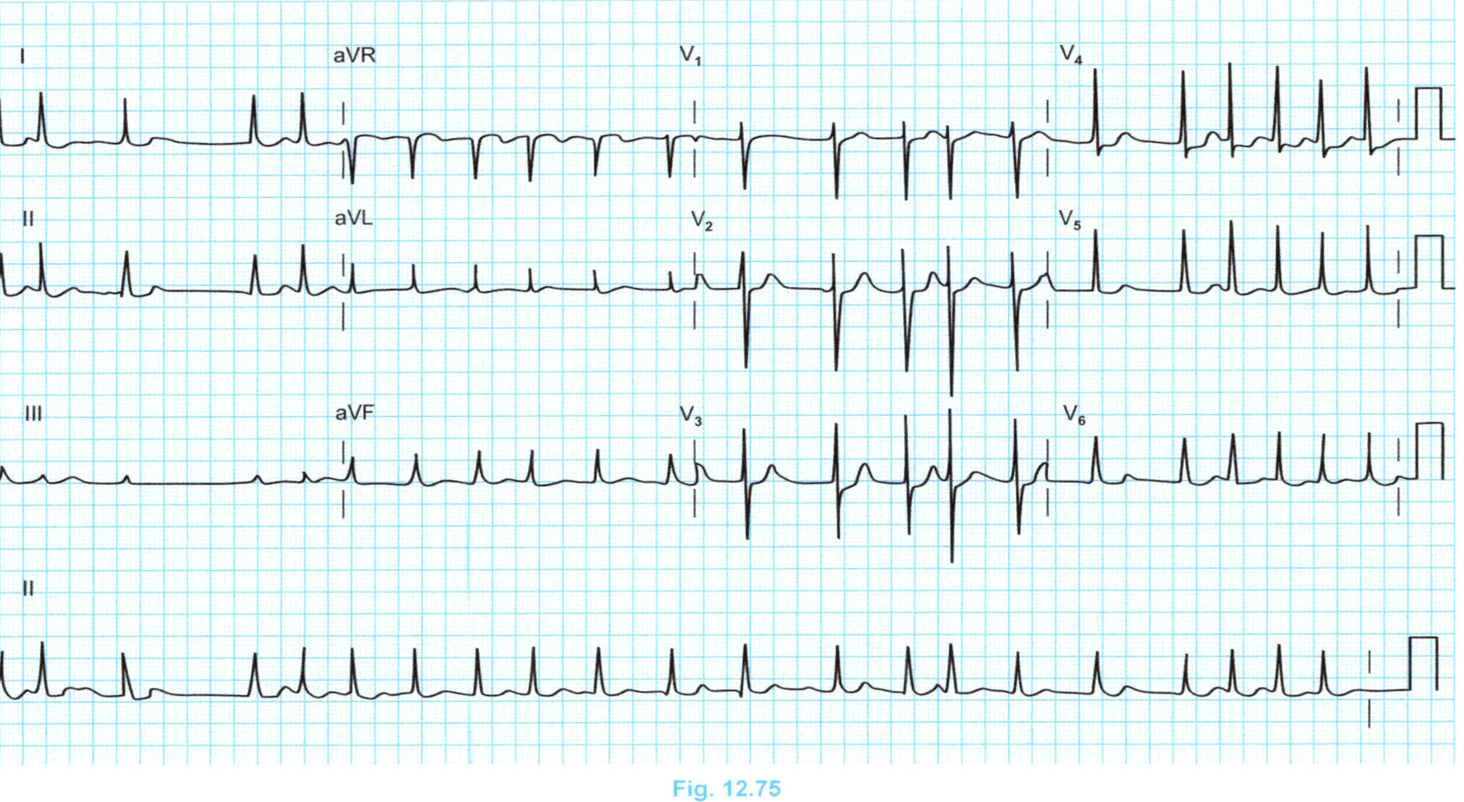

Fig. 12.75

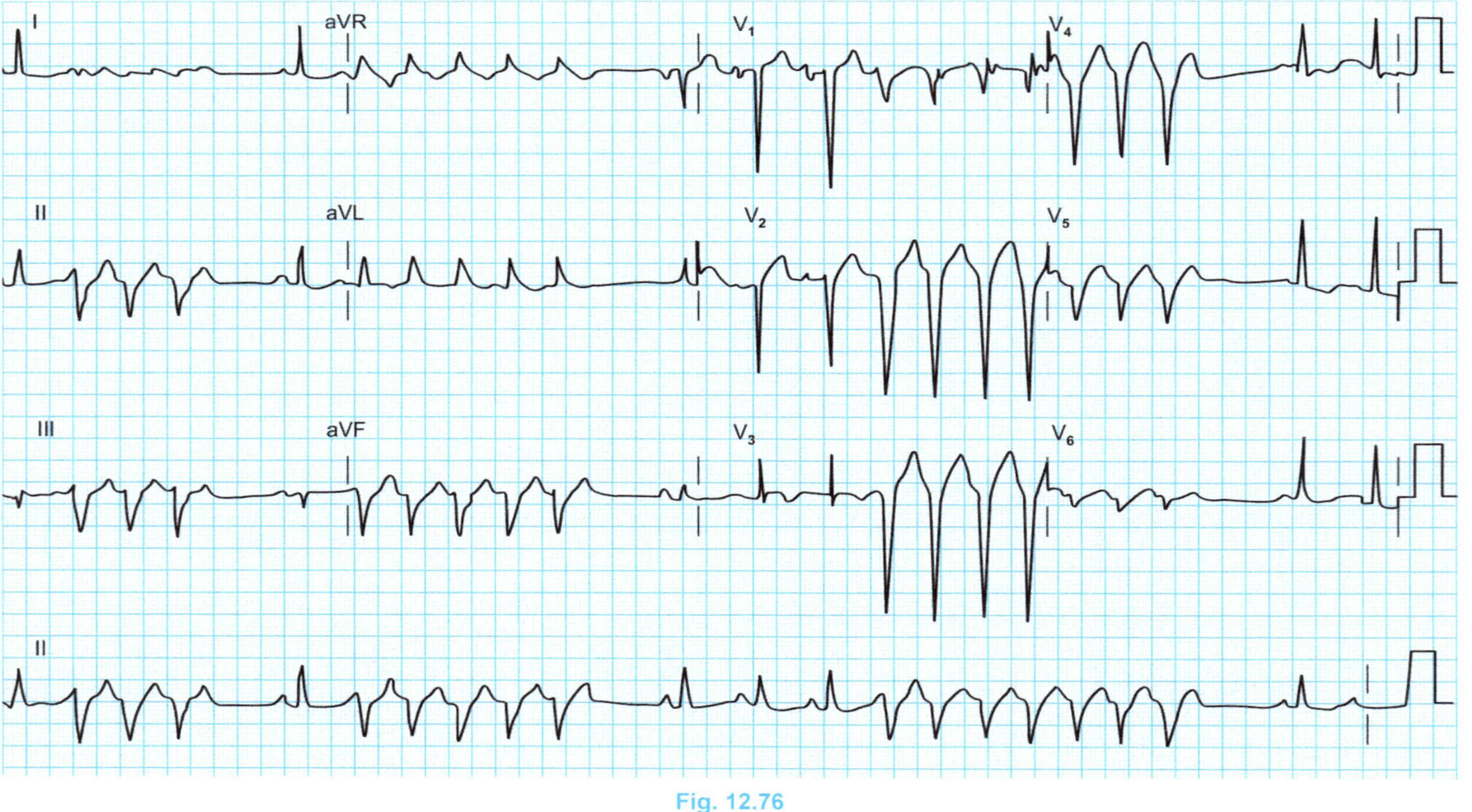

Fig. 12.76

Strip 1 of 2
Strip 2 of 2
12:11:26 PM   235 BPM   Size x1,x1,x1   Ventricular Run
12:12:10 PM   235 BPM   Size x1,x1,x1   Ventricular Run
Ch1
Ch2
Ch3
Ch1
Ch2
Ch3

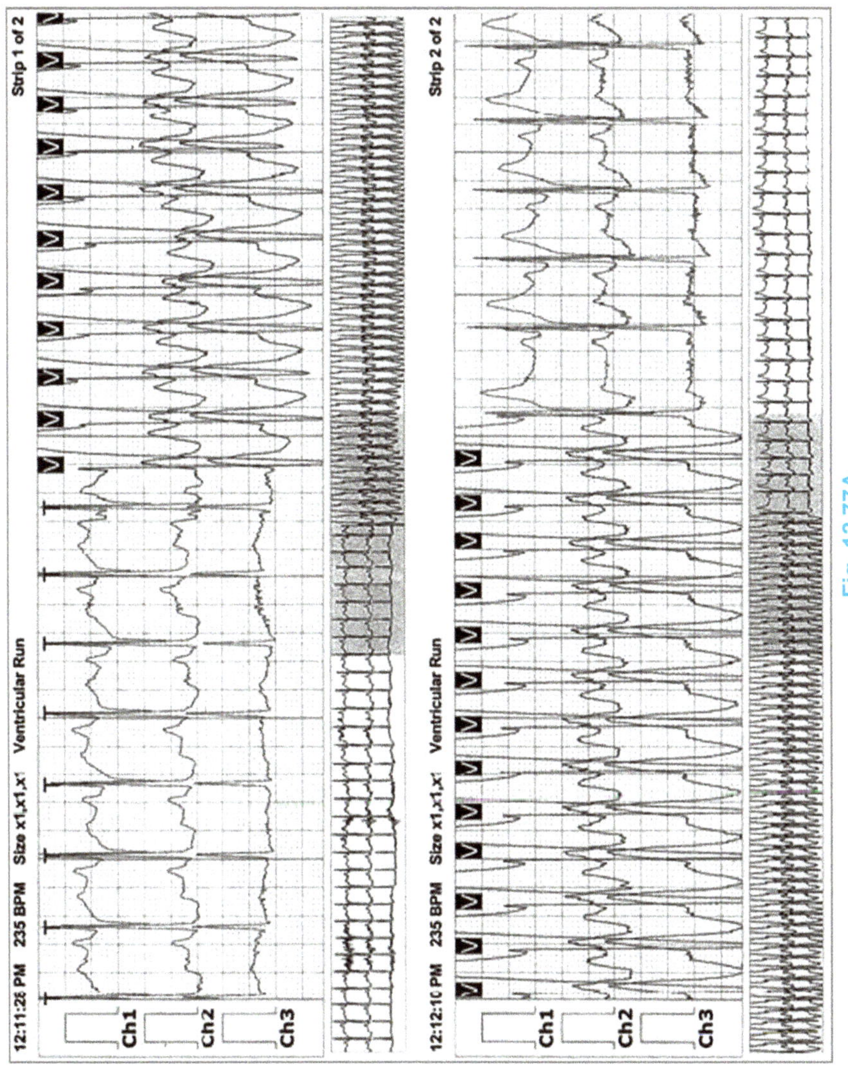

Fig. 12.77A

12:12:01 PM   261 BPM   Size x1,x1,x1   Ventricular Run
Strip 4 of 13
Ch1
Ch2
Ch3
12:12:09 PM   261 BPM   Size x1,x1,x1   Ventricular Run
Strip 5 of 13
Ch1
Ch2
Ch3
12:14:56 PM   98 BPM   Size x1,x1,x1   CHEST DISCOMFORT
Strip 6 of 13
Ch1
Ch2
Ch3

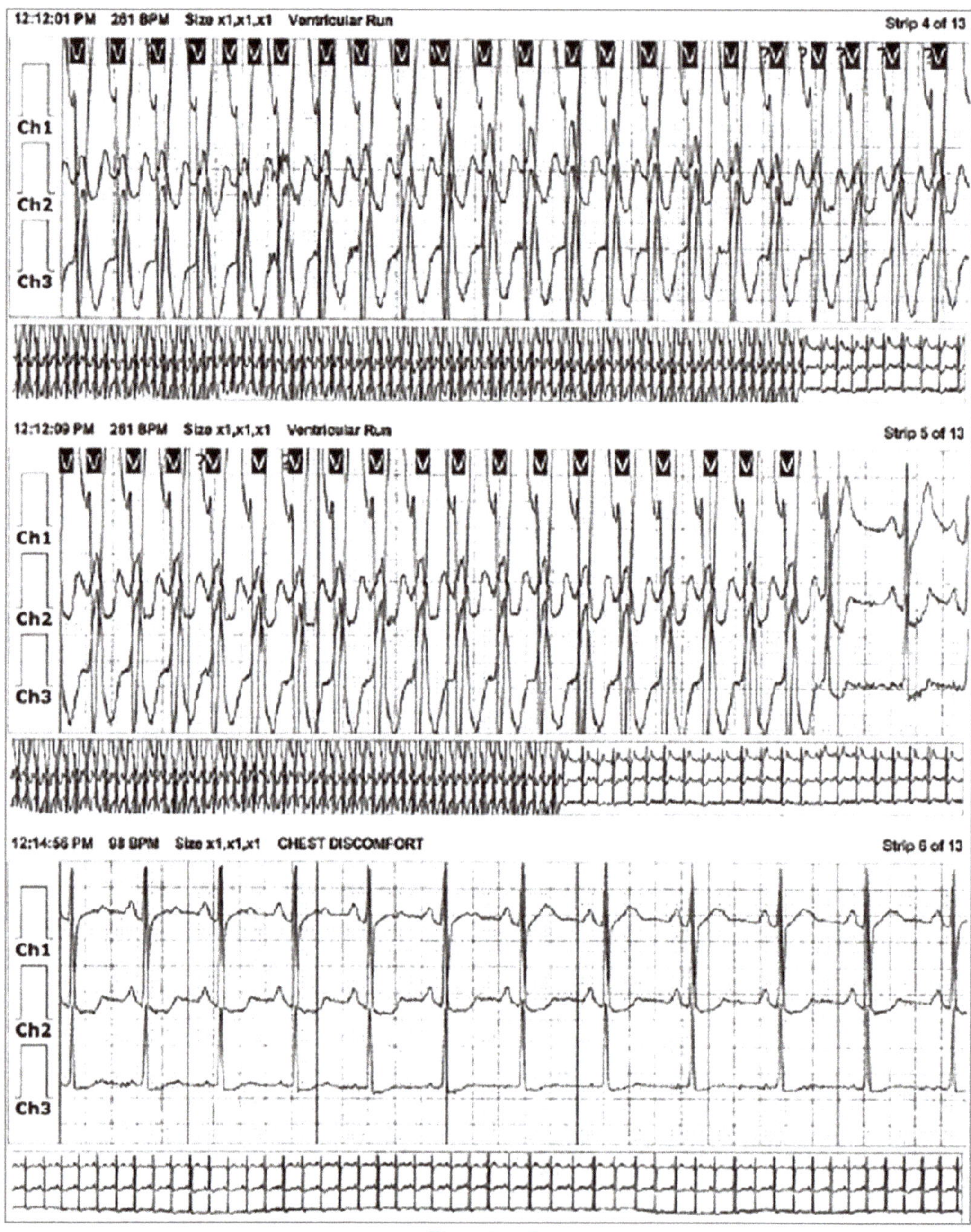

Fig. 12.77B

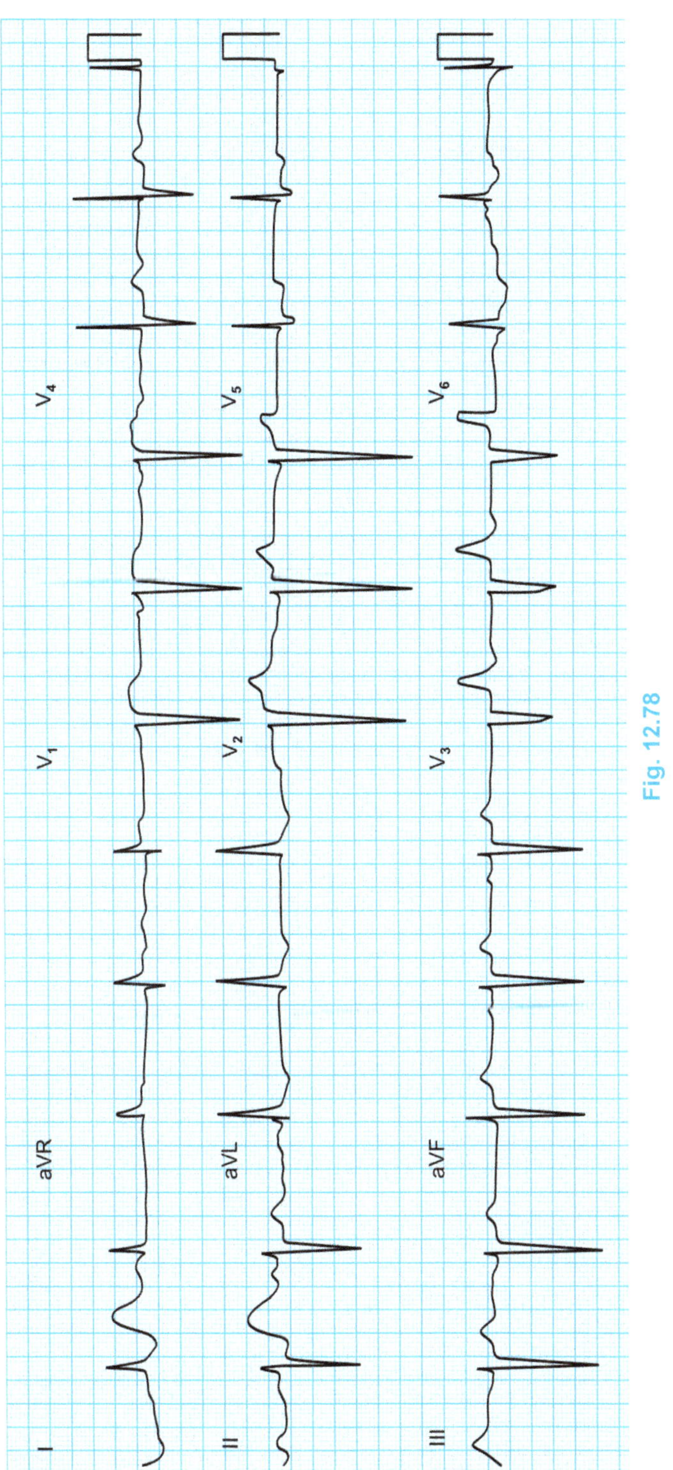

Fig. 12.78

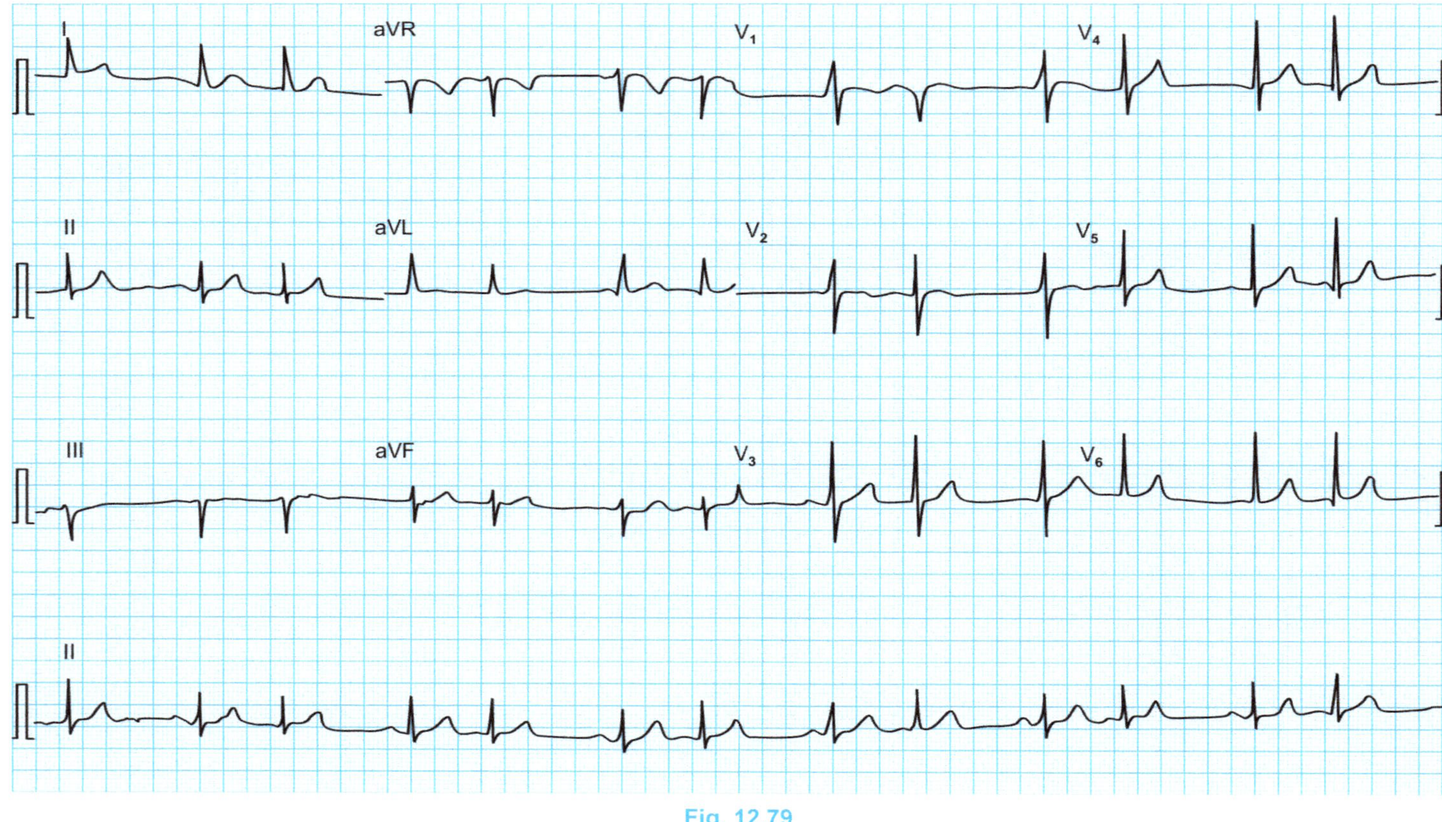

Fig. 12.79

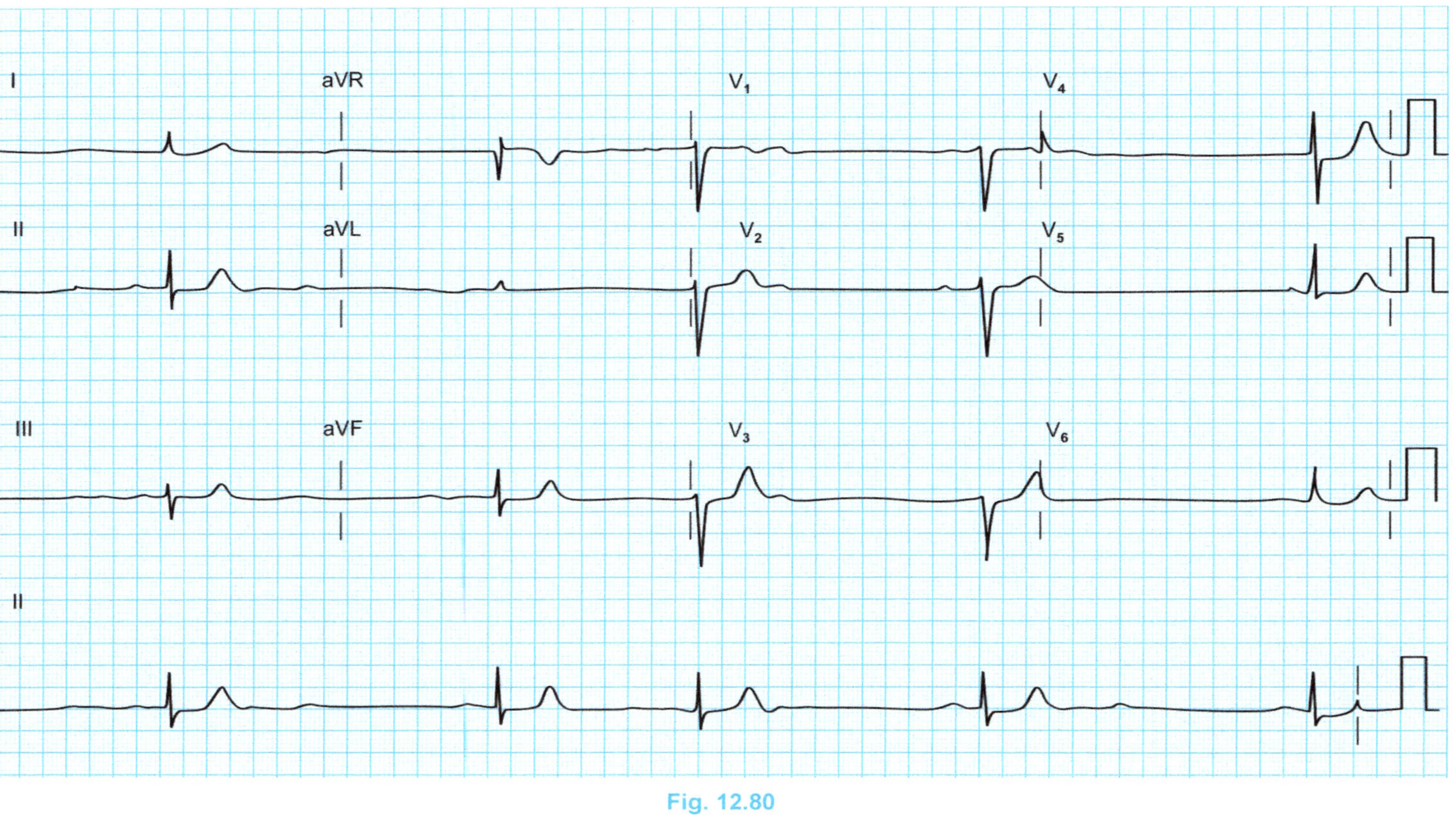

Fig. 12.80

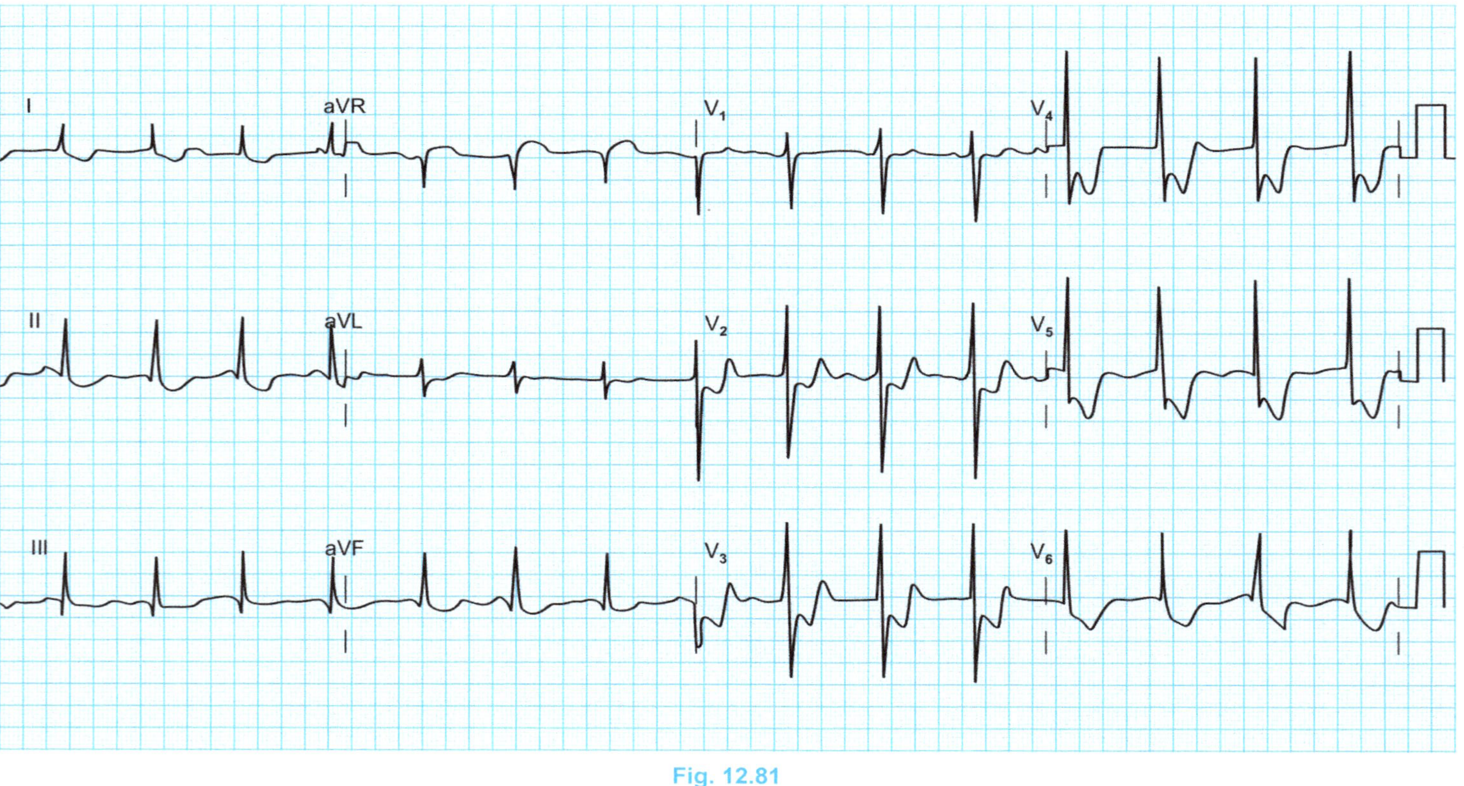

Fig. 12.81

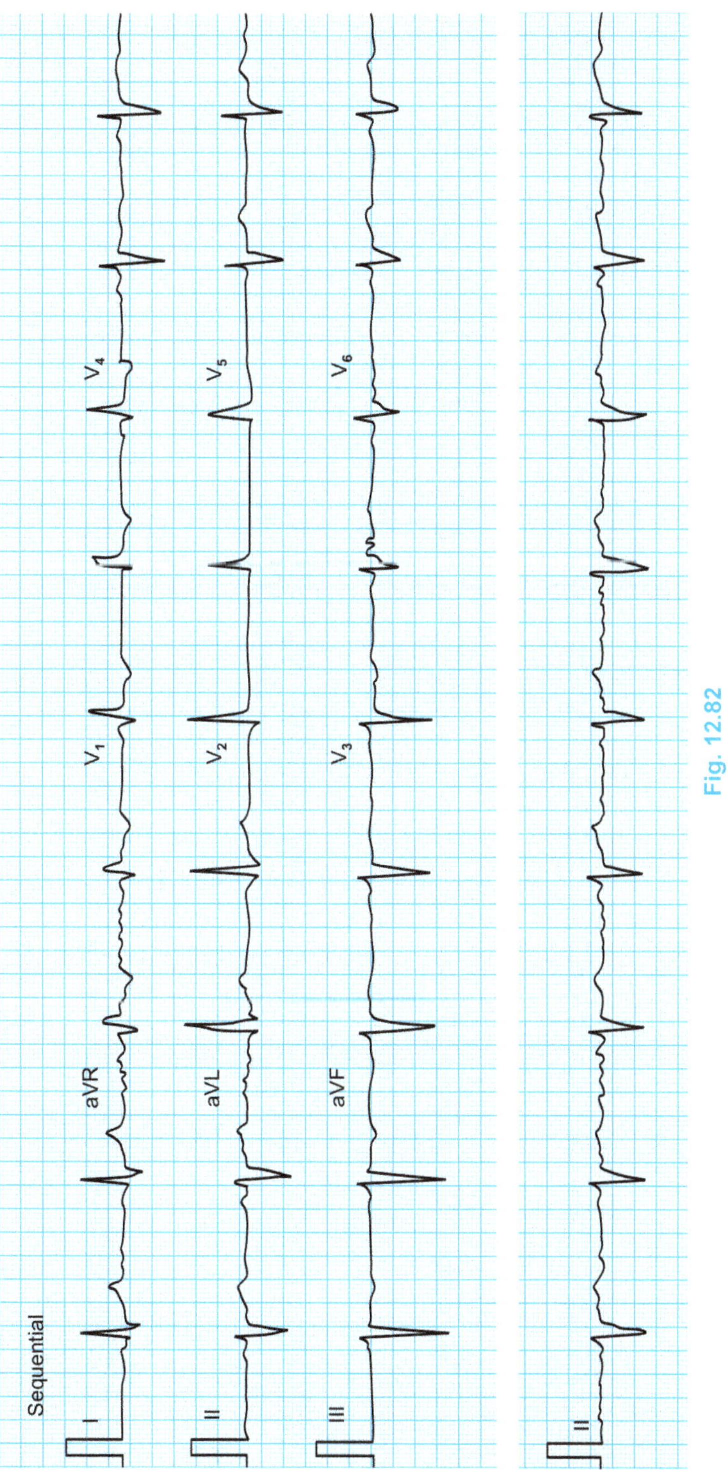

Fig. 12.82

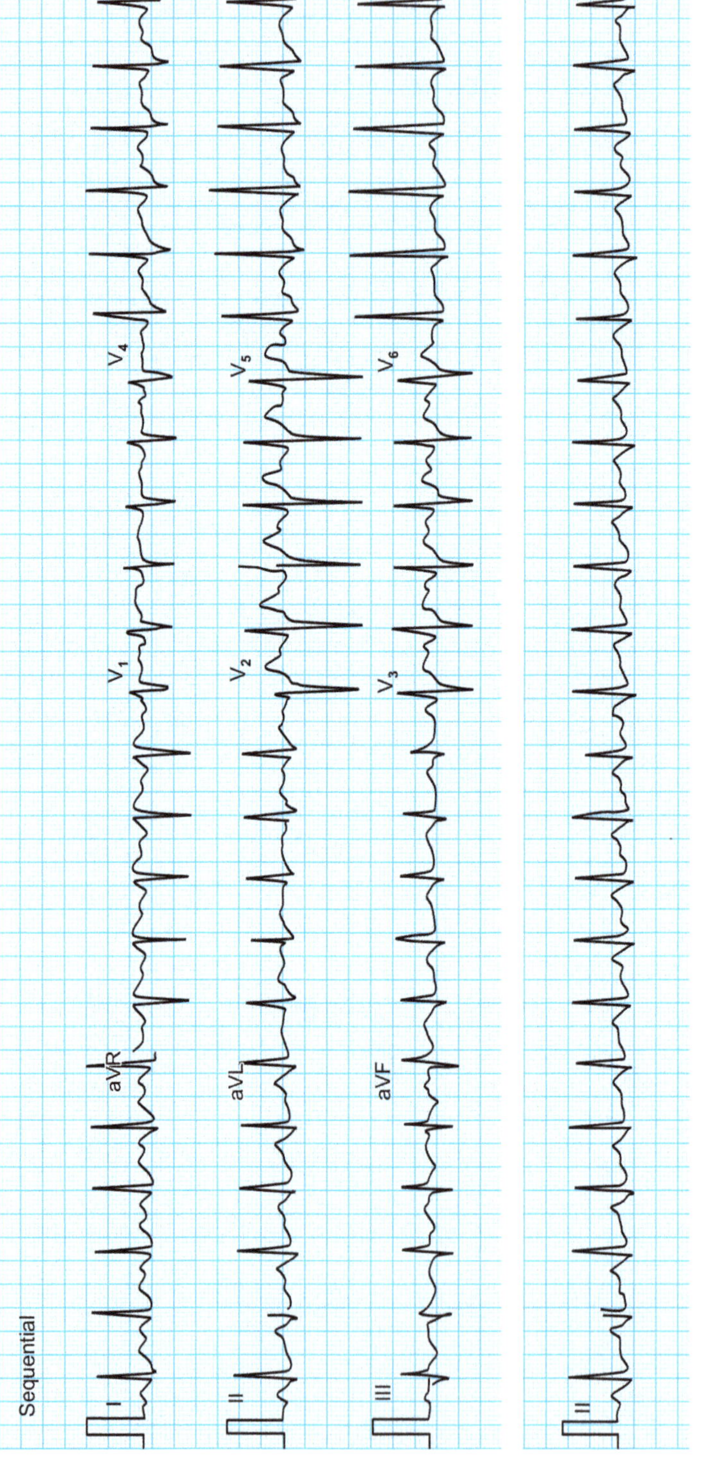

Fig. 12.83

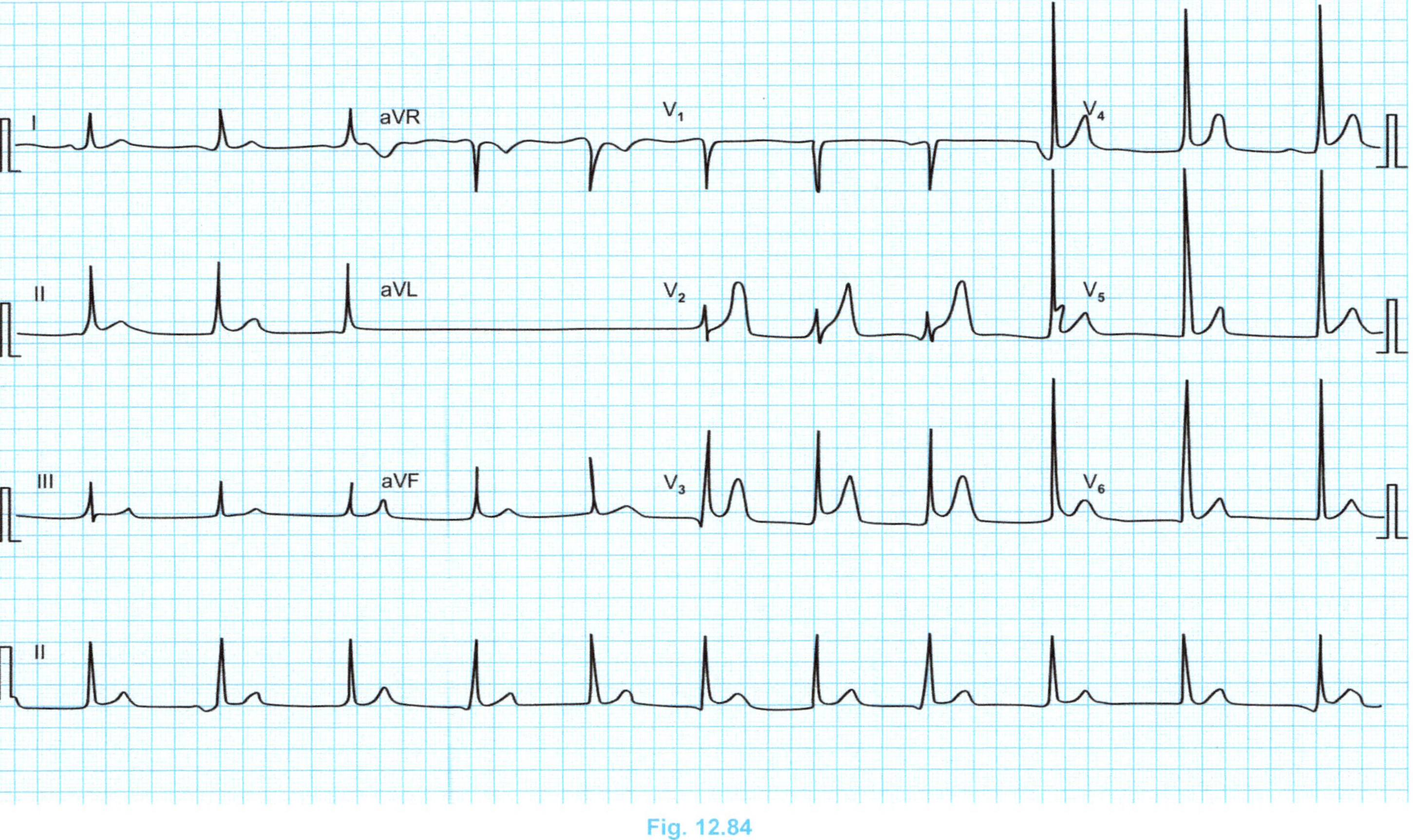

Fig. 12.84

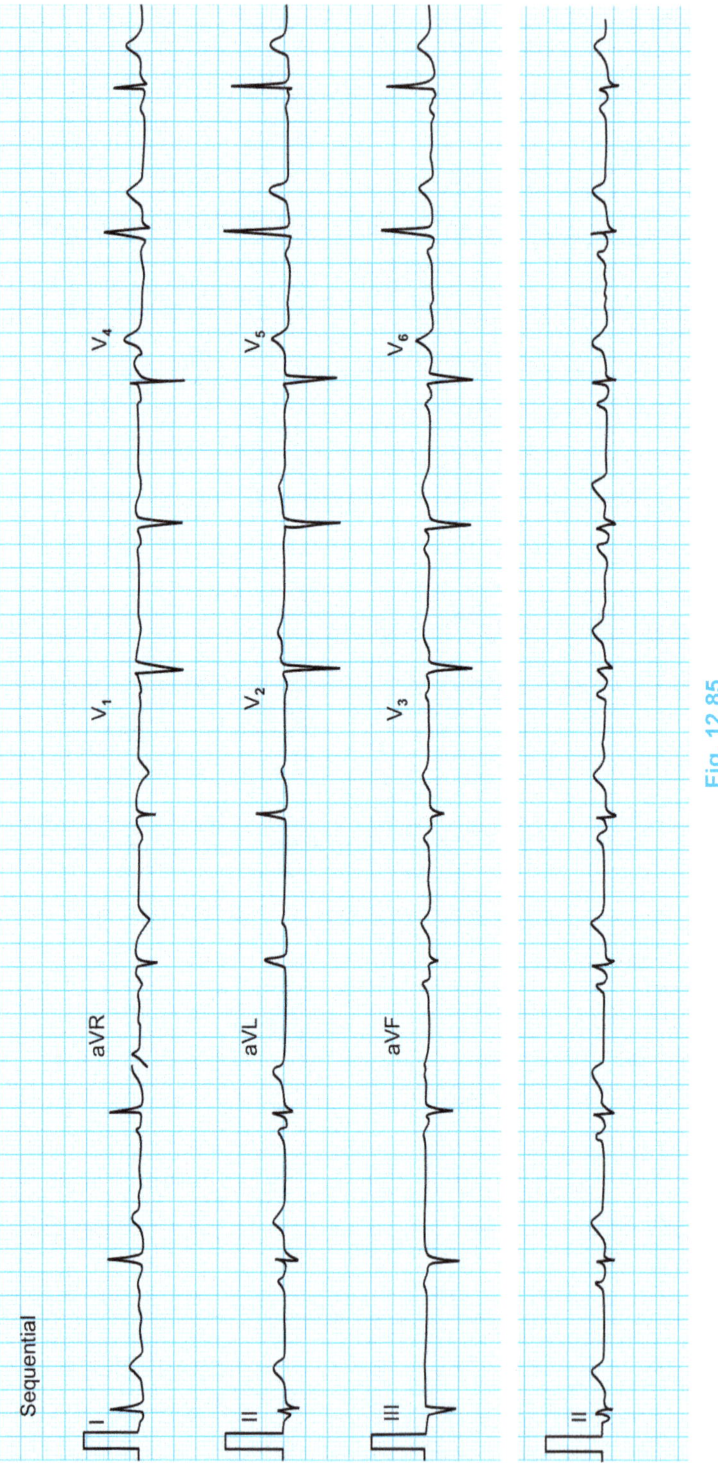

Fig. 12.85

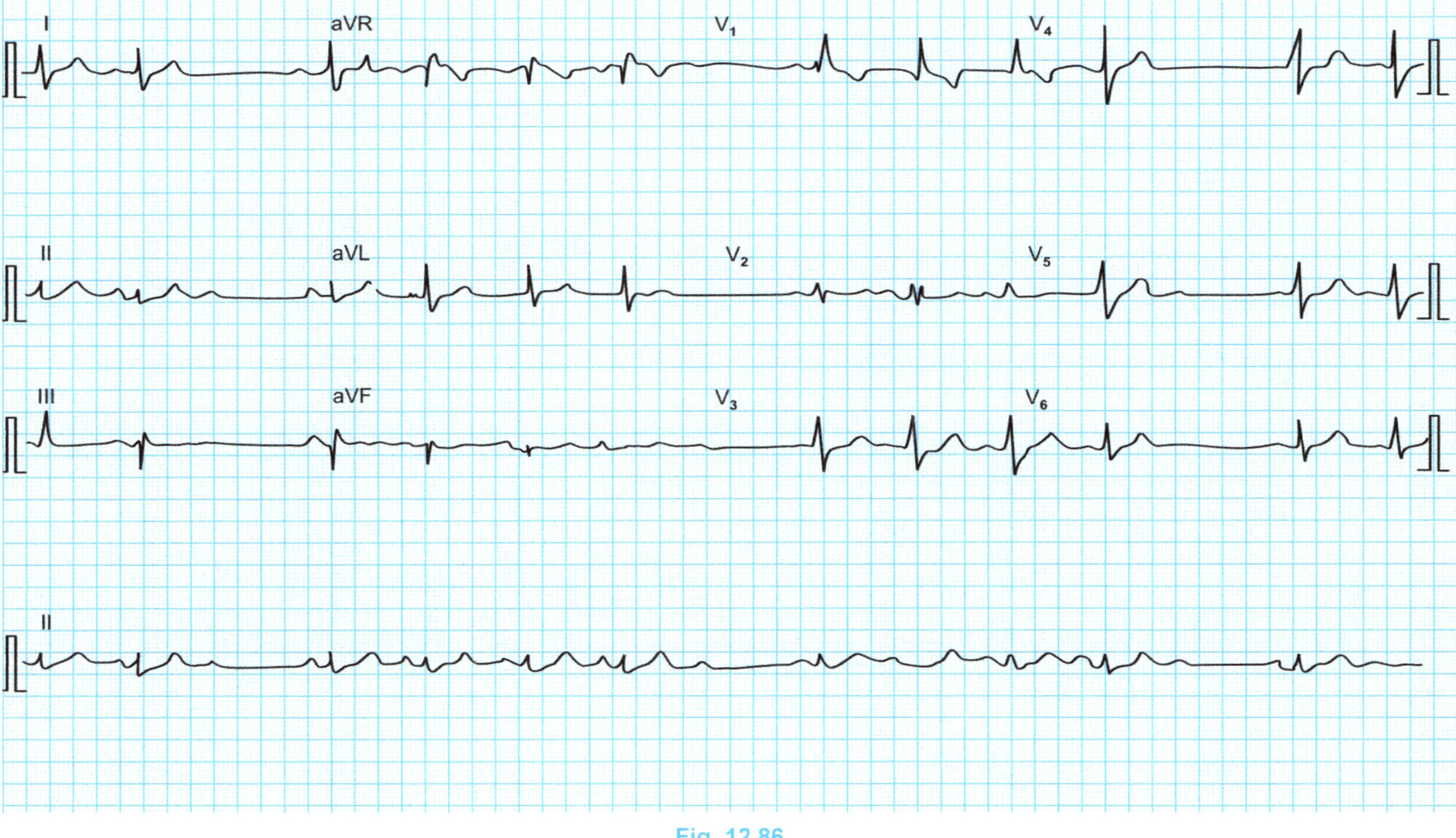

Fig. 12.86

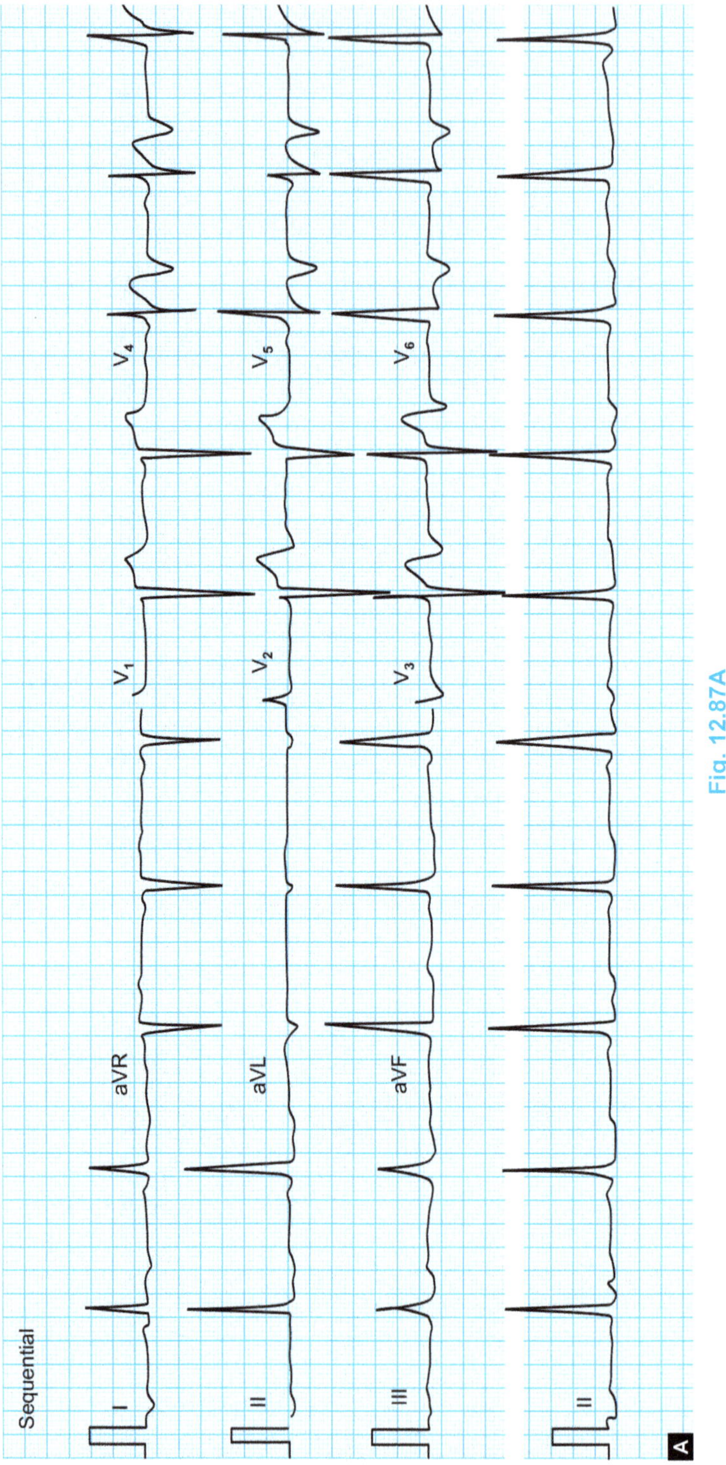

Fig. 12.87A

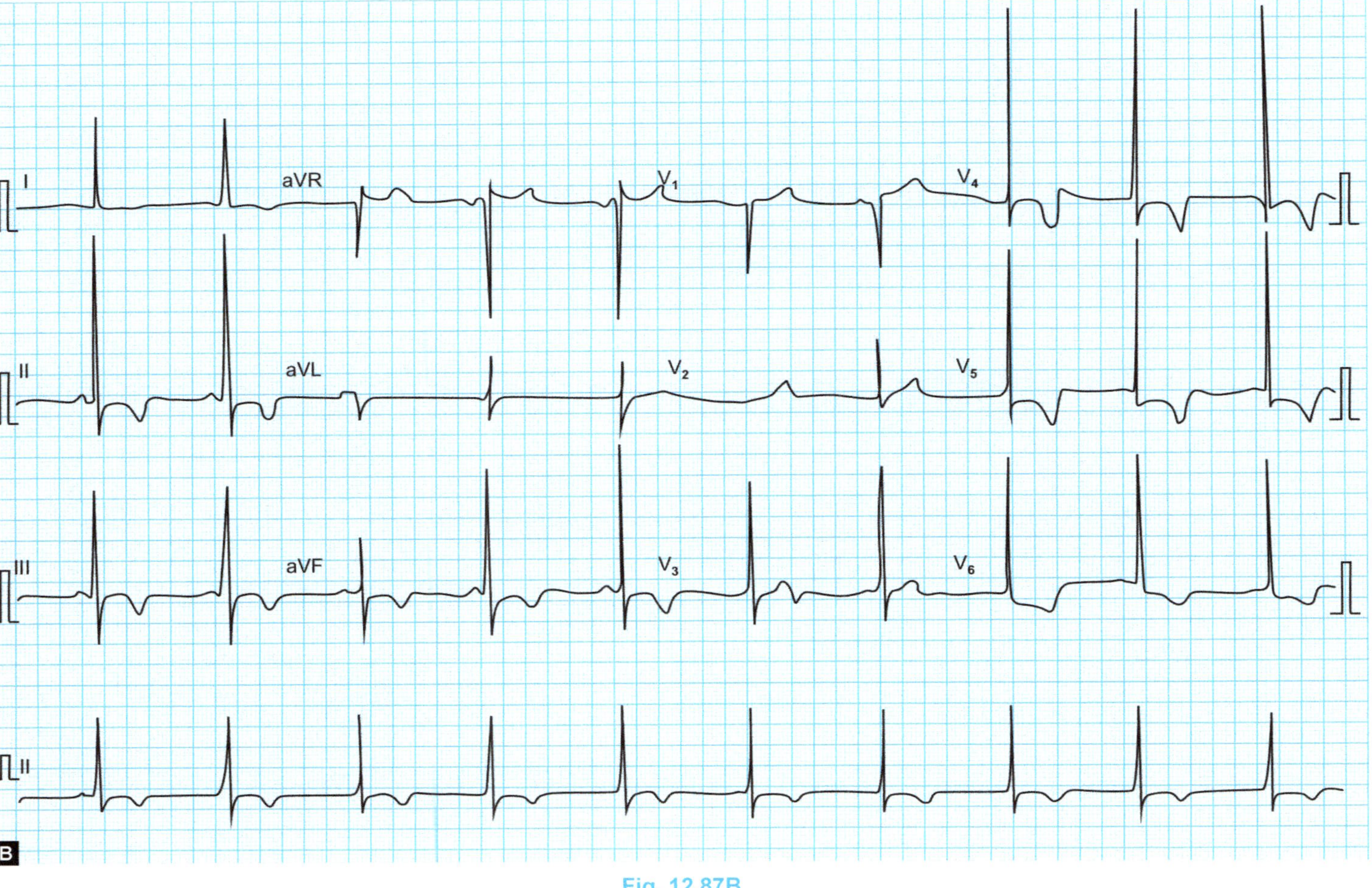

Fig. 12.87B

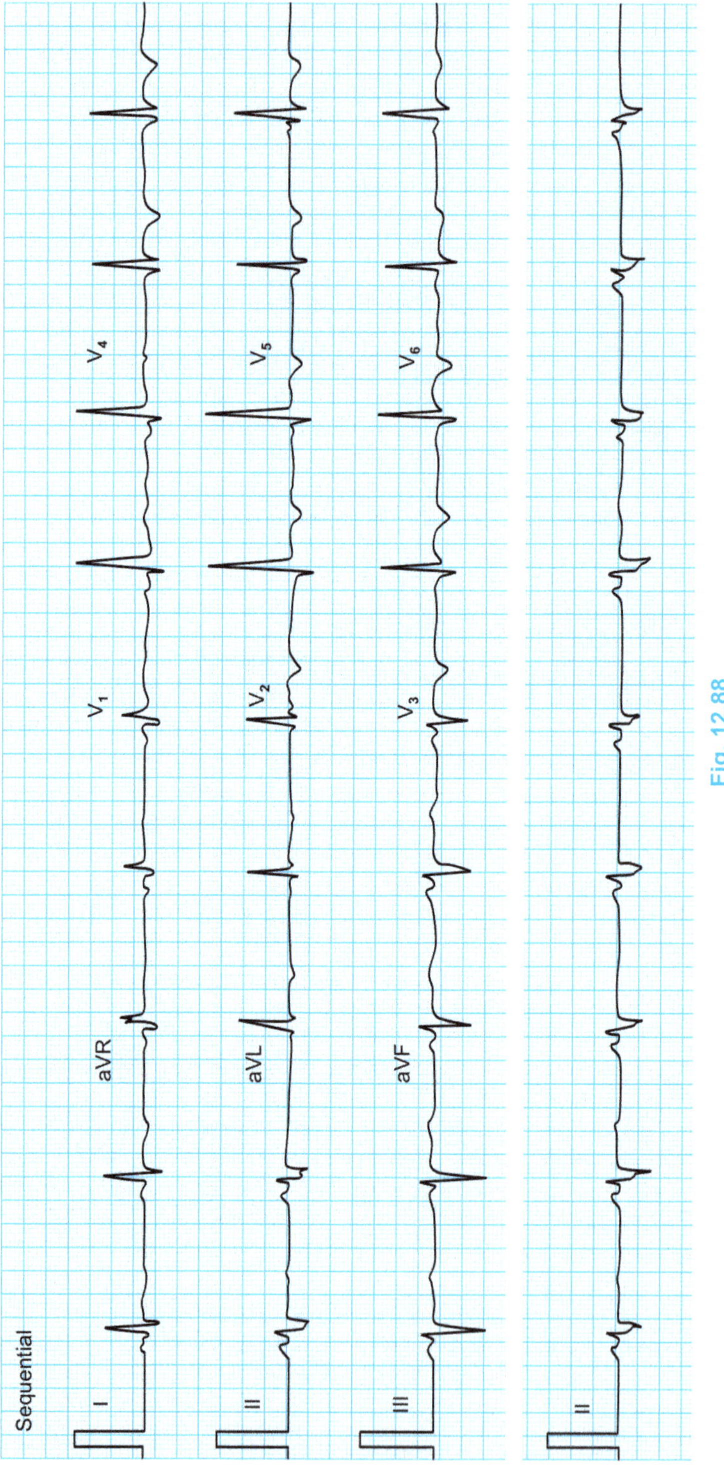

Fig. 12.88

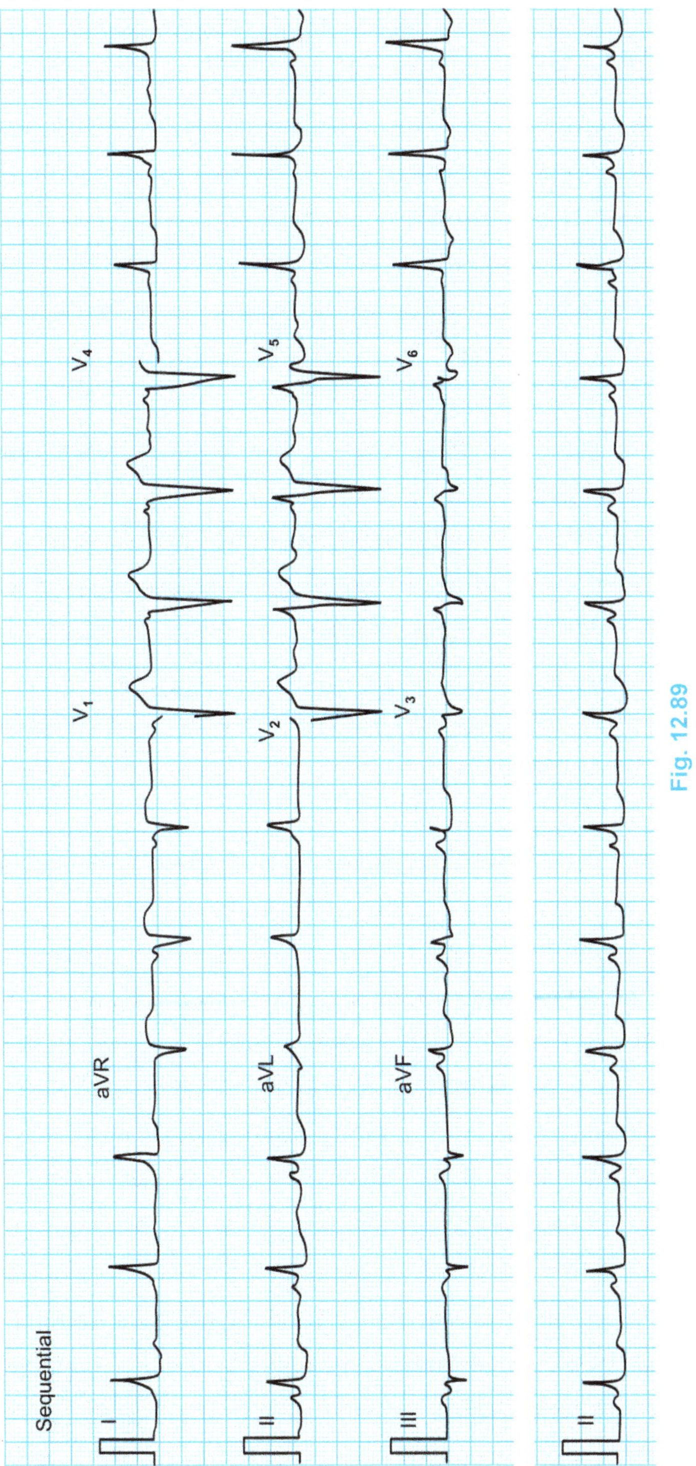

Fig. 12.89

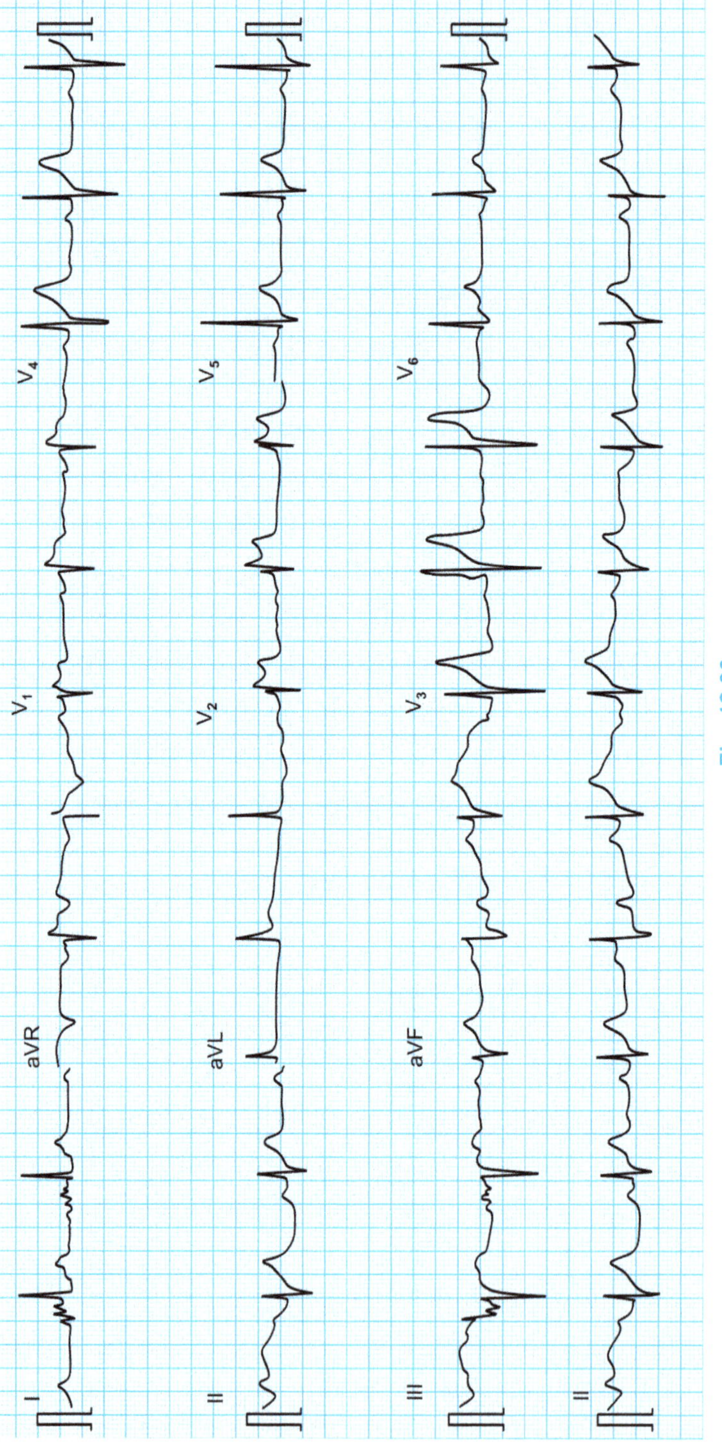

Fig. 12.90

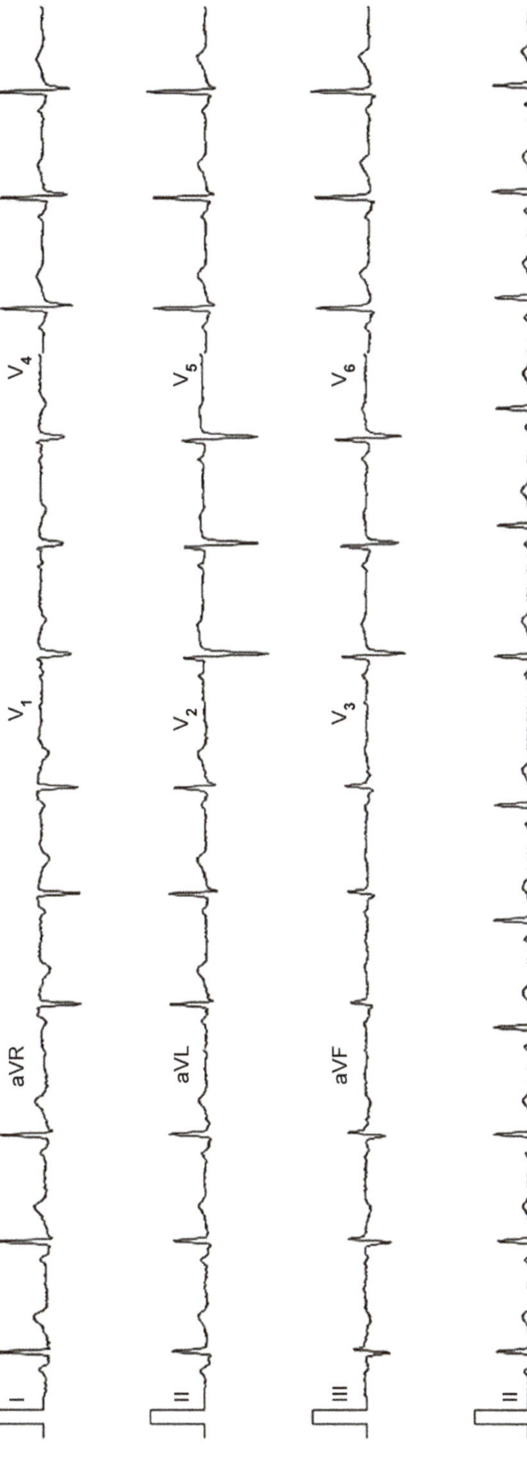

Fig. 12.91

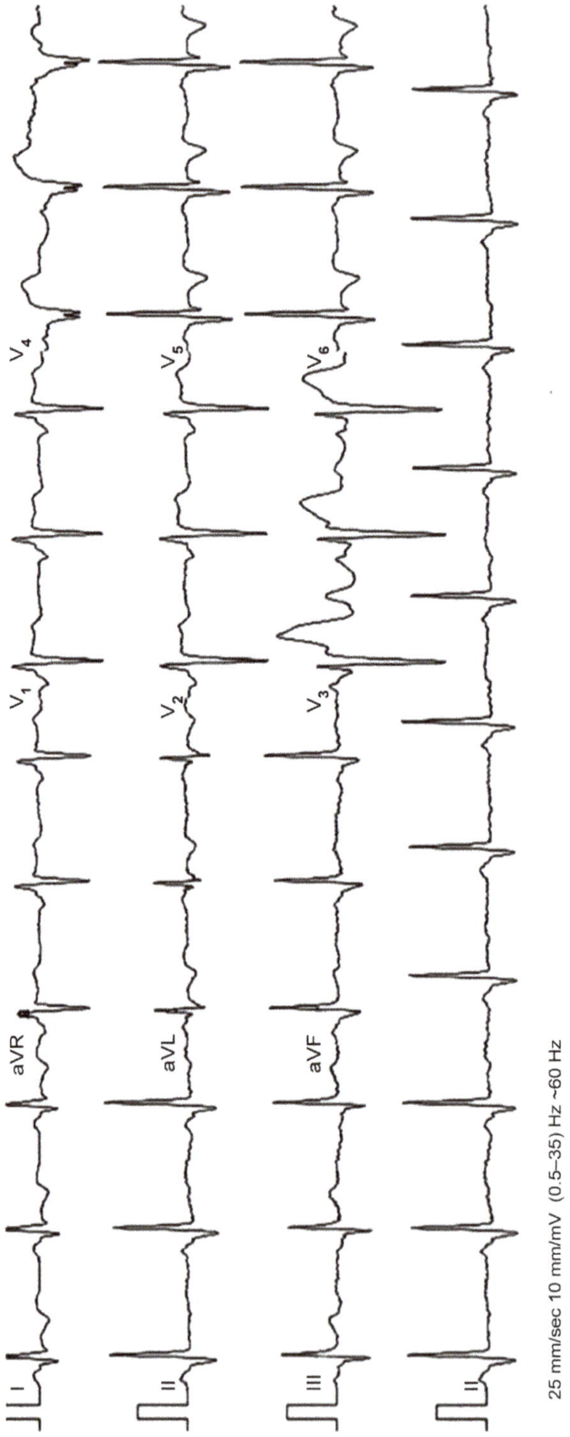

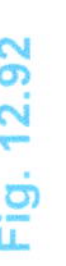

Fig. 12.92

aVR
aVL
aVF
I
II
III
II
V1
V2
V3
V4
V5
V6
25 mm/sec 10 mm/mV (0.5–35) Hz ~60 Hz

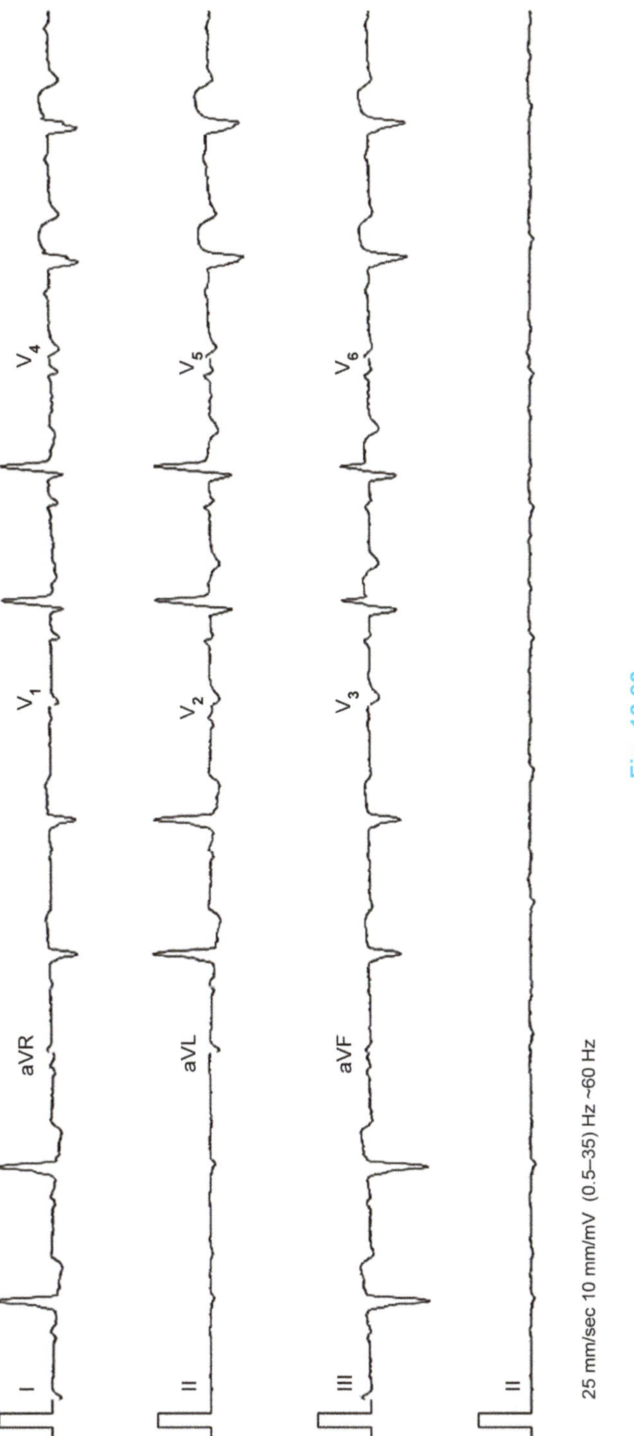

Fig. 12.93

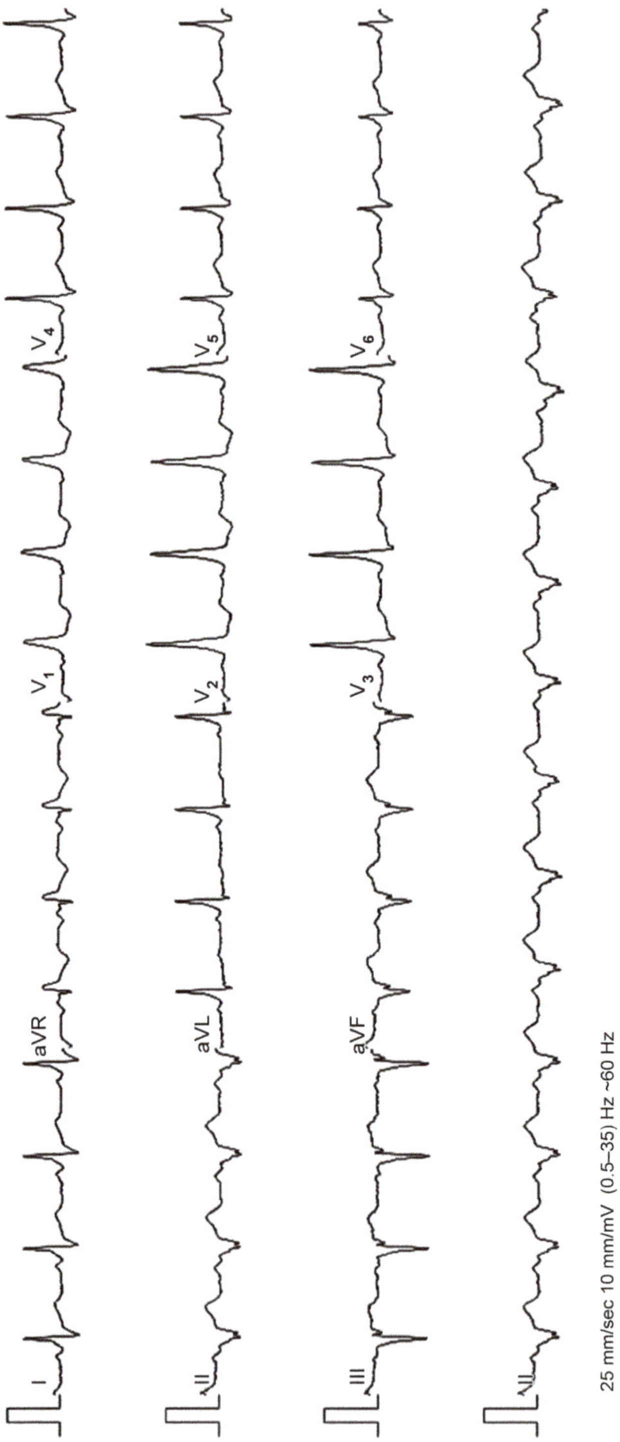

Fig. 12.94

25 mm/sec 10 mm/mV (0.5–35) Hz ~60 Hz

I
II
III
II
aVR
aVL
aVF
V1
V2
V3
V4
V5
V6
25 mm/sec 10 mm/mV (0.5–35) Hz ~60 Hz

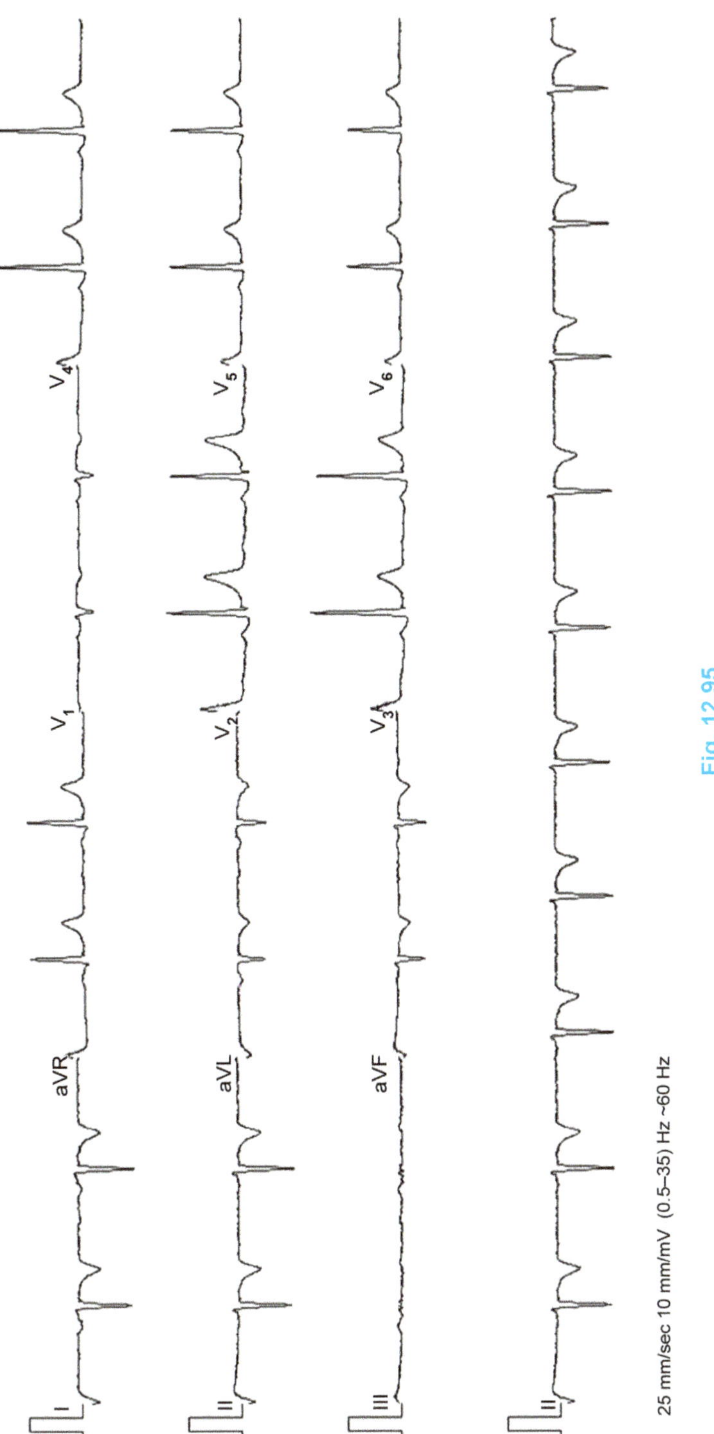

Fig. 12.95

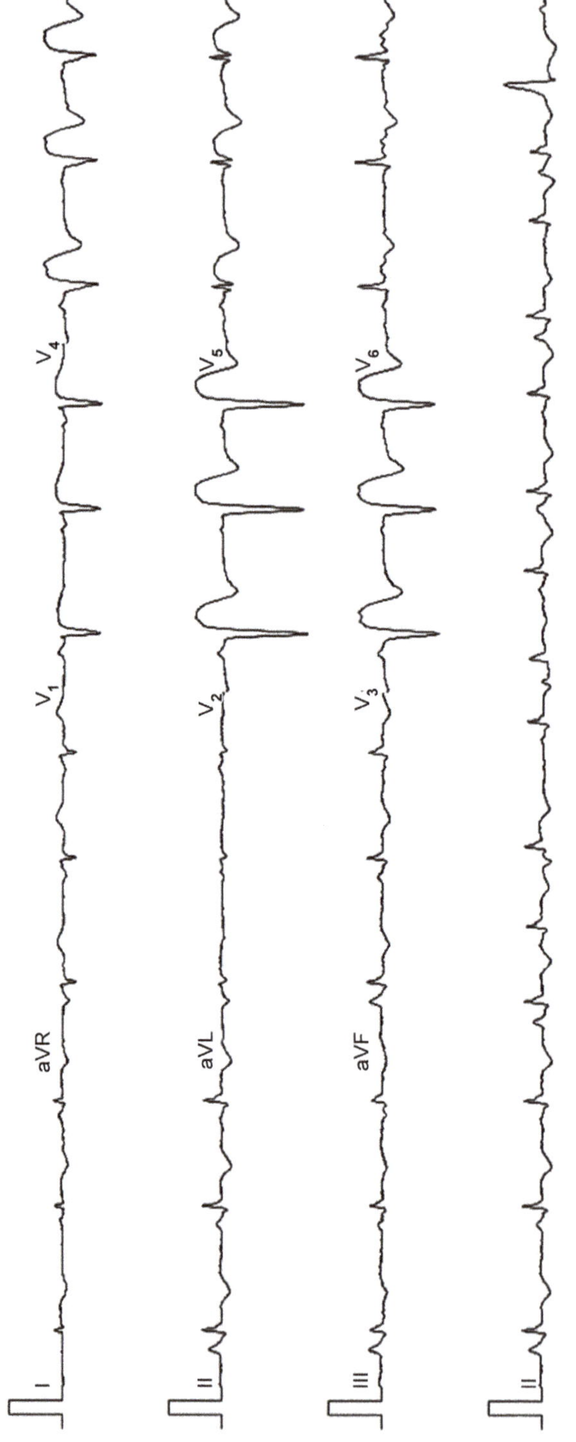

Fig. 12.96

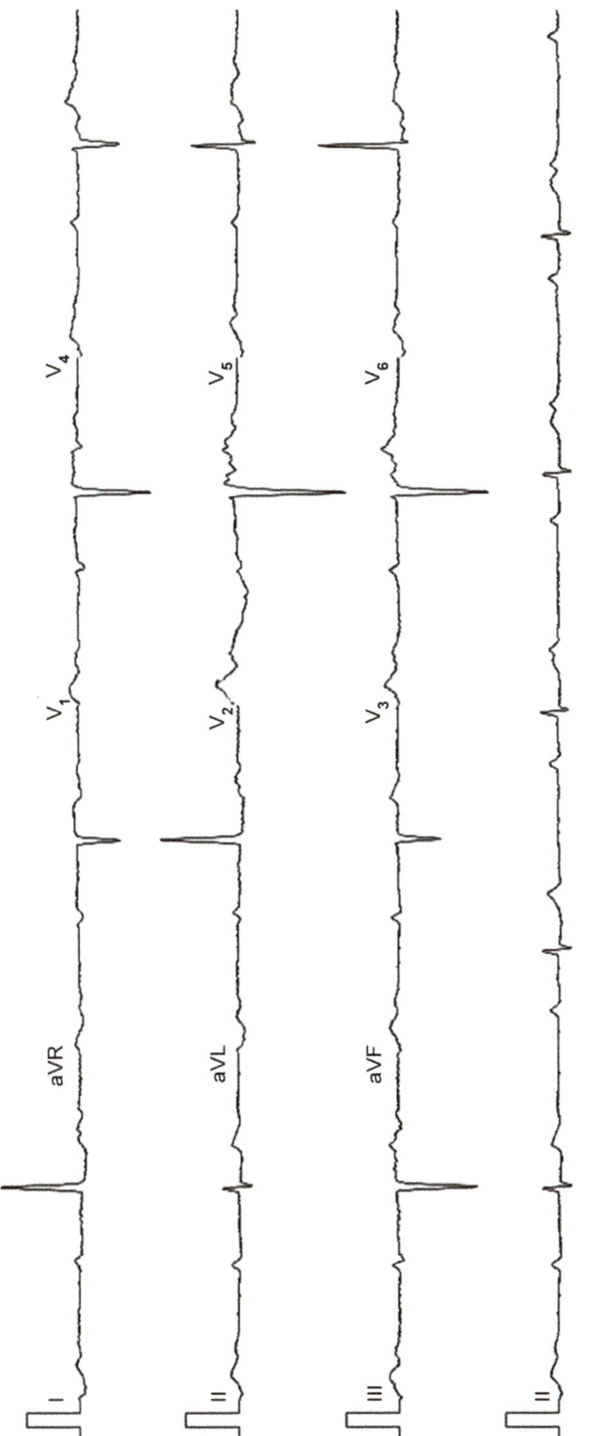

Fig. 12.97

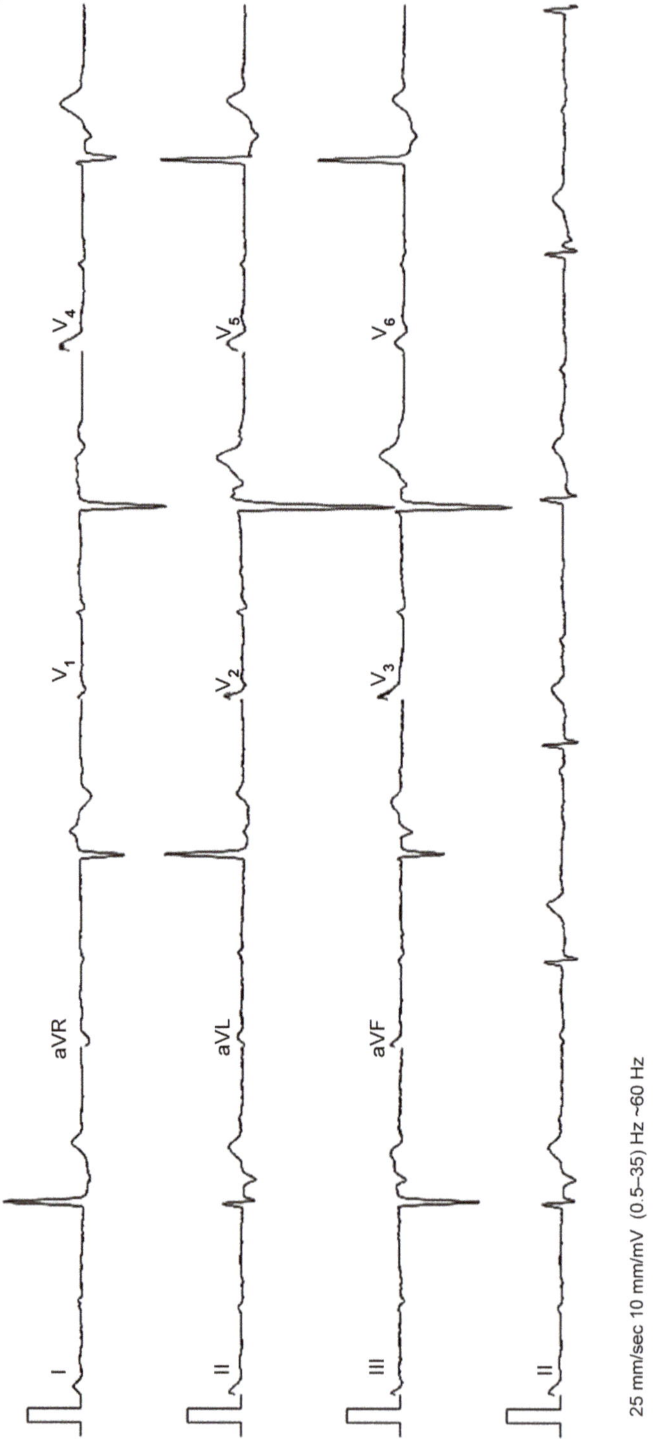
I
aVR
V1
V4
II
aVL
V2
V5
III
aVF
V3
V6
II
25 mm/sec 10 mm/mV (0.5–35) Hz ~60 Hz

Fig. 12.98A

A

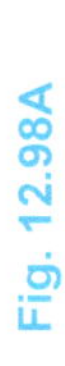

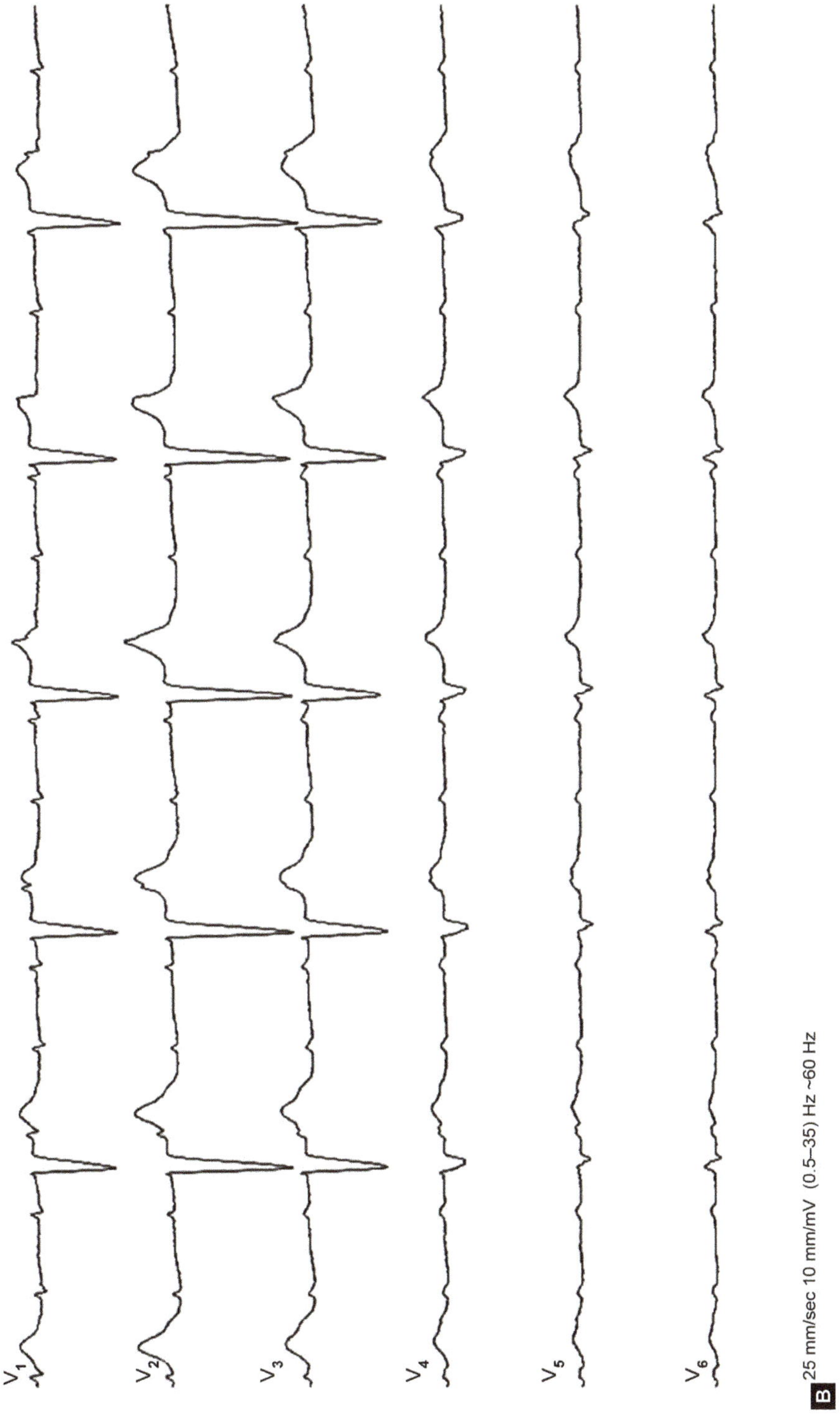

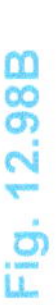

Fig. 12.98B

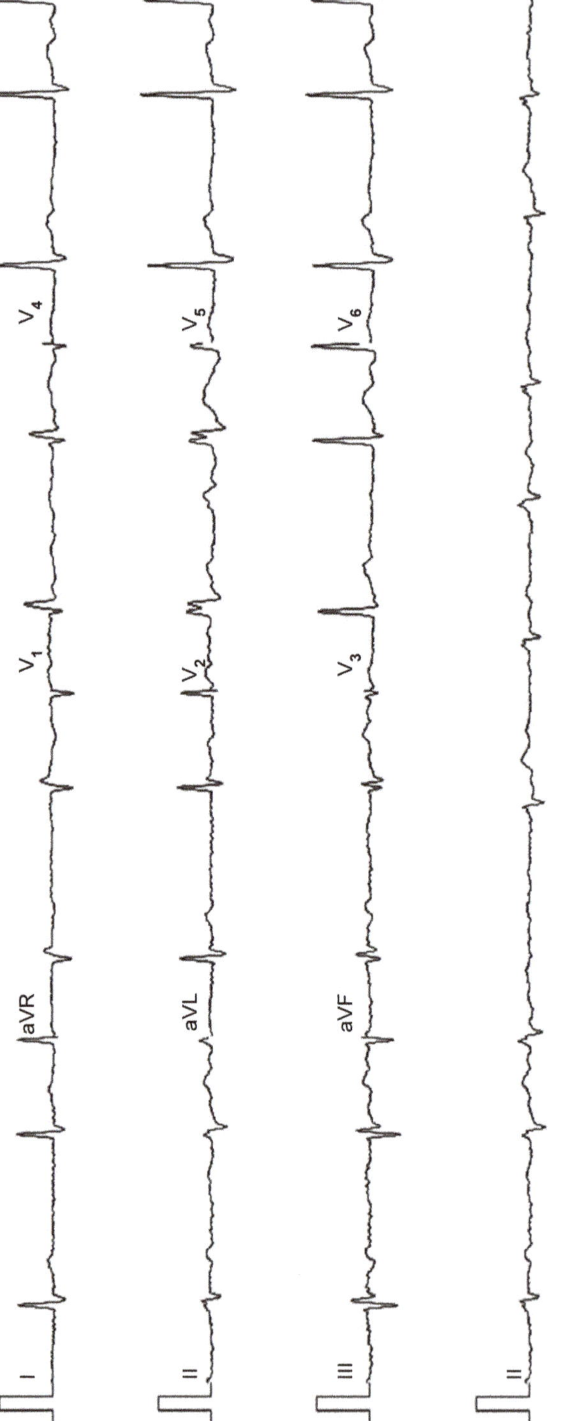

Fig. 12.99

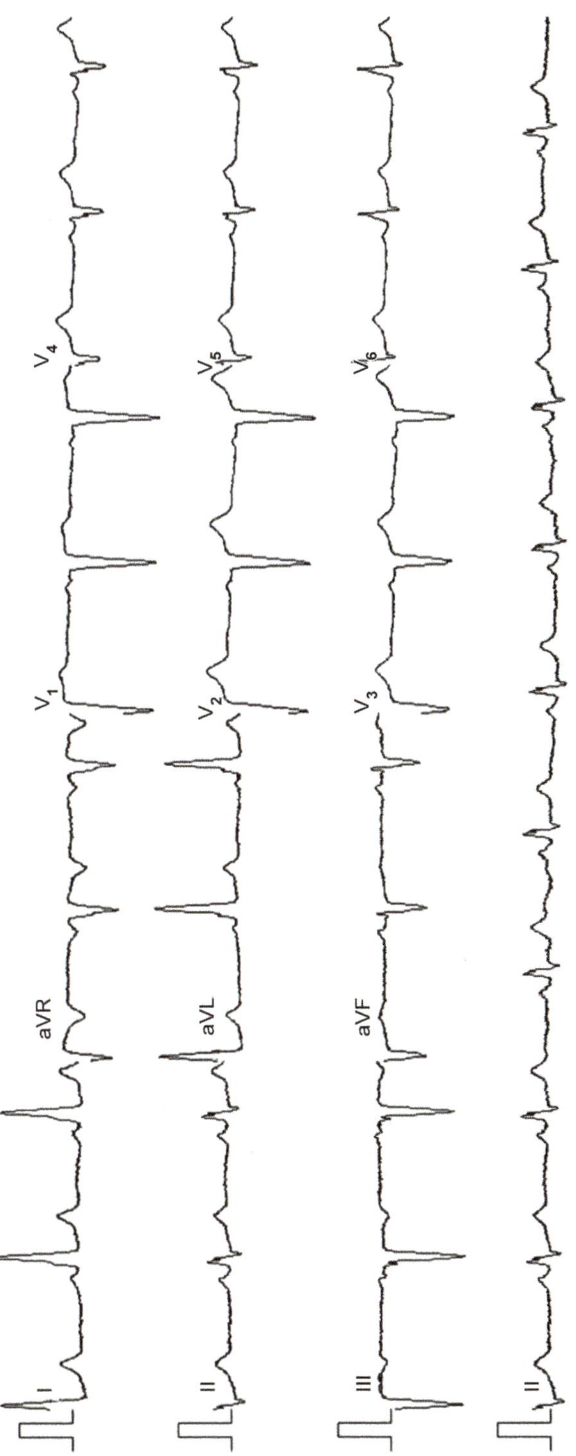

25 mm/sec 10 mm/mV (0.5–35) Hz ~60 Hz

Fig. 12.100

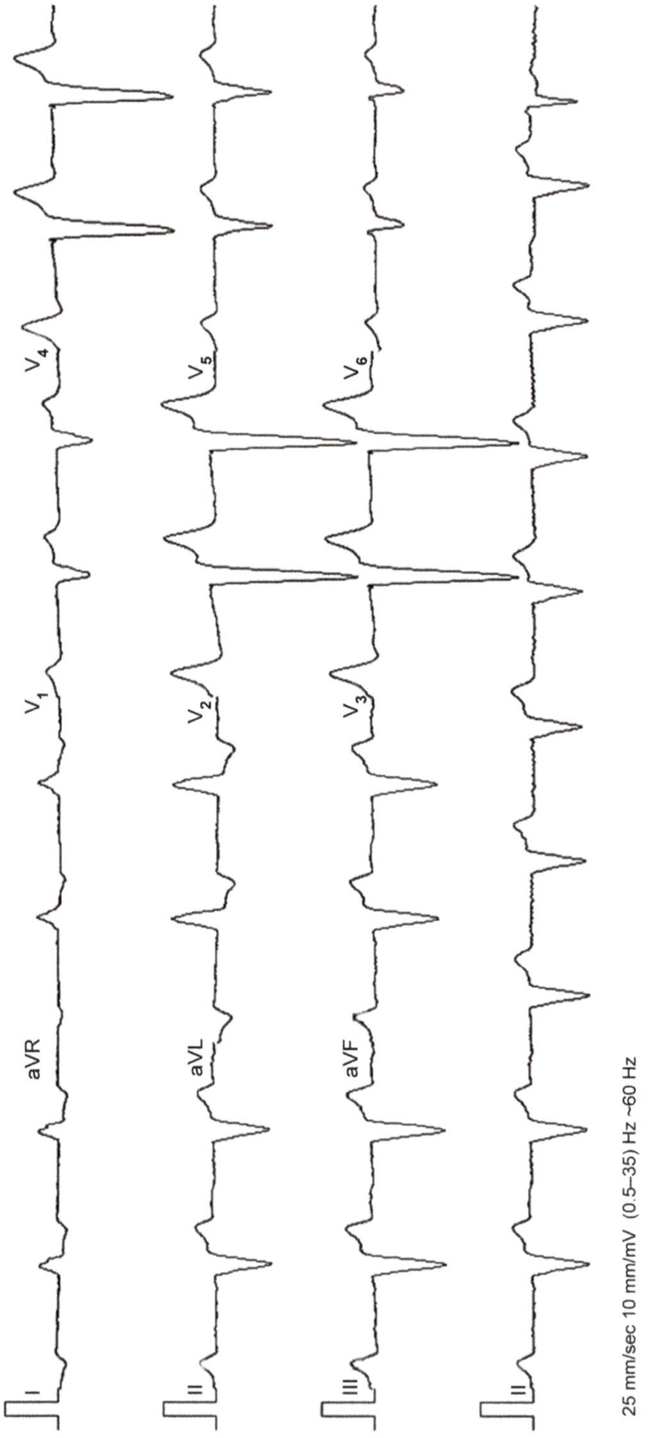
I
aVR
V1
V4
II
aVL
V2
V5
III
aVF
V3
V6
II
25 mm/sec 10 mm/mV (0.5–35) Hz ~60 Hz

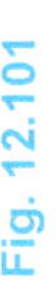

Fig. 12.101

aVR
aVL
aVF
V₁
V₂
V₃
V₄
V₅
V₆
I
II
III
II
25 mm/sec 10 mm/mV (0.5–35) Hz ~60 Hz
A

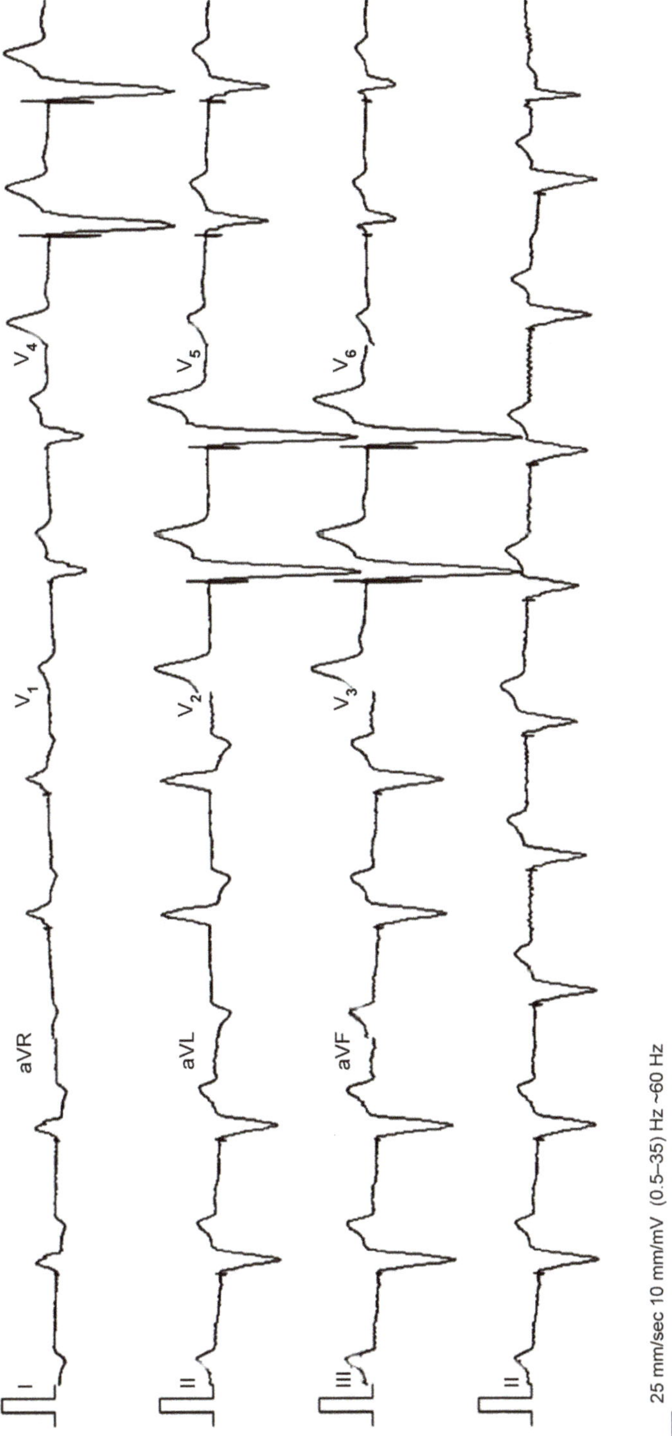

Fig. 12.102A

I
II
III
II
aVR
aVL
aVF
V1
V2
V3
V4
V5
V6
25 mm/sec 10 mm/mV (0.5–35) Hz ~60 Hz

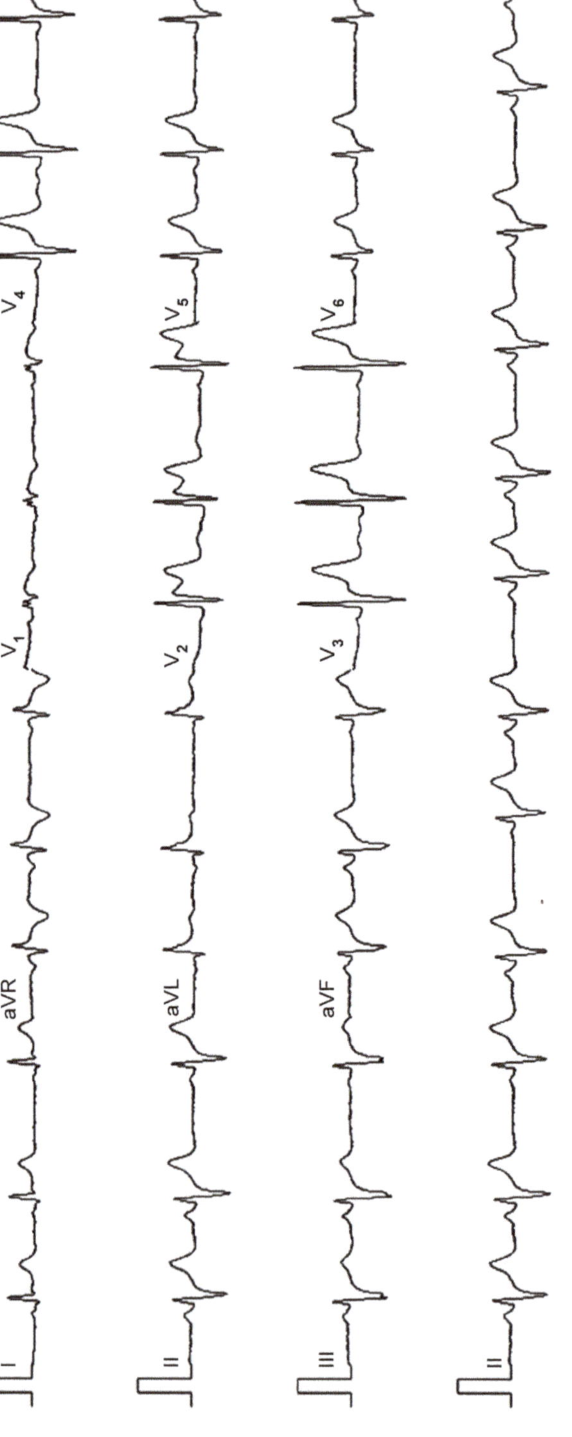

Fig. 12.102B

I
aVR
V₁
V₄
II
aVL
V₂
V₅
III
aVF
V₃
V₆
II
25 mm/sec 10 mm/mV (0.5–35) Hz ~60 Hz

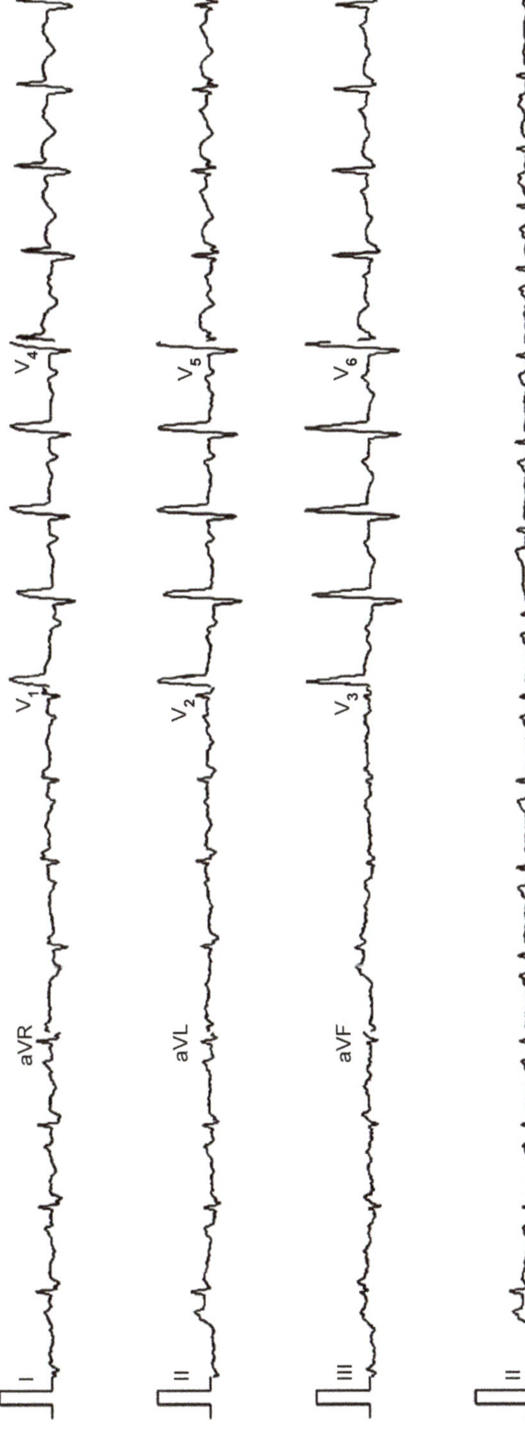

Fig. 12.103

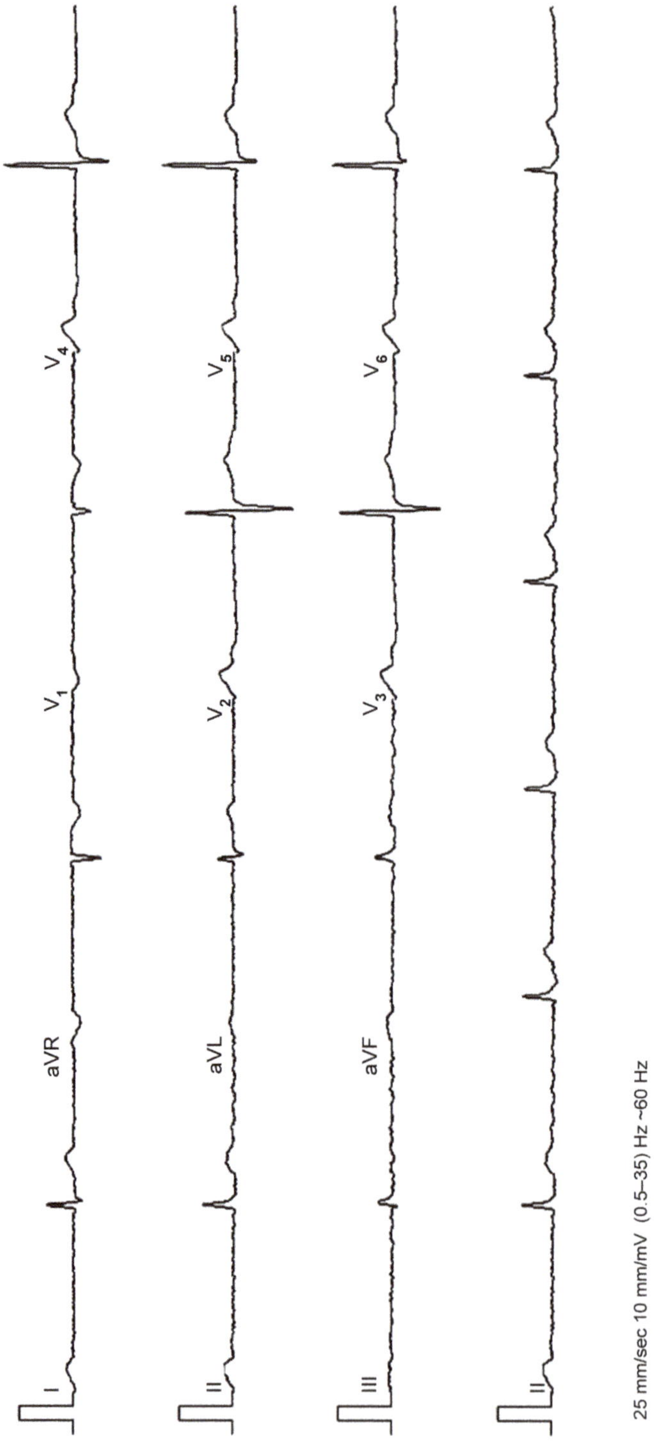
I
aVR
V1
V4
II
aVL
V2
V5
III
aVF
V3
V6
II
25 mm/sec 10 mm/mV (0.5–35) Hz ~60 Hz

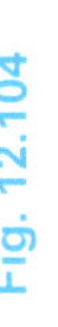

Fig. 12.104

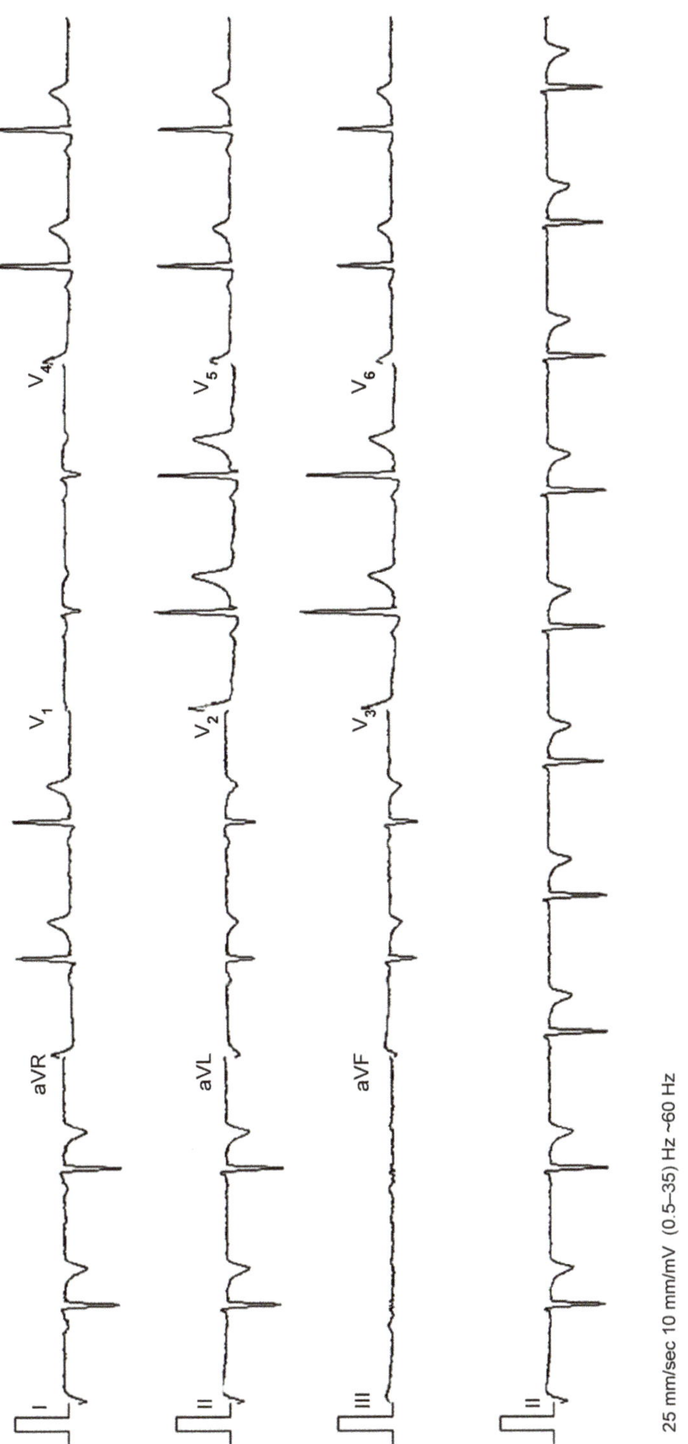

Fig. 12.105

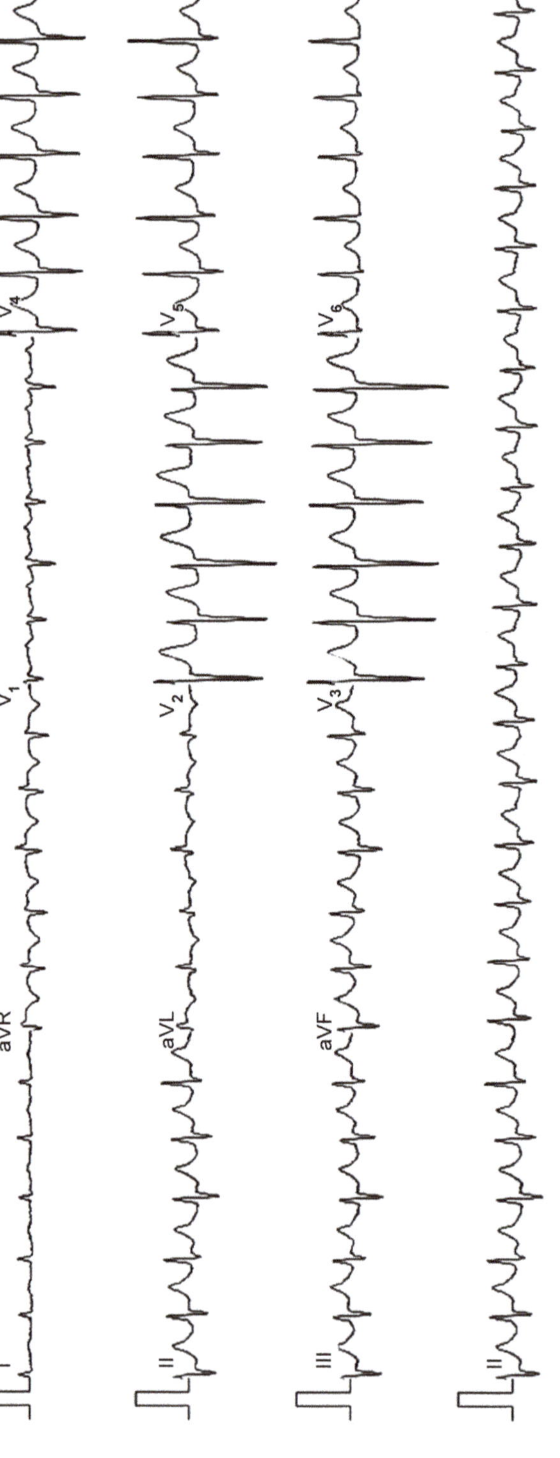

Fig. 12.106

25 mm/sec 10 mm/mV (0.5–35) Hz ~60 Hz

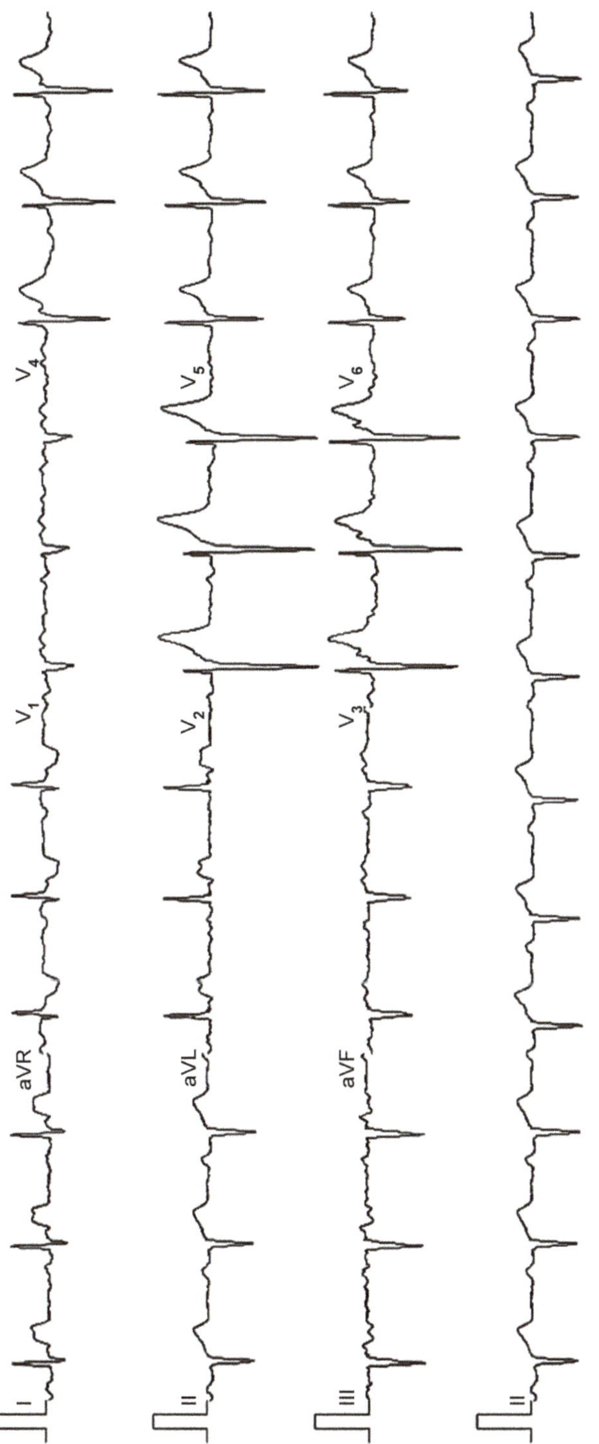

Fig. 12.107

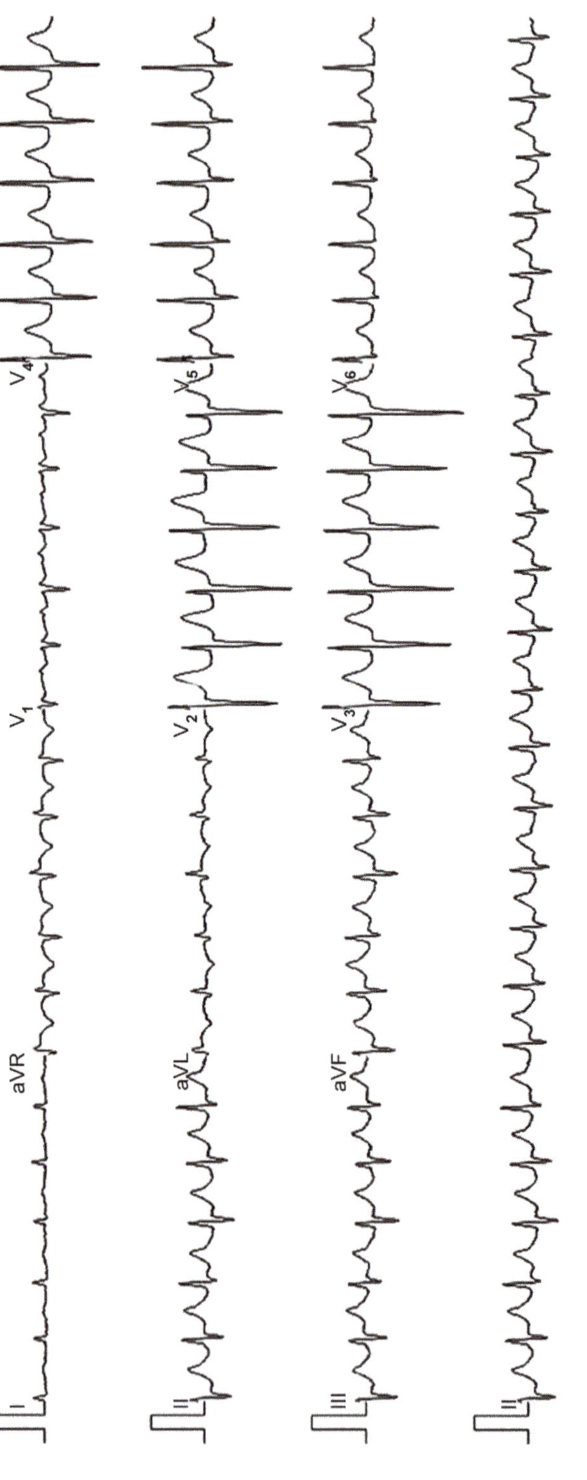

Fig. 12.108A

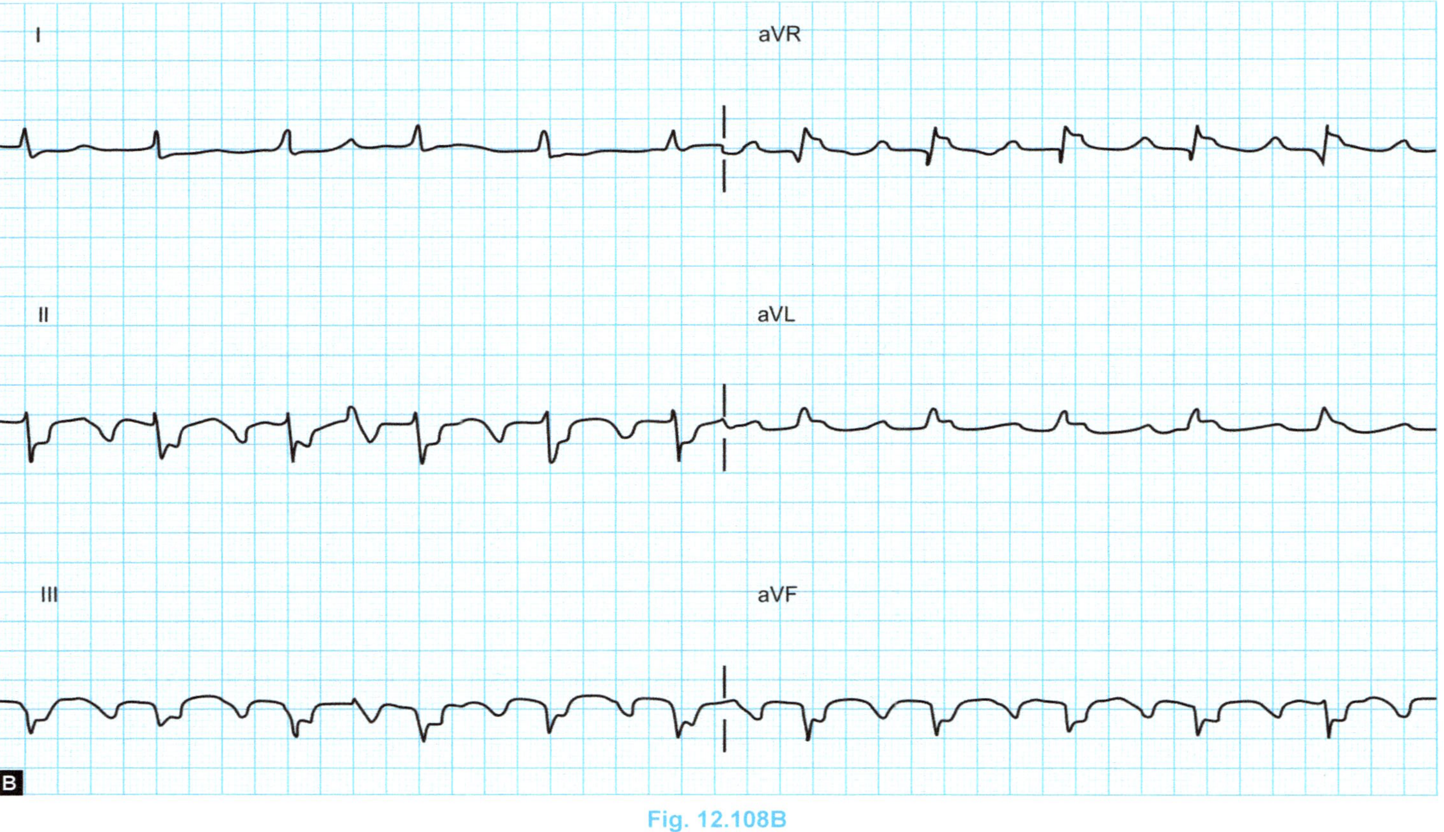

Fig. 12.108B

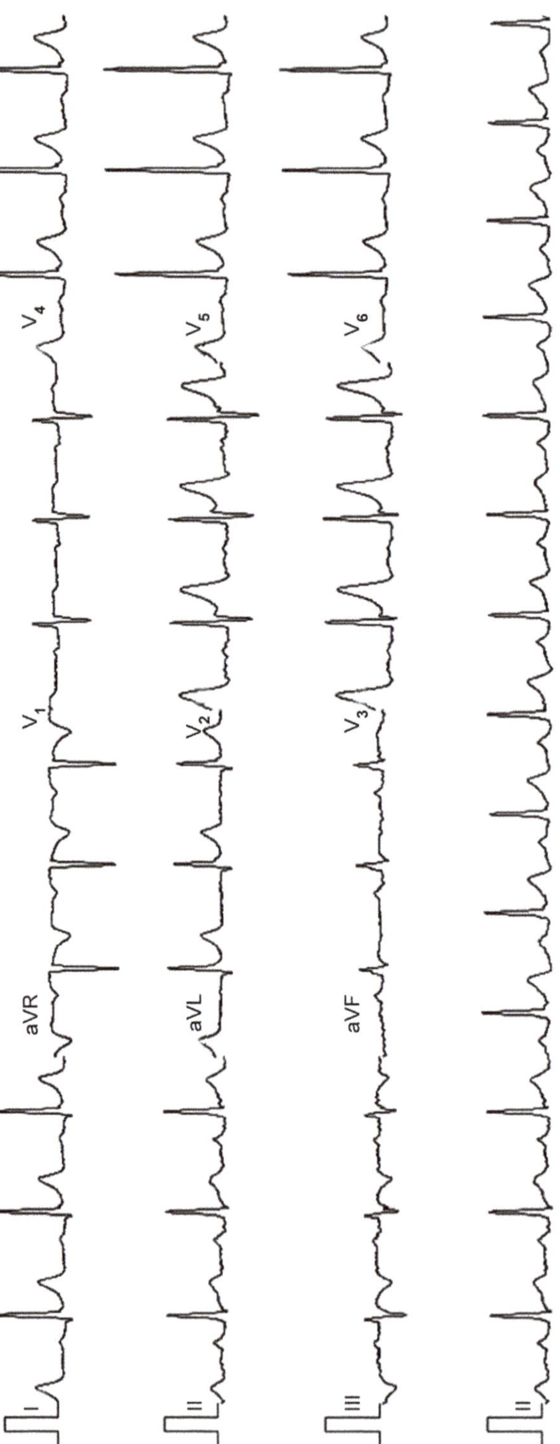

Fig. 12.109

25 mm/sec 10 mm/mV (0.5–35) Hz ~60 Hz

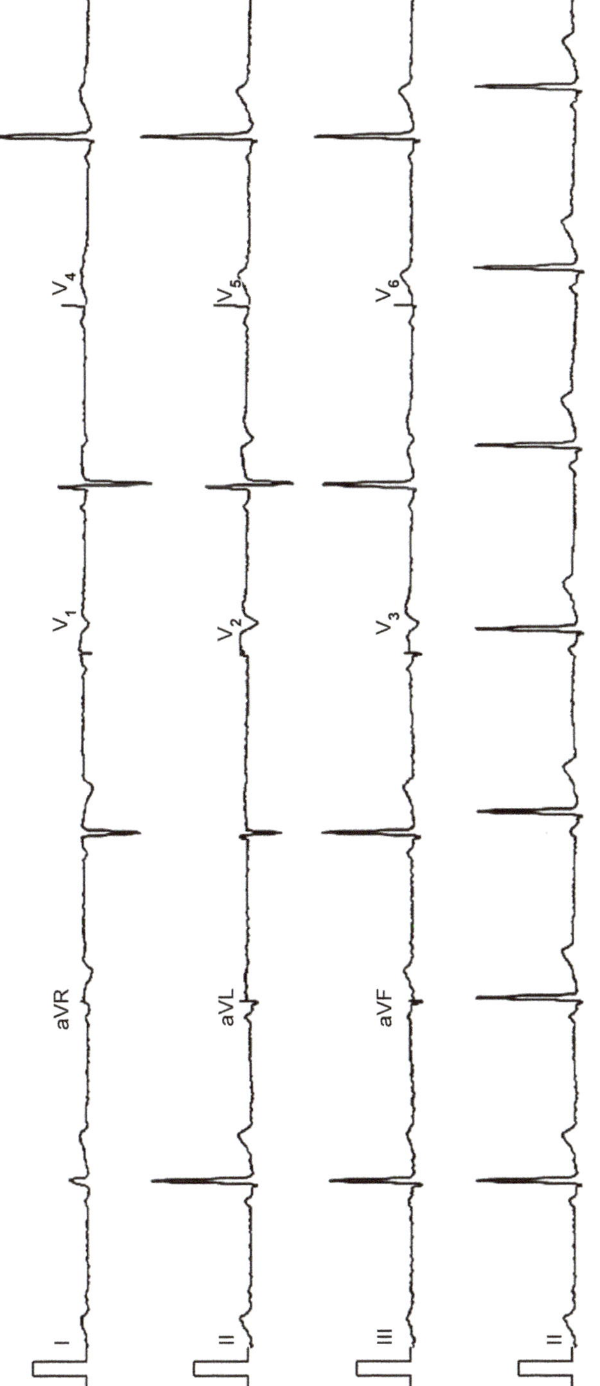

Fig. 12.110

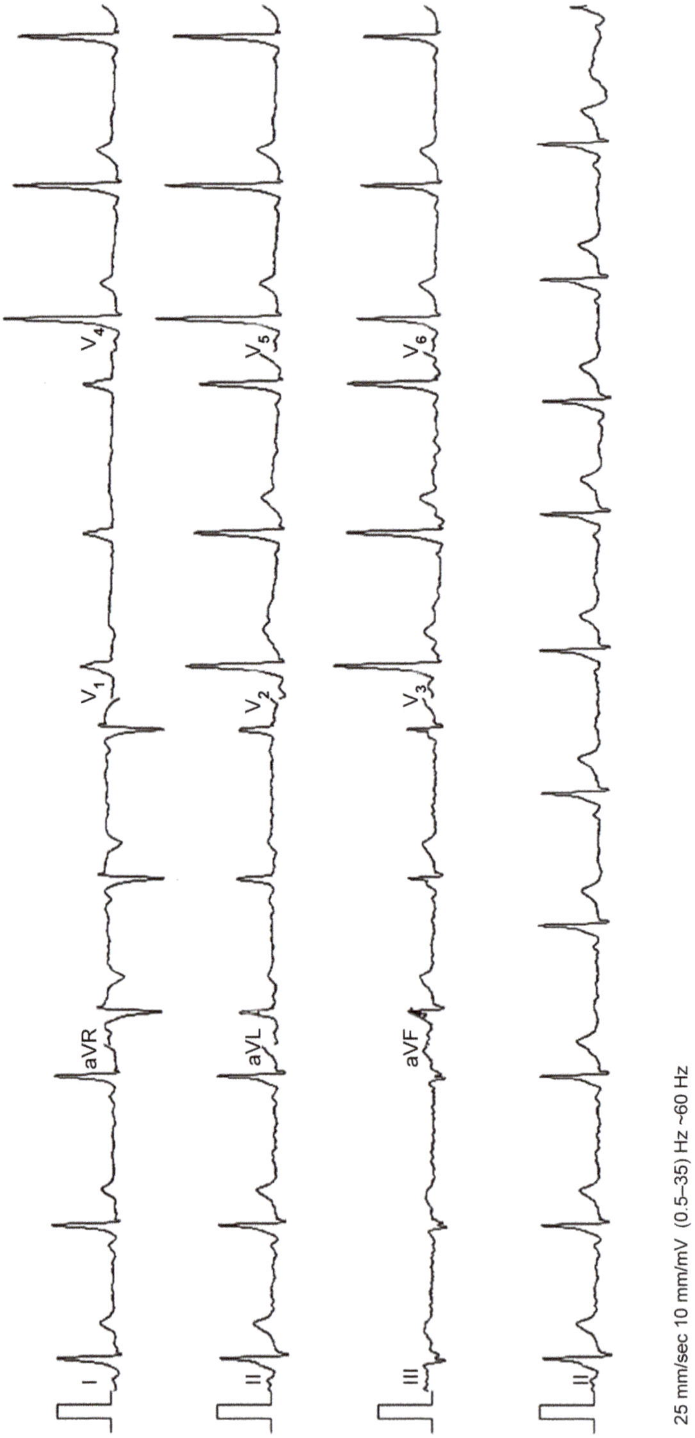
I
II
III
aVR
aVL
aVF
V1
V2
V3
V4
V5
V6
II
25 mm/sec 10 mm/mV (0.5–35) Hz ~60 Hz

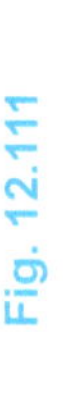

Fig. 12.111

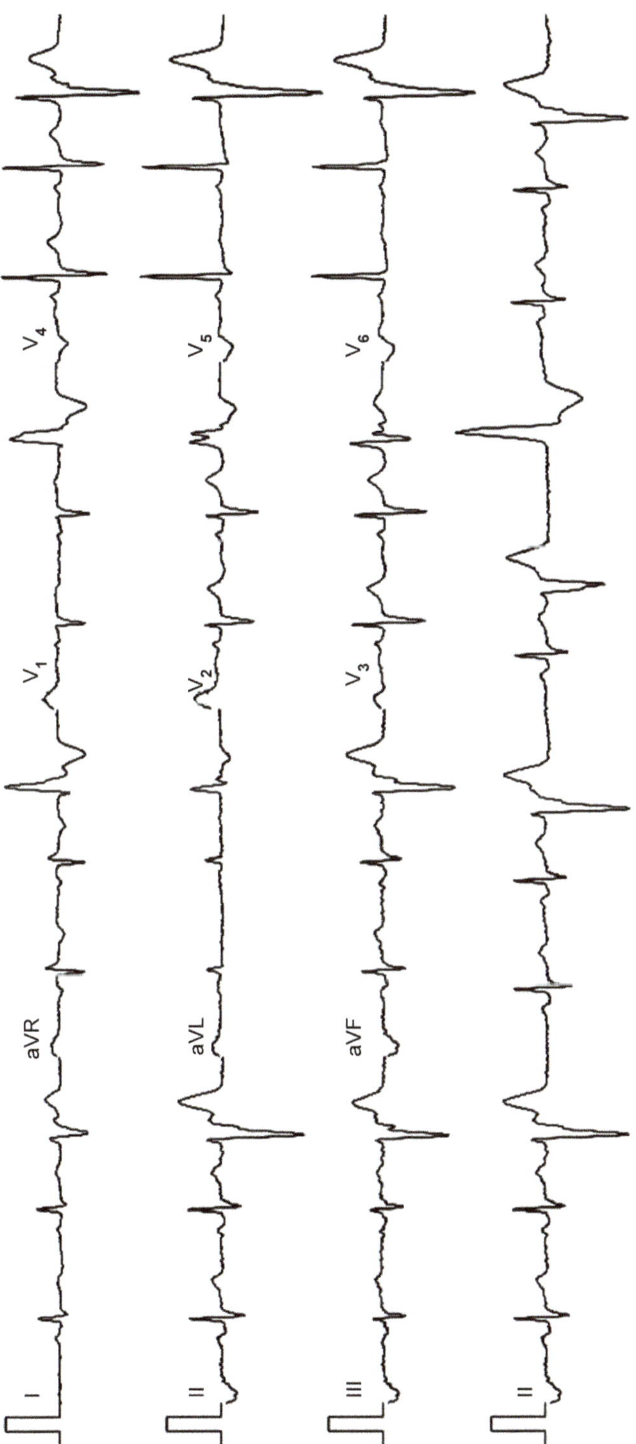

Fig. 12.112

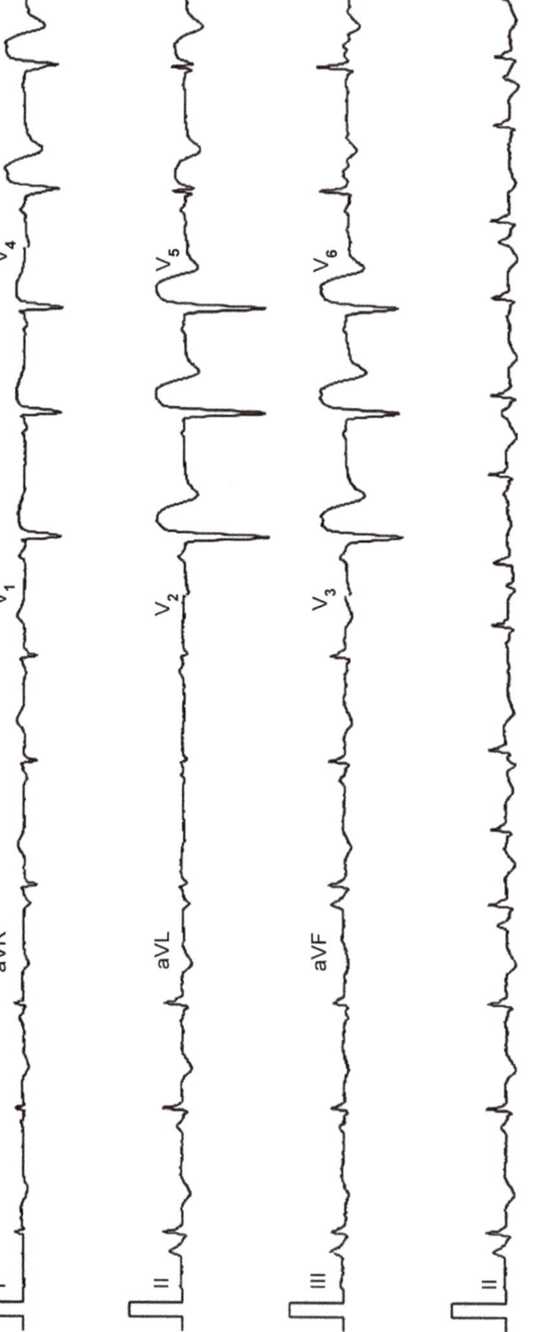

Fig. 12.113

Answers to ECG Self-Assessment Quiz

Fig. 12.1: *Acute pericarditis:* Sinus tachycardia 126 beats/min; typical features: widespread ST elevation and PR segment elevation in aVR, which shows ST segment depression. Note: The J-point level almost equals the height of the T wave in V_6.

Causes of ST segment elevation include:

- Normal variant
- Acute ST segment elevation MI (STEMI)
- Coronary artery spasm: Prinzmetal angina
- Left ventricular aneurysm
- Acute pericarditis
- Left ventricular hypertrophy
- Left bundle branch block
- Acute myocarditis
- Hyperkalemia
- Brugada syndrome; ST elevation V_1-V_3.

Fig. 12.2: Atrial fibrillation with rapid ventricular response 152 beats/min; marked ST segment depression in V_2 to V_6, in keeping with subendocardial ischemia, probable non-ST segment elevation MI.

Fig. 12.3: Acute extensive anterior infarct. Marked ST elevation and pathologic Q-waves in V_1 to V_6. Inferior MI, age indeterminate, and sinus tachycardia 115 beats/min.

Fig. 12.4: *WPW syndrome:* Prominent delta wave, short PR interval, tall R wave in V_2. Note the features in II, III, and aVF mimic inferior MI, and the pattern in V_1 mimics IRBBB.

- Thus, the assessment for WPW syndrome is done early in the interpretive sequence (Step 3) soon after the assessment for bundle branch block.

Fig. 12.5: Hyperkalemia; note the tall tented T waves in V_2-V_4; serum potassium 5.9 mmol/L.

Fig. 12.6: Left ventricular hypertrophy; note also, left atrial hypertrophy. The ST segment depression in lead V_3 suggests the presence of underlying ischemia.

Fig. 12.7: Supraventricular tachycardia; rate 230 beats/min; orthodromic circus movement tachycardia. Patient with WPW syndrome.

Fig. 12.8: **(A)** Note tall R wave in V_1-V_2, small R and deep S in V_6 interpreted by the computer as right ventricular hypertrophy. Findings are caused by incorrect placement of the precordial leads; this is a rare error for technicians; **(B)** Normal ECG; same patient as in (A), correct placement of V leads.

Fig. 12.9: A 2:1 AV block, probably Mobitz type I in view of a normal narrow QRS; approximately 30% of Mobitz type II exhibits a narrow QRS complex. Thus Mobitz type II block cannot be excluded.

The diagnosis of Mobitz type II block is certain when at least two regular and consecutive atrial impulses (P waves) are conducted with a constant PR interval before the occurrence of the dropped beat. Two or more consecutive PR intervals are unchanged before the dropped QRS beat. Note that Wenckebach did not have the use of electrocardiography when he cleverly deduced two forms of blocks from studies of the jugular venous waves in 1906. Mobitz in 1924 using the ECG described type I and type II blocks. Mobitz type I includes Wenckebach phenomenon (with each successive beat, the PR interval gradually lengthens and a beat is dropped). Importantly, not all Mobitz type I AV block reveal Wenckebach phenomenon (*see* Figs. 11.13, 11.14, and 11.15 for Mobitz type II block).

Fig. 12.10: Supraventricular tachycardia (SVT). Rate 155 beats/min. Note the diagnostic pseudo–r′ wave in V_1, and the small distortion of the terminal QRS complex (pseudo–S wave) in leads II, III, aVF. These are typical features of AV nodal reentrant tachycardia (AVNRT) observed in approximately 45% of SVTs.

Fig. 12.11: Atrial fibrillation and ventricular premature beats (VPBs); Note the couplets; and Multiform VPBs. Also left axis. Abnormal ECG.

Fig. 12.12: ST segment elevation V_1, V_2, V_3; normal variant in a 46-year-old man. Note the fishhook pattern in V_2.

Fig. 12.13: Anterior MI, probably in recent past: age indeterminate. Consider LV aneurysm if ST elevation V_2-V_4 has persisted beyond 6 months.

Fig. 12.14: Female aged 68 years old with mild hypertrophic cardiomyopathy confirmed by echocardiography at age of 45 years. Note the significant pathologic Q waves in V_4-V_6, and leads II, III, and aVF. Incorrectly interpreted by computer as old inferolateral MI.

Fig. 12.15: Left bundle branch block.

Fig. 12.16: Wide QRS tachycardia, irregular rhythm: Atrial fibrillation with a ventricular response, 160 beats/min in a patient with Wolff-Parkinson-White syndrome. Clues to WPW syndrome antidromic, pre-excited tachycardia: irregular, wide-complex tachycardia, often with runs at rapid rates exceeding 250 beats/min.

Fig. 12-17: Mimics inferior MI. The ST-T abnormality in lead 1 cannot be explained by an inferior MI. Fishhook-type pattern in II and concave ST segment elevation in III, aVF, are unlike acute MI. Treadmill cardiac nuclear perfusion imaging is normal; echocardiogram shows mild LVH in this 31-year-old male known to have a VSD patch.

Fig. 12.18: LVH, left atrial hypertrophy. Note the shape of the ST segment and deep T wave inversion V_4-V_6 and the extension of these changes to V_3 are in keeping myocardial ischemia and not simply hypertrophy. Also, consider apical HCM.

Fig. 12.19: Mimics dextrocardia. Error by technician: The reversed placement of arm leads is a common error; the reversal of V leads is a rare error and can cause incorrect interpretation of the ECG. Computer interpretation, dextrocardia. In this tracing, $V_1 = V_6$.

Fig. 12.20: Accelerated AV conduction, early transition: normal ECG.

Fig. 12.21: Tracing interpreted by computer as LBBB. Note absence of pacing spikes, because the muscle filter is activated. Deactivation of the computer muscle filter should expose the pacing spikes (*see* Fig. 12.22). The atypical IVCD, the negative concordance V_3-V_6 and in II, III, and aVF are pacing clues.

Fig. 12.22: Electronic pacing; the same patient as in Figure 12.21 but with muscle filter turned off. Capture rate 61 beats/min.

Fig. 12.23: WPW syndrome (type A). Note the tall R waves V_1-V_3.
Causes of tall R wave in V_1 include:

- Normal variants, thin chest wall, detroposition
- Misplacement of chest leads: V_6 placed in V_1 position; fortunately a rare technician's error.
- WPW syndrome: Type A pattern caused by lateral or posterior accessory pathways.
- Right bundle branch block
- Posterior MI; inferoposterior MI
- Right ventricular hypertrophy
- Hypertrophic cardiomyopathy
- Duchenne muscular dystrophy.

Fig. 12.24: Normal ECG; tall peaked precordial T waves in a healthy 35-year-old with normal serum potassium.

Fig. 12.25: Severe myocardial ischemia; probable non-ST elevation MI.
Causes of ST depression include:

- Acute non-ST segment elevation MI (non-Q wave MI)
- Acute myocardial ischemia without infarction (subendocardial ischemia)
- Chronic myocardial ischemia
- Reciprocal ST depression associated with STEMI
- LVH with "strain" pattern
- Conduction defects: LBBB, RBBB, IVCD, WPW
- Digoxin and other drugs
- Hypokalemia
- Cardiomyopathy.

Fig. 12.26: Normal ECG from a healthy 7-year-old. ST-T changes V_1 to V_3 are normal findings.

Fig. 12.27: Hypertrophic cardiomyopathy. An asymptomatic 20-year-old patient; played soccer, rugby, and hockey for the past 5 years. Routine physical revealed a grade II systolic murmur. Echocardiogram: asymmetric LVH; marked septal hypertrophy: septal thickness 36 mm (normal < 11 mm).

Fig. 12.28: Right bundle branch block, left axis—60°, left anterior fascicular block (hemiblock).

Fig. 12.29: Normal variant ST elevation V_2-V_5 in a 24-year-old male. Note the J-point fishhook in V_3. Normal variant ST elevation is common in males and rare in females. Many cardiologists and interpreters refer to the ST change as "early repolarization".

Fig. 12.30: Old inferior MI: Deep wide Q wave changes in II, III, and aVF have persisted for more than 15 years. Also, features of LVH and anterolateral ischemia are present.

Fig. 12.31: Atrial flutter. *Note:* a ventricular rate of 150 beats/min is a clue to atrial flutter with 2:1 AV conduction; the prominent sawtooth pattern in II, III, and aVF is typically absent in I, V_5, and V_6.

Fig. 12.32: Brugada syndrome. Note the atypical incomplete RBBB pattern with a curious coved ST segment elevation in V_1, V_2, and saddle-back type elevation in V_3. A 40-year-old Algerian male who collapsed; following an episode of syncope; an ICD was placed. Brugada and WPW syndrome should be considered along with assessments of blocks and is thus put as Step 3 of the 11-step strategies. Readers may wonder why interpreters should be on the watch for these rare conditions. They can cause death in young individuals, and these deaths and/or hospitalizations can be prevented.

Fig. 12.33: Nonsustained ventricular tachycardia in a 38-year-old male presenting with chest pain at 3:14:41 AM.

Fig. 12.34: Ventricular premature beats, triplets. ECG at 3:13:29 AM on presentation to the ER. Same patient as in Figure 12.33; ECG taken a minute later.

Fig. 12.35: Acute inferior myocardial infarction. Note the reciprocal depression in leads I and aVL. Right bundle branch block.

Fig. 12.36: Extensive anterior infarct probably in recent past; age indeterminate; left anterior fascicular block (hemiblock).

Fig. 12.37: WPW mimics inferior MI.

Fig. 12.38: Atrial fibrillation, normal ventricular rate.

Fig. 12.39: Severe myocardial ischemia. A 52-year-old female with angiographic proven severe obstructed coronary artery disease. Current ECG similar to 4 years prior and unchanged over 6 years. Received PTCA and stent at age of 48 years.

Fig. 12.40: Electronic pacing; capture rate 66 beats/min. Note the premature beat in V_1 is followed by a correctly timed paced QRS and indicates that the pacemaker is sensing correctly. The paced beat after the premature beat occurs at the correct pacing interval equal to the distance between the pacing spikes.

Fig. 12.41: RBBB and Q waves II, III, and aVF: Probable old inferior MI.

Fig. 12.42: A 41-year-old African male with long-standing restrictive cardiomyopathy. T wave changes caused by myocardial disease mimic LVH and ischemia. Borderline IVCD.

Fig. 12.43: Old anterior MI. Left atrial abnormality; APB, left axis, left anterior fascicular block (hemiblock).

Fig. 12.44: VPBs, bigeminy.

Fig. 12.45: A 2:1 AV block. Note the P-P intervals are constant. Computer interpreted as nonconducted APBs. ECG from a 44-year-old female with some shortness of breath, no presyncope. ECG tracing November 30, 2005. Note the heart rate, 43 beats/min, is identical in a tracing done 1 year later, shown in Figure 12.9. If the heart rate is less than 45 beats/min, screen for bradycardias.

The differential diagnosis for marked bradycardia, slow rate of less than 45 beats/min include:
- Sinus bradycardia
- Nonconducted APBs (bigeminy)
- Sinoatrial block (SA block)
- A variety of AV block (2:1 AV block, 3:1 block, complete AV block, and atrial fibrillation or flutter with complete AV block during which the ventricular rate becomes regular because of an idioventricular rhythm).

Fig. 12.46: Acute MI. Marked diffuse ST segment depression; note the ST elevation in aVR and little less so in V_1, a clue to the diagnosis of left main coronary artery occlusion.

Fig. 12.47: Right atrial hypertrophy.

Fig. 12.48: Atrial flutter. Note: Usually there is little visible evidence of flutter waves in lead I; V_5 and V_6 also tend to be silent or may reveal negative P-like waves.

Fig. 12.49: LBBB in a man with mitral valve bioprosthesis more than 20 years duration, marked precordial rocky motion caused by left ventricular aneurysm.

Fig. 12.50: LVH, and ischemia, axis 50, left anterior hemiblock, IRBBB, in a 65-year-old man with severe aortic regurgitation.

Fig. 12.51: Old anterior and lateral MI; left atrial hypertrophy; left axis—60°, small q in I, small r in III: left anterior hemiblock.

Fig. 12.52: Complete heart block. Rate 38 beats/min.

Fig. 12.53: Junctional tachycardia, rate 148 beats/min. Note: P wave inverted in II, III, and aVF, positive in aVR, and aVL.

Fig. 12.54: Atrial premature beats, with runs, also, junctional escape beats in V_4-V_6.

Fig. 12.55: RBBB with abnormal Q waves V_1, V_2, V_3: old anterior MI; APB, left axis—75°, left anterior fascicular block (hemiblock).

Fig. 12.56: Left atrial hypertrophy: Bifid P lead II, left atrial abnormality shown in V_1. Right axis, small r wave in lead I, small q in lead III: indicates probable left posterior hemiblock.

Fig. 12.57: Sinus bradycardia 44 beats/min. Left ventricular hypertrophy and left atrial hypertrophy. A 50-year-old Vietnamese female with well controlled very mild hypertension for 10 years; semi-giant T wave inversion V_5-V_6 is likely caused by apical hypertrophic cardiomyopathy as unlikely to be caused by very mild controlled hypertension. Echocardiogram shows some apical hypertrophy.

Fig. 12.58: RBBB; small Q in I, small r in III, and left axis—70° = left anterior fascicular block (hemiblock), and atrial premature beat.

Fig. 12.59: Nonspecific ST-T wave changes and LVH. ECG 1-12-06 from a 69-year-old man. Very active exercise. From 1996 to 2004, he was able to walk 10 km without pain. ECG 1998, nonspecific ST-T wave changes: mild LVH and probable ischemia. During 2005, atypical chest ache, not related to exertion. Angiograms October 2005, 95% proximal LAD occlusion. Stented successfully. ECG during 2006 similar to 2004 through 2005. Note serious coronary disease with nonspecific ST-T wave changes.

Fig. 12.60: Acute anterior MI. ST elevation V_1 through V_4 (STEMI).

Fig. 12.61: WPW syndrome mimicking RBBB; ECG from a 26-year-old male. A good reason to assess for WPW early in the interpretive sequence (Step 3) done soon after the assessment for RBBB and LBBB.

Fig. 12.62: Acute inferior MI (STEMI); abnormally shaped high ST segment in inferior leads. Note the reciprocal depression in leads I, aVL, V_1, and V_2.

Fig. 12.63: Ventricular tachycardia.

Fig. 12.64: Anteroseptal MI; age indeterminate. ECG from a 60-year-old man; ECG done during annual assessment, silent MI; the patient had a normal ECG 1 year earlier.

Fig. 12.65: Extensive anterior MI in a 50-year-old female. Note: ST elevation in 8 leads.

Fig. 12.66: A 2:1 AV block, IRBBB; erroneously read by computer as APBs nonconducted. Note: With second degree AV (type I or type II block), the PP interval remains constant and the P wave morphology is unchanged. Note the P waves stuck to the T waves are not premature in time, and with nonconducted APBs, the PP interval will vary. Nonconducted APBs should not be mistaken for second-degree AV block and vice versa. A 2:1 AV block can be either type I or type II.

Fig. 12.67: Accelerated junctional rhythm; IRBBB.

Fig. 12.68: Sinus tachycardia 125 beats/min; APB.

Fig. 12.69: Acute anterior MI (SEMI). Sinus bradycardia 49; ECG from a 39-year-old male.

Fig. 12.70: Old inferior MI. Note the Q waves in II, III, and aVF may be interpreted as "nondiagnostic inferior Q waves noted." The tracing is similar to 5 years prior. ECG from a 55-year-old female with severe hyperlipidemia (total cholesterol > 8 mmol/L, 300 mg/dL from age 20–30). She had a proven inferior MI at the age of 32 years with typical inferior Qs. Subsequent angina and CABG. Stable for the past 15 years. LDL maintained less than 2.5 mmol/L past 20 years. Wide inferior Q waves have become narrower and less deep over a 5-year period postinfarction.

Fig. 12.71: Atrial flutter.

Fig. 12.72: Acute anterior MI (STEMI).

Fig. 12.73: Old inferior MI. Note the Q waves in II, III, and aVF are distinct and diagnostic (*see* Fig. 12.70).

Fig. 12.74: Apical hypertrophic cardiomyopathy. Note the giant T wave inversion in keeping with apical HCM seen mainly in Japanese people. Despite the sinister looking ECG with giant T waves and high precordial QRS voltage, an outflow tract gradient does not develop and the prognosis is good compared with obstructive HCM. ECG from an 80-year-old Vietnamese woman with minimal cardiac symptoms over 10 years, during which time the ECG remained similar.

Fig. 12.75: Atrial fibrillation, ventricular rate 140 beats/min.

Fig. 12.76: Nonsustained ventricular tachycardia.

Figs. 12.77A and B: (A and B) Wide complex regular tachycardia, rapid rate 235–260 beats/min. Computer incorrectly interpreted Holter record as ventricular runs. Note in (B) the tachycardia is triggered by an APB. The wide complex rapid rate suggests preexcited antidromic tachycardia. An accessory pathway was documented and ablation was successful in this 28-year-old patient with 3-year duration of recurrent palpitations. He had presented once to ER with atrial fibrillation, ventricular rate 160 beats/min.

Fig. 12.78: Hypertrophic cardiomyopathy. Poor R wave progression V_2-V_3, nonspecific ST-T wave changes, borderline IVCD, left anterior hemiblock, and left atrial hypertrophy.
A constellation of abnormal findings in a 51-year-old female with shortness of breath. Echocardiogram showed asymmetric septal hypertrophy, septal thickness 1.7 cm, posterior wall 1.4 cm, left atrium 5.0 cm, systolic anterior motion (SAM) of the mitral valve with leaflets touching the septum, resting outflow gradient 75 mm Hg, increasing to 146 mm Hg after amyl nitrate.

Fig. 12.79: APBs. Atrial bigeminy.

Fig. 12.80: Complete AV block. Ventricular rate 28 beats/min.

Fig. 12.81: ECG from a 74-year-old man who presented with chest pain. The marked diffuse ST segment depression in 10 leads accompanied by ST elevation in aVR greater than in V_1 suggested probable acute left main coronary occlusion and proved true on coronary angiograms.

Fig. 12.82: RBBB: note the prolonged duration of the S wave in lead 1, V_5, V_6, >30 ms. Left axis—60°; left anterior fascicular block.

Fig. 12.83: Sinus tachycardia 140 beats/min. Nondiagnostic inferior Q waves noted in a 31-year-old male with chest infection.

Fig. 12.84: ST segment elevation V_2-V_5 (fish hook feature in V_3): normal variant in a 30-year-old male.

Fig. 12.85: Tracing from a healthy 60-year-old female. Poor R wave progression V_2, V_3 is a not uncommon finding caused by lead placement of V_2, V_3 in females. Mimics a probable old anteroseptal MI.

Fig. 12.86: Sinus rhythm, RBBB; atrial premature beats nonconducted: These are a common cause of an unexpected pause. It is preferable to use the term nonconducted APB rather than blocked APB.

Fig. 12.87A: ECG from a 47-year-old man. Age corrected Sokolow index (SV1 + RV5 or V_6 = 57 mm, 5.7 mV). The abnormal ST–T change in V_3 and the abnormal coving of the ST segment in V_4-V_6 should prompt a diagnosis of ischemia. See Figure 12.87B: definitely LVH.

Fig. 12.87B: LVH proven in a 50-year-old female with long duration hypertension. Note the so-called typical "strain pattern" in V_4 to V_6: asymmetric ST segment depression; the T wave has a gradual descending and a steep ascending limb, a hallmark of LVH.

Fig. 12.88: RBBB, pathologic Q waves in V_1-V_4 indicates definite old anteroseptal MI.
In the presence of RBBB a Q wave in V_1-V_2 may occur in the absence of MI. Also, the tracing shows left anterior fascicular block.

Fig. 12.89: Figure 12.82. WPW syndrome: changes mimic incomplete LBBB. The atypical bundle branch block or conduction delay should prompt search for short PR and delta waves (1, 11, and aVL).

Fig. 12.90: RSR′ in V_1–V_2 suggests incomplete RBBB, but there is no slurred or widened S wave (the S wave is not of prolonged duration) in leads 1, V_5 or V_6 to indicate true RBBB. This should alert the interpreter to assess for atypical RBBB, a feature of Brugada syndrome.

Scrutiny of the ST segment in V_1, V_2 reveals a coved and saddle-back deformity, characteristic features of the syndrome.

Fig. 12.91: Sinus rhythm; nondiagnostic inferior Q waves noted; 25 < Q < 35 ms in aVF; with Q in II, III; Q/R > 1/5 in aVF; Clinical correlation required; Borderline ECG. Tiny Q waves in II, III, aVF; Diagnosis: Nondiagnostic inferior Q-waves.

Fig. 12 92: Deep wide Q waves II, II aVF, = old inferior MI; Deep wide Q waves V_4–V_6, lead 1 aVL = lateral MI; Diagnosis; old inferolateral MI.

Fig. 12.93: Q waves V_1–V_6: old anterior MI. Deep wide Q waves leads III; aVF: old inferior MI; wide QRS complexes; right bundle branch block.

Fig. 12 94: WPW mimic inferior MI; also mimics right bundle branch black (RBBB).

Fig. 12.95: QS in V_1–V_3; Old anteroseptal infarct. Abnormal ECG.

Fig. 12.96: Reversed arm leads.

Fig. 12 97: Acute anterior MI.

Figs. 12.98A and B: Same patient: complete heart block; third-degree AV block (Daggette).

Fig. 12.99: Atrial fibrillation with normal mean ventricular response with long RR intervals; QRS = 147 ms; RSR′ in V_1; S > 30 ms in I V_5–V_6 = RBBB.

Fig. 12.100: WPW: Not anteroseptal MI.

Fig. 12.101: Atypical IVCD; Consider pacing.

Figs. 12.102A and B: Baseline and muscle filter off revealing pacemaker spikes. (B) Nondiagnostic inferior Q-waves.

Fig. 12.103: Atypical I RBBB with saddle back ST segment deformity V_2 Diagnosis: Brugada syndrome.

Fig. 12.104: Sinus rhythm; APBs: atrial premature beats; Q wave in V_3, V_4; QRS = 147 ms; RSR′ in V_1, V_2; S>30 ms in I V_5, V_6. Diagnosis: Old anteroseptal infarct. RBBB.

Fig. 12.105: Known atrial fibrillation in past; now atrial fibrillation with very slow regular rhythm = : complete AV block with AV junctional escape pacemaker (rhythm)

Fig. 12.106: Arm electrodes interchanged: reversed arm leads.

Fig. 12.107: Regular tachycardia supraventricular tachycardia (SV) and atrioventricular nodal reentrant tachycardia (ANVRT): Rate 140 beats/min.

Figs. 12.108A and B: (A) A 42-year-old male sinus rhythm ECG (2017) left axis. LAFB; left anterior fascicular block (hemiblock). This ECG can be misinterpreted as old inferior MI similar to 2014 when at age of 39 years (B), no heart problems; routine ECG 2014, sinus bradycardia, left axis deviation, consistent with LAFB.

Fig. 12.109: Atrial tachycardia. The P-waves are barely discernible in lead I and are inverted in II, III, and aVF. There is 2:1 atrioventricular block. The atrial rate is 264 beats/min; ventricular rate is 132 beats/min. Note the isoelectric baseline between the P-wave and the QRS complex.

Fig. 12.110: Computer diagnosis: mid-precordial ST elevation, consider acute ischemia; Corrected to: S-T segment elevation V_2, V_3 normal variant; ECG within normal limits.

Fig. 12.111: An 18-year-old female; sinus bradycardia; T inversion V_1–V_3 consider juvenile and/or feminine pattern. ECG within normal limits.

Fig. 12.112: Tall R waves V_1, V_2. Diagnosis: WPW syndrome.

Fig. 12.113: Multiform VPBs, couplets. Extensive recent (past 24 hours) anterior infarct: QS in V_2, V_3, V_4; $25 < Q < 35$ ms in V_5, V_6.

New Placements of Limb Lead Provide Superior Quality ECGs

More than 60 million electrocardiograms (ECGs) are done annually. The ECG is the oldest cardiologic test, but even 100 years after its inception, it continues as the most commonly used cardiologic test. Despite the advent of expensive and sophisticated alternatives, the ECG remains the most reliable tool for the confirmation of acute myocardial infarction (MI). The ECG—not creatine kinase-MB (CK-MB), troponins, echocardiogram, or single photon emission computed tomography (SPECT) or positron emission tomography (PET) scan—dictates the timely administration of lifesaving percutaneous coronary intervention (PCI) or thrombolytic therapy. There is no test to rival the ECG for the diagnosis of arrhythmias, which is a common and bothersome clinical cardiologic problem. Also, the clinical diagnosis of pericarditis and myocardial ischemia is made mainly from ECG findings.

Many out of hospital laboratories perform ECGs and often artifacts, distortions of wave form make the tracing difficult or impossible to interpret. The ECG may be reported as "artifacts preclude accurate interpretation".

Modified lead placements were used for several years in some clinics in Wales and parts of the United Kingdom and Europe. After several years of use and obtaining superior quality tracings, clinicians in Wales performed a study to verify accuracy of modified leads. Jowett et al. indicated that "The appeal of this easily applied lead system has resulted in extensive use in our hospital, both in emergency and nonemergency situations". Their study of 100 patients resulted in the disappearance of five of six inferior infarcts that were previously observed on the standard ECG.

Jowett et al. obtained better quality ECGs and emphasized the advantages of modified leads, but did not recommend them for routine use.

The author conducted a study of 1,200 patient and indicated that Jowett placement of electrodes placed on the acromion process and lower abdomen qualified as torso leads. The acromion process is part of the scapular and thus, part of the trunk. It is not surprising therefore that this torso electrode position used by Jowett et al. caused the disappearance of five of six inferior infarcts. Placement of limb electrodes on the torso destroys Einthoven's hypothesis: the equilateral triangle concept.

Figure 13.1 gives the new electrode placement (NEP) for the limb leads. Figures 13.2 to 13.4 give results of NEPs in the Khan study (2015). The NEPs were adjusted throughout a small pilot study and finally tested in 1,200 patients.

Artifacts disappeared, ECG recordings were of superior quality and no loss of inferior infarcts or appearance of lateral infarct signs occurred. Atrial fibrillation and other arrhythmias showed no differences in the ECGs done with standard and with the new placement method.

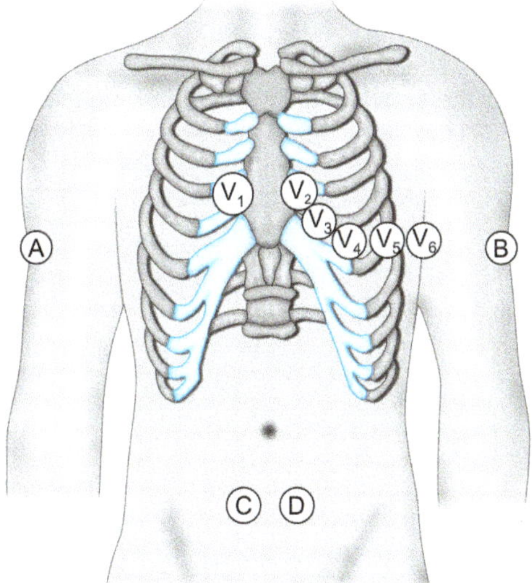

Fig. 13.1: The arm electrodes (A and B) are placed on the mid-arm, on the lateral aspect of the biceps, immediately below the V_4 horizontal line. The abdominal electrodes (C and D) placed 7.6 cm (~3 inches) below the umbilical horizontal line, and 5 cm (~2 inches) on either side of the umbilical vertical line. The distance between these two electrodes to be 10 cm (~4 inches).
Source: Adapted with permission from Khan MG. A new electrode placement method for obtaining 12 lead ECGs. Open Heart. 2015;2(1):e000226.

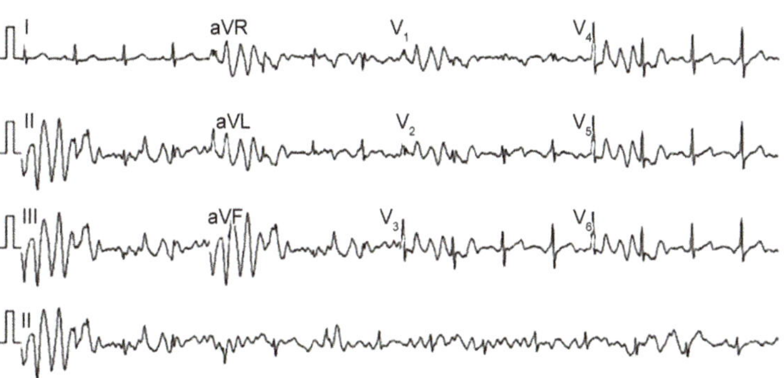

Fig. 13.2A

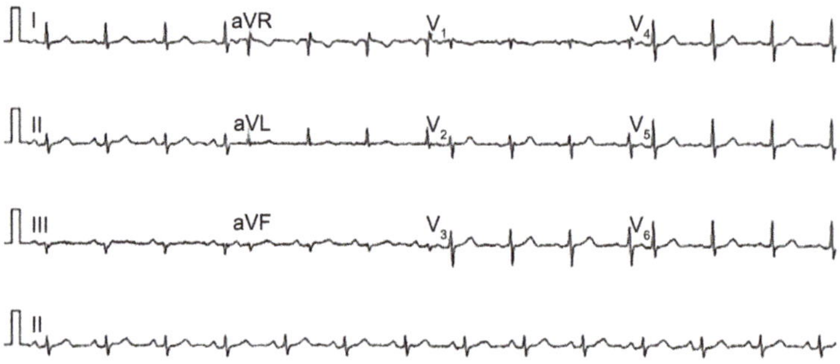

Fig. 13.2B

Figs. 13.2A and B: (A) Standard 12-lead ECG showing artifacts; (B) New electrode placement ECG, carried out within 30 seconds of the standard tracing reveals no artifacts.
Source: Adapted with permission from Khan MG. A new electrode placement method for obtaining 12-lead ECGs. Open Heart. 2015;2(1):e000226.

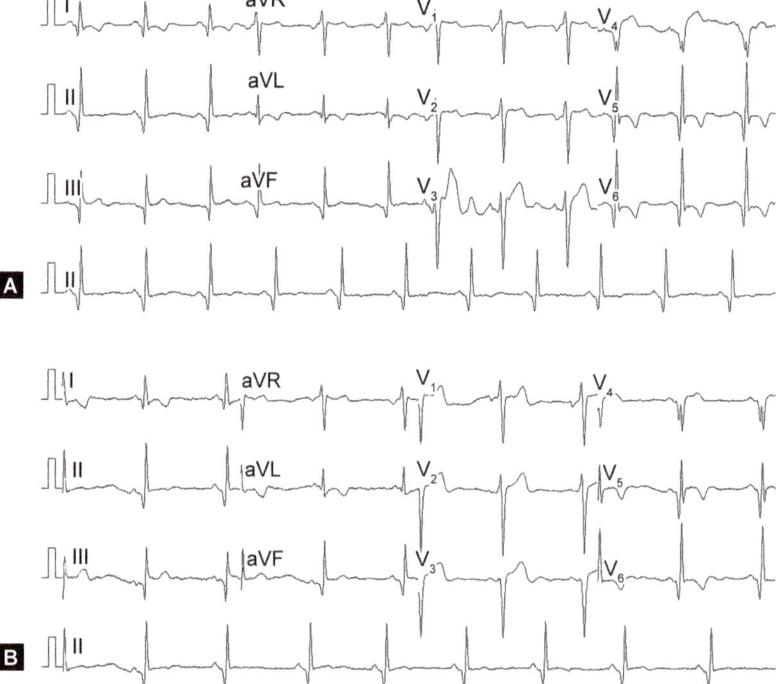

Figs. 13.3A and B: (A) Standard lead ECG: deep wide Q waves in leads II, III, aVF: old inferior, and anterolateral myocardial infarction, artifacts in V_3, V_4. (B) New electrode placement ECG, old inferolateral infarct; the tracing is similar to the standard recording, but with clearing of artifacts in V_3 and V_4. The R wave amplitude in all 12 leads is the same in the standard and the new electrode placement ECG.
Source: Adapted with permission from Khan MG. A new electrode placement method for obtaining 12-lead ECGs. Open Heart. 2015;2(1):e000226.

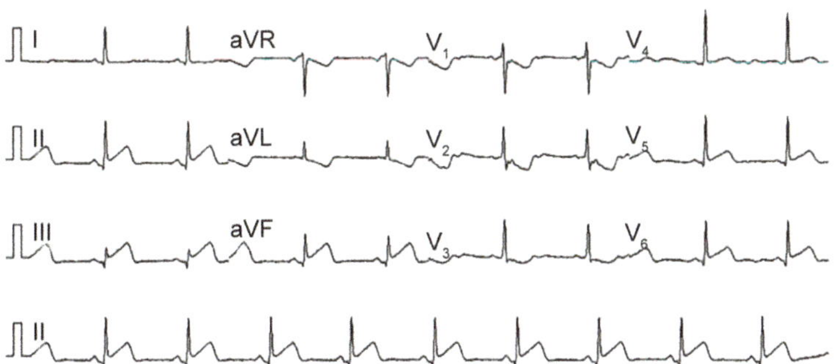

Fig. 13.4: New electrode placement ECG from a female, aged 57 years old with acute chest pain, shows abnormal ST elevation in leads II, III, aVF, V_5, V_6: typical findings of acute inferior MI with lateral involvement, ST segment elevation MI. Reciprocal depression V_1-V_2, aVL is not diagnostic but helps confirm the diagnosis of acute MI.
Source: Adapted with permission from Khan MG. A new electrode placement method for obtaining 12-lead ECGs. Open Heart. 2015;2(1):e000226.

The article is a BMJ Open Heart access and can be consulted (Khan 2015).

The study emphasizes:

- The new placements give recordings with better quality, and no recalls of patients.
- Not having to remove hosiery or other leg garment is convenient and allows more rapid acquisition of ECGs.
- Time saved is important for therapy, and for hospital and nonhospital laboratories.
- Generates the need to study the NEP in patients with probable acute coronary syndrome where timely PCI or thrombolysis can save lives.
- The forearms are freed for intravenous or radial artery access and further ECGs needed during procedures can be obtained.

BIBLIOGRAPHY

1. Jowett NI, Turner AM, Cole A, et al. Modified electrode placement must be recorded when performing 12-lead electrocardiograms. Postgrad Med J. 2005;81:122-5.
2. Khan GM. A new electrode placement method for obtaining 12-lead ECGs. Open Heart. 2015;2(1):e000226.
3. Takuma K, Hori S, Sasaki J, et al. An alternative limb lead system for electrocardiographs in emergency patients. Am J Emerg Med. 1995;13:514-7.

Page numbers followed by *f* refer to figure and *t* refer to table.